Navigating the Maze of Nursing Research
An Interactive Learning Adventure

Navigating the Maze of Nursing Research
An Interactive Learning Adventure

Sally Borbasi RN PhD
Associate Professor
School of Nursing and Midwifery
Flinders University
Adelaide, South Australia

Debra Jackson RN PhD
Associate Professor
School of Nursing, Family and
Community Health
University of Western Sydney
New South Wales

Rae W Langford, EdD, RN
Private Practice
Research and Statistics Consultant
Rehabilitation Nurse Consultant
Legal Nurse Consultant
Houston, Texas

Mosby

Sydney   Edinburgh   London   New York   Philadelphia   St Louis   Toronto

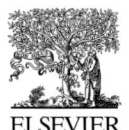
ELSEVIER

Mosby
is an imprint of Elsevier

Elsevier Australia
30–52 Smidmore Street, Marrickville, NSW 2204

This edition © 2004
Elsevier Australia (a division of Reed International Books Australia Pty Ltd)
ACN 001 002 357

This publication is copyright. Except as expressly provided in the Copyright Act 1968 and the Copyright Amendment (Digital Agenda) Act 2000, no part of this publication may be reproduced, stored in any retrieval system or transmitted by any means (including electronic, mechanical, microcopying, photocopying, recording or otherwise) without prior written permission from the publisher.

Every effort has been made to contact copyright holders of material reproduced in this book. In the few instances where this has not been possible, the publishers invite such copyright holders to contact them.

National Library of Australia Cataloguing-in-Publication Data

Borbasi, Sally.
    Navigating the maze of nursing research : an interactive
    learning adventure.

    Includes index.
    ISBN 0 7295 3730 7.

    1. Nursing—Research—Methodology. 2. Nursing—Research.
    I. Langford, Rae. II. Jackson, Debra.
    III. Title.

    610.73072

Publisher: Vaughn Curtis
Publishing Editor: Meg O'Hanlon
Developmental Editor: Rhiain Hull
Publishing Services Manager: Helena Klijn
Edited by Kay Waters
Cover and text design by Modern Art Production Group
Index by Max McMaster
Printed and bound by Kyodo Printing Singapore

Contents

From the Authors vi
To the Reader vii

Section 1: Finding It Fast and Reading It Well — 1

1. Getting the Most Out of the Library 2
2. Surfing the Internet 24
3. Reading Faster, Reading Smarter: Managing Information Wisely ... 48

Section 2: Talking the Talk — 65

4. Research: What, Why, Where and Who? 66
5. Quantitative Research: Summing It Up 88
6. Qualitative Research: The Whole Picture 128
7. Reading Research: Critical Approaches to Effective Understanding ... 154

Section 3: Walking the Walk — 177

8. Reading and Using Research in Maternal–Infant Care 178
9. Reading and Using Research in the Care of Children and Adolescents ... 200
10. Reading and Using Research in the Care of Adults 222
11. Reading and Using Research in the Care of Older Adults ... 248
12. Use It or Lose It: Putting Research Into Action 270

Glossary 287
Index 297
Student Challenges 310

From the Authors

Let us introduce ourselves. We have all been faculty members for a number of years. Sally and Debra work in different states in Australia, and Rae is based in the United States. We have all taught research and statistics at the baccalaureate, masters and doctoral levels for nursing students. We all work to varying degrees with practising nurses to make research less mystifying and more readily applicable to clinical practice. During these times we have experimented with a number of ways to more clearly distinguish and optimise learning experiences for students at various levels, and to make research come alive for students and practitioners alike. This learning package is in part a result of that experimentation stemming largely from Rae's work in the United States. In this edition Debra and Sally have adapted Rae's original work to meet the needs of students from Australia and New Zealand.

Many of the games, puzzles and challenges have been tested with undergraduate students, who have found them fun and challenging. Many have commented that this approach makes research seem more real and relevant, and helps them to feel more confident in reading and making sense of research articles. We have had faculty members in clinical courses ask what we are doing because their students are suddenly discussing and applying research findings in their clinical situations.

The goal of this learning package is to equip students with skills that enable them to quickly find, critically read and readily identify possible uses for relevant clinical research. It uses an interactive, multimodal approach that gets students actively involved in the learning process and provides multiple opportunities to practise and integrate newly acquired skills. We hope you find this approach as useful as our students and we have.

Sally Borbasi
Debra Jackson
Rae W. Langford

Reviewers

Australia and New Zealand

Beverley Bird
School of Nursing, Faculty of Medicine
Nursing and Health Sciences
Monash University, Melbourne, Australia

Sue Gasquione
Lecturer, School of Health Science
Faculty of Health and Environmental Sciences
Unitec Institute of Technology, Auckland, New Zealand

Joyce Jenkin
Nurse Librarian, Peninsula Library
Monash University, Melbourne, Australia

Cherie Wells
School of Nursing, Faculty of Community and Health
Otago Polytechnic, Dunedin, New Zealand

Beverley Wood
Senior Lecturer, Coordinator of International Studies
School of Nursing and Midwifery
La Trobe University, Melbourne, Australia

USA

Margaret M Anderson
Associate Professor, BSN/MSN Programs
Chair, Department of Nursing
Northern Kentucky University, Highland Heights, Kentucky

Betsy Barnes-McDowell
Associate Professor, School of Nursing
Lander University, Greenwood, South Carolina

To the Reader

An Important Message from Your Authors!

Did you know that warming patients before clean surgery reduces the incidence of postoperative wound infection? (Read *Lancet* 2001;358:876–880.)

Do you think automated cuffs provide accurate measurements of blood pressure? (Read about it in *International Journal of Nursing Practice* 2001;7(4):246–250.)

Does drinking cranberry juice reduce recurrent urinary tract infections in women? (Find out in the *British Medical Journal* 2001;322(7302):1571–1573.)

Do you know that colorectal surgery patients benefit more from a combination of low-dose unfractionated heparin (LDH) plus compression stockings than LDH alone? (Check out the *Cochrane Library* 2003;1.)

Do you know whether the provision of CPR training to spouses of patients recovering from an acute cardiac event decreases their anxiety? (Find out more in *Research in Nursing and Health* 2000;23(4):270–278.)

Do you know the long-term effects of injection drug use? (Find out in *Research in Nursing and Health* 2001;24:423–432.)

Do you know an effective intervention to reduce depressive feelings and symptoms in patients with cancer? (Read *Oncology Nursing Forum* 2002;29:73–84.)

Does knowing that chronic pain affects the way individuals view their bodies, their relationships with others and their sense of time help you to understand them better? (Read more in the *Western Journal of Nursing Research* 2000;22:683–699.)

Answers to these questions are just a sample of the wealth of information that waits at your fingertips to help you improve the nursing care that you give every day. If you want to be *the best nurse you can be* then find out what judicious use of nursing research can do for you.

What does *research* have to do with this, you ask? Well, your professional association, the Australian Nursing Council, considers research so vital to the profession of nursing that it expects *all* registered nurses, regardless of educational preparation, to be research consumers. What is a *research consumer*? A research consumer is able to read research articles, evaluate their relevance and apply the findings to the practice of nursing.

This is where this learning package (textbook, CD-ROM and website) fits in. This package is designed to enhance your skills so that you can effectively read, understand, evaluate and apply research findings in your everyday clinical practice. It encourages you to examine what you do in the clinical area and to pose such questions as: 'Is this the best intervention?' or 'Is this the best way to carry out this intervention?'. It seeks to involve you as an active participant in this learning process. Student activities and critical thinking opportunities are featured throughout the text, along with interactive exercises, puzzles and games on the CD-ROM. The more you participate in the various activities, exercises and discussions about the identified research content, the more confident and competent you will become in using research as a tool to improve your practice.

This learning package is also designed to enhance your skills in finding information fast, and reading and using that information effectively. Section 1 is devoted to honing your library and internet skills, reading skills and abstracting skills. Section 2 gives you the vocabulary necessary to read and understand research studies by introducing you to the two main types of research: quantitative and qualitative. Section 3 gives you step-by-step guidance in applying research findings to a variety of clinical situations. It also explores ways to use research results in order to change the way you practise and to influence the systems you practise in.

Special Features of This Book

- Student Quotes You can probably identify with other students' feelings about nursing research.
- Abstracts Just as a research article has an abstract, an introductory paragraph that summarises the article, so too does each chapter of the book.
- Learning Objectives These describe what you should be able to do after reading each chapter and working through the exercises.
- Chapter Outline Each chapter contains a list of the major headings to give you an idea of the topics covered.
- Key Terms A list of the terms that are important to know is provided for each chapter.
- Student Challenges Try these exercises to apply what you are reading and learning.
- Hints and other boxed information Be sure to remember these useful tips and notes!
- Resource Kits These provide a list of materials to refer to for further information.
- Glossary A list of all the key terms in the book is provided at the back of the book for your convenience.

How to Use Your Learning Package

You have three integrated tools to help you make your way through this maze.
- Textbook As you read the textbook, you will be referred to activities on the CD-ROM and to websites accessible through links on the book's Evolve website. In the page margins you will see icons referring you to the activities on the CD-ROM and the website activities found on the Evolve site.

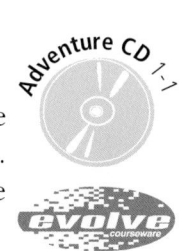

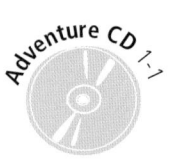

- CD-ROM The CD-ROM provides over forty interactive exercises that cover all twelve chapters of the book. It includes activities such as word scramble, multiple choice, cryptograms and many other fun and challenging exercises. A special icon appears in the margin of the book when there is a corresponding CD-ROM exercise, signalling you to go to the CD-ROM.

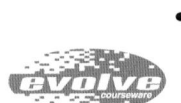

- Evolve website This website, located at http://evolve.elsevier.com, provides links to internet sites that correspond to activities on the CD, and other websites relevant to nursing research. Each activity in the book that sends you to the internet is indicated by this symbol. Also included on the website are Frequently Asked Questions about nursing research, Teaching Tips for faculty members, and other pertinent information.

You may find that you not only learn how to effectively use research in your nursing practice, but that you also increase your ability to read and think critically, to analyse situations, and to better use and manage available resources. We invite you now to begin the first step in your journey to navigate the maze that is nursing research.

Finding It Fast and Reading It Well

Section 1

Taking Advantage of the Information Explosion and the Miracles of Modern Technology
... Be Prepared

We live in a time where information is available on just about any subject you can dream up, and more is produced every day. Unfortunately, many of us fail to take advantage of this wealth of information and have little idea about how to find and use it when we do need it. Maybe we are overwhelmed by the abundance of information and cope by ignoring it all. Unfortunately, ignoring the problem breeds ignorance. To be information literate is essential to our personal and professional well-being, but how do we achieve this? We must recognise when we need information and hone the skills necessary to find, evaluate and use that information. Both the library and the internet offer excellent readily available resources. This section discusses how to use the library and the internet and describes how to read and summarise essential information effectively. It will help you develop skills to take advantage of and harness the information explosion.

http://evolve.elsevier.com/AU/Borbasi/maze

Learning Objectives

After reading this chapter and following critical reflection the student will be able to:

1. Describe the organisation and functions of libraries.
2. Identify relevant library components and services.
3. Locate components and services in a specified library setting.
4. Discuss the purpose of library filing/classification systems.
5. Distinguish between manual and computerised information retrieval systems.
6. Discuss the differences between cataloguing and indexing systems.
7. Compare and contrast sample indexes available to access nursing and health care-related information.
8. Describe how to conduct an information search using library resources.
9. Conduct a search at a specified library setting, using available library search tools.
10. Evaluate the results of a search effort for an identified topic.

Chapter Outline

Do You Need This Chapter?
What Is a Library?
Types of libraries
Classification schemes
What's in the Library?
How Do You Use the Library?
Catalogues
    Manual catalogues
    Electronic catalogues
Indexes and abstracts
    Manual indexes and abstracts
    Electronic indexes and abstracts
Comparing manual and electronic indexes
How Do You Successfully Search for Information?
Clearly define your mission
Choose appropriate resources
Choose appropriate indexes
Define your search parameters
Place limits on your search
View your search results

Chapter 1
Getting the Most Out of the Library

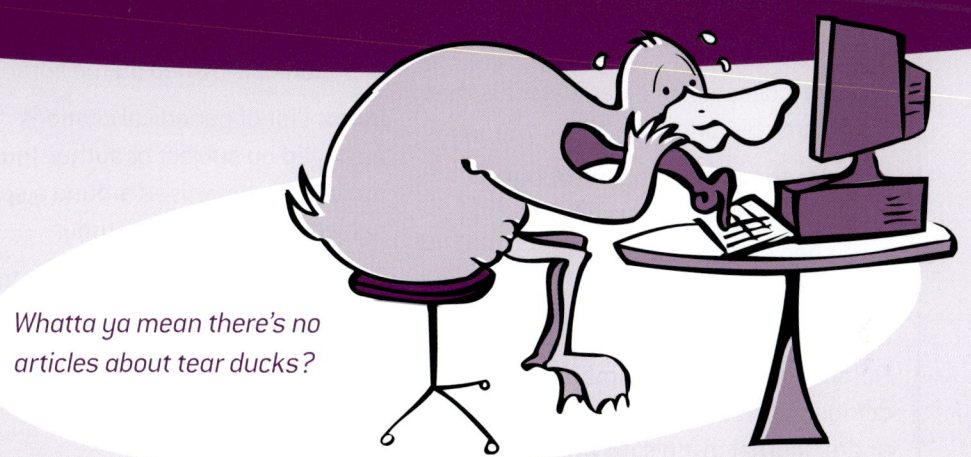

Whatta ya mean there's no articles about tear ducks?

Student Quote

'The library used to be so overwhelming. I'd avoid going because I could never find what I needed anyway. Who knew it could be so useful?'

Abstract

Libraries collect, store and organise information and make it readily accessible for use. Materials are organised using a classification system and are arranged on shelves by call numbers. Materials are located by using catalogues and indexes. These filing systems are now available mostly in electronic form, with some libraries still using print form for their older collections. Successful searches for information about a particular subject demand certain skills. These include the ability to define the topic of interest, select appropriate search resources, refine search skills, and selectively review and evaluate the materials produced by a search.

Key Terms

Library Lingo

abstract Summary of the essential characteristics of something more extensive (e.g. a summary of a research article).

abstracts Special type of indexes that include citations and summaries of articles.

archive Collection of older materials that have some historical value.

book (monograph) Volume about a single subject or related subjects published once (later editions may update material).

call number (classification number) Number or letter-and-number combination assigned to each book and/or journal to indicate where it is shelved in a library.

catalogue List of materials made available by the library with a citation and call number (location details). Materials are usually physically located in the library but not always so.

CD-ROM Compact disc containing one or more electronic databases, programs or images.

circulating Describes materials that may be checked out of the library.

citation Bibliographical information about books or journals (e.g. author, title, source, date of publication).

collection All materials owned by a library.

database Collection of related information such as a catalogue, index or abstract.

dissertation (see also thesis) Research paper written by a graduate student as part of the degree requirement.

electronic database Database that is accessed for a search by computer.

holdings The specific volumes or issues of periodicals owned by the library.

index List of periodical citations arranged by subject or author. Indexes are usually organised around a specific subject area or field of study.

information literacy The ability to recognise the need for information, and identify, locate, access, evaluate and apply the needed information (Australian Library and Information Association).

interlibrary loan Library service that allows books and copies of articles to be borrowed from other libraries for use.

journal (periodical) Published collection of articles, usually of a scholarly nature.

microfiche Materials that have been reduced and placed on photographic film (e.g. microform, microfilm).

online (1) Describes materials that are computerised and accessed by other computers (e.g. a computer network). (2) Having an active connection to the internet.

periodical Journal or magazine.

> **reference collection** Noncirculating materials that are meant to be used for reference rather than read through (e.g. indexes, encyclopaedias, dictionaries).
>
> **search** Use of indexes, abstracts and catalogues to find information about a specified subject.
>
> **shelves (stacks)** Library bookshelves.
>
> **special reserve (closed reserve)** Materials that cannot be checked out of the library.
>
> **thesis** Research treatise written by a graduate student as part or all of the degree requirement.
>
> **volume** Single book or bound sequence of issues of a periodical.

We've heard many nurses admit that they have not darkened the door of a library since they finished school. We've taught senior students who have no library skills. We're afraid some of them don't even know where the library is located. Why? The first excuse given usually has to do with lack of time or with the library's shortcomings (e.g. 'They never have what I want' or 'I can never get any help'). Further exploration with students and practising nurses alike, however, usually reveals feelings of being overwhelmed, of not knowing where to start or who to ask. In short, a trip to the library is a frustrating and unpleasant experience. Today, of course, with the explosion of information available online, many students may not have to physically enter a library; today an increasing number of the resources provided by libraries can be accessed at home via a computer. Whether you need to visit your library in person or access it from home, if you find the thought of libraries a little intimidating or if you need a refresher course in how libraries work, this chapter is for you.

Do You Need This Chapter?

Take the following quiz to find out if you need to read this chapter:
1   Do you know what libraries are available in your area?
2   Do you know what kinds of materials they have and what kinds of services they offer?
3   Do you know where they are located, when they are open, and who can use them?
4   Do you have library privileges? Are they current?
5   Have you used a library in the last month?
6   Do you find it easy to locate what you are looking for when you do use a library?
7   Can you operate computerised search systems? (Hint: If you don't know what a search system is, you need this chapter.)
8   Do you know how much it costs to make a photocopy of a reference?

9 Could you identify a reference librarian if he or she weren't behind the reference desk?
10 Do the librarians know you by name at the loans desk?

If you answered 'yes' to most of these questions you may want to just skim this chapter. However, if you've ever said to a lecturer or colleague, 'There wasn't any information about *(fill in the blank)* available', then you definitely need to read this chapter and complete the Student Challenges.

What Is a Library?

A library is a place (nowadays this can be virtual or physical) where large amounts of information are available on various subjects. More specifically, a library is a **collection** of materials organised for ease of use. The key terms here are 'collection' and 'organised'. We usually think of a library collection as consisting of **books (monographs)** and journals, but today's libraries offer numerous electronic resources as well. A library might also be a collection of art, maps or audiovisual materials. What is collected often determines the library type.

> A library is a collection of materials that have been organised for use.

Types of libraries

There are three basic types of libraries that may prove helpful to you: public libraries, academic libraries and special libraries. Public libraries are provided through public funds for public use. They collect information of interest to the community being served. These may be local or national libraries and they may have several hundred to several hundred thousand available items. If you live in a large urban area, there are probably a number of small public libraries located in the suburbs, with a main library located in the city centre. The main library houses the most extensive part of the available collection of materials.

Academic libraries are connected with academic institutions above the secondary level and collect information of interest to faculty (academic staff) and students. The types of materials collected are strongly associated with the major degree areas offered at that academic institution. The size of the student body and the sources of funding influence the size and quality of the collection. Many large universities have more than one library on campus or more than one campus with a library. One of these is usually designated as the main library, and the others tend to be specialty or branch libraries.

Special libraries are formed by organisations with specialised information needs. They collect information on specific topics dictated by the needs of the organisation that funds them. These may include business and corporate libraries, or professional libraries, such as law or hospital libraries. The information collected is based on the needs of the special population being served. If you are located in an acute care centre, you may have access to the institution's library, which is usually a cross between an academic and a specialty library.

Classification schemes

Shelves of haphazardly collected books do not constitute a library. Fortunately, libraries don't keep their books organised like we do at home. Can you imagine going into a library and the librarian saying, 'You want a copy of *Contexts of Nursing: An Introduction?* Let's see, I seem to remember that it has a green and purple cover ... I know it's around here somewhere'. Libraries actually use very precise systems to organise all the information they collect. These organising systems are called classification schemes. Libraries use two major classification schemes: the Dewey Decimal Classification (DDC) and the Library of Congress classification.

The DDC was devised in 1876 by an American librarian named Melvil Dewey. He used a system of categories and decimal numbers to indicate subjects of books. This meant that one place in the library would contain all the books on a particular subject category. Dewey devised 10 main categories that are numbered in segments of 100. These main categories each contain 10 subcategories with number segments of 10. These subcategories are infinitely expandable to additional subcategories using a combination of numbers, decimal sets and letters. This classification scheme was 12 pages long in 1876. By 1986 it was 3500 pages long and continues to expand (ALA 1986).

The Library of Congress system also classifies information by subject matter using main categories and subcategories. However, its 21 main categories are designated by letters of the alphabet. Subcategories are formed by adding a second letter and/or a series of numbers. This system is more flexible and more readily revised than Dewey's system (Feather & Sturges 1997).

Both systems use number–letter combinations to label their collections. These labels are called **call numbers**. Some libraries put call numbers on all their materials, while others label only books. Each book has a unique call number, and ranges of call numbers are clearly marked on library shelves to make a particular book or a range of books about a specific subject easy to locate. As a rule of thumb, in Australia most public and academic libraries use the DDC. Specialty libraries may use a scheme adapted to handle large volumes of materials in relatively few subject areas. Medical libraries may use the National Library of Medicine® classification system, adapted from the Library of Congress system.

All the material in the library is carefully organised to make it easy to find and use.

What's in the Library?

Every library is arranged differently, but they usually have common features. The main section of the library typically contains a loans desk (circulation desk), an information desk, a reference desk and an area set aside for computer terminals where you can search for catalogues, indexes and abstracts. Other key areas include a **reference collection**, a current periodicals section, a bound periodicals section and the shelves. Most libraries also have a media or audiovisual centre, microfiche section, reserve section and special collections.

The *loans desk* is where you borrow books and other **circulating** materials to use outside the library setting. The *information desk* is the place to go when you don't know where to look for needed materials or when you have questions about various library services and resources.

> **HINT** Many libraries have pamphlets on library use and locations of materials. Read them. However, if you can't find what you need within 10 minutes, don't hesitate to ask a librarian.

In addition, most academic libraries offer instructive tours of the library and will willingly demonstrate how to access various databases and so on.

The reference desk is staffed by a reference librarian who can help you find specialised or hard-to-find resources. Some libraries combine the functions of the information and reference desks. Some floor area is set aside for the catalogue and indexing systems, which serve as search tools (via computers). These systems list all the library's materials and let you know where to find them.

The reference collection contains materials such as encyclopaedias, dictionaries, statistical reports, directories, handbooks and other materials that are handy for quick reference. Some libraries also put periodical indexes and abstracts here. These materials are referred to as 'for reference only' because they are intended for use on the premises and may not be checked out or removed from the general reference area.

The current **periodicals** section has the newer issues of journals and magazines displayed and organised alphabetically by title or call number. These issues frequently start with the first issue of the current year and contain all the issues for the year to date. The *bound periodicals* section contains journals and magazines for previous years. They have been bound together in a book form called a **volume**. The number of years contained in a volume depends on the size of the journal and number of issues published annually. Typically, one year of a journal constitutes a volume, and the specific volumes or issues of periodicals the library owns are referred to as its **holdings**. This section is usually arranged by call number (e.g. DDC) but in some libraries it is arranged alphabetically by periodical title.

The **stacks** are the library's main bookshelves. They usually contain books and occupy the most space in a library. In Australia and New Zealand, they may more commonly be referred to as **shelves**.

> **HINT** Some libraries store bound periodicals in the shelves rather than in a periodical section. If this is the case, the periodicals are given a call number and are stored by subject.

The media or audiovisual centre contains films, videotapes, audiotapes and computer software. Some libraries also house CD-ROMs here. The microfiche section contains microfilm and microform and the machines that allow you to read them. Microfilm and microfiche are inexpensive methods of storing large amounts of printed material in a small space. You may find back issues of newspapers, magazines, theses, maps and other materials stored on microfiche.

The reserve section contains materials placed aside by the library staff or faculty for special use. These materials typically can only be checked out for a few hours or one or two days, or may not be checked out at all. These materials are often heavily used, and so a reserve system allows a greater number of people to access them.

Special collections, or **archives**, contain rare materials that would not be replaced easily. These might include collections of such things as government and professional documents; old, rare or one-of-a-kind books; or materials of historical importance. Access to these materials may be restricted, and they may not be borrowed.

Chances are that you have at least visited your university or a health centre library. However, if you have only a sketchy idea about where things are located and how things are operated, please take time to do the following Student Challenge. It can save you a lot of time and energy when you need to use the library and want to locate the materials or services you need quickly.

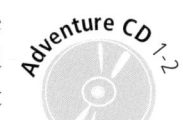

Student Challenge

Exploring Library Layouts

Make a trip to your university or health centre library. Allow an hour for this experience.

- Wander around, explore and browse.
- Pick up any handouts that are available to users as helpful hints or guides.
- Sit for a while and people watch.
- Skim the brochures you've collected.

Become comfortable with the space and with the idea of being there, then do the following tasks:

1. Make a map of the physical layout. (Hint: The library may have a ready-made map for users.) Locate and physically visit each of the following areas:
   a. loans desk, information desk, reserve desk, reference desk
   b. search tool section (e.g. indexes, abstracts and catalogues). Find the available computerised and manual versions. (Manual versions are rapidly disappearing.)
   c. list of periodical holdings
   d. current periodicals
   e. bound periodicals
   f. bookshelves
   g. reference collection
   h. special collections and archives
   i. government documents
   j. theses and dissertations
   k. media centre
   l. audiovisual aids (microfilm, microfiche, videotapes, audiotapes, audio CDs, CD-ROMs, DVDs)
   m. copy machines, change machines, vending machines
   n. study areas, lounges, toilets, telephones
   o. computers for word processing
   p. any other services

2. Find out about library operations.
   a. What are the library's opening hours?
   b. When are library staff available to help?
   c. Are library tours and/or classes in library use available?
   d. What are the policies for borrowing and return of materials?
   e. How do you get borrowing and interlibrary loan privileges?
   f. Is this library connected with other libraries you can use?
   g. Can you access computer search tools from computers in other locations on campus or from your home computer?

3. How is the library collection classified?

4. Where are the nursing materials located? Nursing books? Nursing journals? Professional documents, such as those from the Australian Council of Nurses

> (ANC) or the Royal College of Nursing Australia (RCNA)? New Zealand Nurses Organisation (NZNO)? Statistics about nurses and nursing?
> 5 What nursing journals do they hold? What nursing research journals do they hold?

How Do You Use the Library?

To find specific materials and retrieve the information you seek, you must understand the library's filing system. This means knowing how to use catalogues, abstracts and indexes to help you locate the materials you're interested in. These resources will usually be in computerised form. If your library does offer a manual system you may want to sit down and skim it to get a feel for how a catalogue or index is organised. However, doing a search in the twenty-first century, you will generally find that the computer is not only much quicker and more versatile, but is fast becoming the only modality on offer.

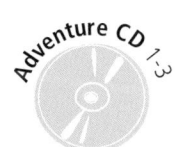

Catalogues

The catalogue lists books and usually other materials that are available in a specific library. Books are listed with bibliographical information, call numbers and borrowed status. Title, author or subject matter can be used to locate a book. The titles of periodicals and other library materials, such as government or professional documents, may also be listed, but information about the specific content contained in those periodicals or documents is usually not in the catalogue.

Manual catalogues

If the library has a manual cataloguing system, every book is listed on an index card and stored alphabetically in wooden file drawers. There are at least three cards for each book: one is listed and filed by book title (Figure 1-1), one by the author's last name, and one or more by the subject matter of the book. Some libraries have separate filing cabinets for each type of card—a title, an author catalogue and a subject catalogue. Others integrate all the cards in one large cataloguing system. Each card lists all bibliographical information plus the call number and related classification subject headings.

Not many libraries still have all their books on a manual card system. Most use a computerised system of some kind. A few libraries will have both systems in place, with older books on the manual system and newer books on the computer system.

Full Bib Display

AMICUS NO:	23695320 23695320 23695320
TITLE:	Nursing research : methods, critical appraisal and utilisation /Zevia Schneider ... [et al.].
EDITION:	2nd ed.
PUBLISHER:	Sydney : Mosby Publishers, [2002], c2003.
DESCRIPT'N:	xiii, 487 p. : ill. ; 25 cm.
ISBN:	1) 0729536653 :
	2) 0729536653 :
CONTENTS:	Section I. Research and Practice: 1. Research and professional practice; 2. Approaches to research; 3. Searching literature Appendix A. Women recovering from first-time myocardial infarction (MI): a feminist qualitative study / Debra Jackson, et al
NOTE(S):	1) Includes index.
	2) Previous ed.: Artarmon, N.S.W. : Mosby Publishers, 1999.
	3) Bibliography: p. [452]-478.
SUBJECT:	1) Nursing -- Research.
	2) Nursing Research.
AUTHOR(S):	Schneider, Zevia.
ABNRID:	000023695320

Figure 1-1 *Sample card catalogue on an index card, listed by book title*

Electronic catalogues

A computerised cataloguing system may be on **CD-ROM** (compact disc-read only memory) or directly **online**. A CD-ROM catalogue disc looks just like a music compact disc but it contains information on books or other materials located in the library. You access that information by putting the CD-ROM disc into the CD-ROM drive of a personal computer located in the reference or main section of the library. Directions will pop up on the screen that tell you how to search for a book by title, author or subject matter.

Online catalogues require you to use a computer terminal or personal computer that has a connection to the computerised **database**, which lists books and other library materials. The entries and directions look similar to those on the CD-ROM. The advantage of computerised systems (CD-ROM, online) over manual systems is that you can do a subject or title search using any of several key words, which affords you more flexibility. Online systems offer the added advantage of providing the latest information on all new materials coming into the library. CD-ROMs must be replaced with new versions and may be as much as a year behind in listing new materials. Online systems usually also carry additional information such as whether a book is on the shelves or has been borrowed and, if so, when it is due back. They may also give you information about resources in other nearby libraries.

Using your library's computerised catalogue, do the following challenge.

Student Challenge

Scanning Computer Catalogues*

1. Sit down at one of the computer terminals in the library.
2. Examine and try the different options available on the computer screen.
3. Use the online catalogue to locate one of your nursing textbooks by using a key word in the title.
4. Try locating it by author.
5. Try locating it by subject matter.
6. Which way was easiest for you? Did any of these give you problems? How did you solve them?
7. Go and locate the book in the library. What information did you use to find the book?

*Note: Catalogues list book citations; indexes list periodical citations.

Indexes and abstracts

Indexes list citations to periodicals and other publications such as newspapers and government or professional documents. **Abstracts** are simply indexes that also include a short summary of each citation. These citations are arranged by subject matter and/or author. Several different indexes exist for a wide variety of specialty areas. The library will not hold all the materials cited in a particular index, but it may have access to them through **interlibrary loan**. Look for a list of the indexes and abstracts available in a particular library to aid in your search abilities. Some common and useful indexes and abstracts are listed in Box 1-1.

BOX 1-1 Sample of Indexes/Abstracts

Subject-Specific Indexes/Abstracts
Australian Education Index (AEI)
Australasian Medical Index (AMI)
Aboriginal and Torres Strait Islander Health Bibliography (ATSIHEALTH)
British Nursing Index (BNI)
Cumulative Index to Nursing and Allied Health Literature (CINAHL)
Current Index to Journals in Education (ERIC)
Hospital and Health Administration Index
Index Medicus® (MEDLINE®)
Index New Zealand on Te Puna (INNZ)

International Nursing Index
International Pharmaceutical Abstracts
PsycINFO
Social Sciences Citation Index (SSCI)
Science Citation Index (SCI)
Sociological Abstracts
Social Work Abstracts

Magazines
Australian Journals Online (AJOL): the National Library of Australia's database of Australian electronic journals, newspapers, magazines, webzines, newsletters and email fanzines (http://www.nla.gov.au/ajol/).

Newspapers (Australian Indexes)
Sydney Morning Herald (INFOQUICK): a comprehensive index to articles about Australia and Australians, published in the *Sydney Morning Herald* and associated publications: *Sun Herald, Eastern Herald, Northern Herald* and *Good Weekend* from 1998 onwards (http://www.slnsw.gov.au/infoquick/welcome.htm).
INFOKOORI: an index of Australian Indigenous Affairs—an index to the *Koori Mail*, a national fortnightly newspaper published in Lismore, NSW, for Aboriginal and Torres Strait Islander people (http://www.slnsw.gov.au/koori/koori.htm).

Government Documents
Australian Public Affairs Information Service (APAIS)
Australian Monthly Economic and Social Indicators (MESI)
Parliament of Australia Database: an index to Australian Parliamentary Hansards, Bills, explanatory memoranda, Journals, Votes and Proceedings, Notice Papers, Committee publications and library journal articles.

Dissertations (Theses)
Australian Digital Theses project, http://adt.caul.edu.au/
Dissertation Abstracts

Computers
Gale Directory of Databases

Two indexes—*Cumulative Index to Nursing and Allied Health Literature* (CINAHL) and *Index Medicus* (MEDLINE)—serve as major search tools for materials in nursing and medicine. CINAHL contains indexed citations for over 1200 journals in nursing, medicine and 15 other allied health disciplines. Over 500 of the journals have abstracts—short summaries of articles—included with the article citation.

CINAHL also indexes material from consumer health and alternative therapy sources. Abstracts of nursing **dissertations/theses**, educational software and audiovisuals are included. *Index Medicus* contains indexed citations from over 3900 journals in medicine, nursing, dentistry, veterinary medicine and preclinical sciences. Author-generated abstracts are available for articles in most of these journals (PubMed 1999). CINAHL covers nursing, allied health and psychosocial issues better than *Index Medicus*, but coverage of medicine is more comprehensive in *Index Medicus*. Most major nursing journals can be found in either index.

Manual indexes and abstracts

Indexes are available in both computerised and printed formats. The printed indexes and abstracts are bound in large volumes arranged by different areas of specialty. They are usually stored on tables so you can use them in the same location that you find them. While they have mostly been replaced by computerised systems, a few libraries may have printed indexes for older periodicals (i.e. before the mid-1980s) and computerised indexes for newer periodicals. If your library has printed indexes, to become familiar with them, try the following Student Challenge.

Student Challenge

Perusing Printed Indexes

1. Select a printed volume of any one of the indexes available in your library.
2. Skim through it. What do you see?
3. Locate the listing of subject heads. (Hint: The listing of subject heads is located at the front of the index.)
4. Examine it. Try finding a topic or two in this listing.
5. Was the topic there? If you couldn't find it, did you try a synonym for the word you were looking for?
6. Look through the listings. Note that some major headings have pages and pages of listings, while subheadings have fewer listings.

Electronic indexes and abstracts

Electronic databases are available either on CD-ROM or online. They offer access to a wider range of information than their print counterparts. For example, CINAHL online offers proceedings from nursing conferences, standards of practice, and many statistics about nurses and nursing in addition to the indexed journals, professional publications and nursing dissertations. Electronic indexes may have different names, such as MEDLINE, which is the electronic version of *Index Medicus*.

Many electronic indexes combine two or more print index titles. For example, ERIC is an education electronic database that incorporates the *Current Index to Journals in Education* (CIJE) and *Resources in Education* (RIE) print indexes. Various electronic databases are available, and each operates in a slightly different fashion. The introductory computer screen and help feature will guide you in your search, but if these aren't sufficient, be sure to consult a reference librarian for additional help.

> **HINT** When you click on the 'help' button, it gives you information that corresponds to functions you are currently trying to perform. This is known as 'context-specific help'.

CD-ROMs usually contain one or two indexes per disc for a certain year span. These discs are replaced each time an update occurs. Updates may range from once a month to once a year. Thus, you might use a MEDLINE Professional CD-ROM disc to view the *Index Medicus* for 1994 to the present. MEDLINE Professional is updated every two months. The library may have their CD-ROM collection already stored on the computer. If so, simply click on the CD-ROM listings and then click on MEDLINE to get access to that particular index.

Online systems allow you instant access to a wide range of electronic indexes and abstracts. These indexes are kept on a master computer in a central site and are accessed by the computers in your library and in many cases from home or other computer sites. You will find a listing of available online indexes by viewing a listing on the screen of one of your library computers. The advantages of an online system over a CD-ROM are that updates occur more frequently, and user-timely messages may be posted on the site.

Try the following Student Challenge to get a feel for using electronic indexes and how they differ from computerised catalogues.

Student Challenge

Examining Electronic Indexes

Sit down at one of the computer terminals in the library.

1. Does the same terminal allow you to do catalogue and index searches? If so, how do you go from one type of search to the other?
2. Look at all the indexes available either on CD-ROM or online. Which ones look like they would be relevant to nursing or health care?
3. Explore at least two indexes that you consider relevant to nursing. Can you locate a description of the index? Can you find a list of the journals that are indexed?

Comparing manual and electronic indexes

If you have access to the printed version you will notice some differences between printed and electronic indexes. In an electronic database, you see only those things you have specifically requested by the search parameters you set up. However, you don't have to know the specialised vocabulary on which the index is based. The computer will guide you in the terms to use. You can search for key words or parts of words or combinations of words in any part of the article. You can do a cross search by entering several terms at once and instructing the computer on how to use these terms. You can place limits on the search by instructing the computer to look only for certain groups of articles, certain types of journals, or certain publication dates. After you enter these parameters, the search results appear with the touch of a button. You can change the limits or terms instantly and rerun your search as many times as you wish. This makes the search process more flexible, less time consuming and generally more productive. More recent technological advances have produced online journals and the ability to download full-text versions of journal articles. This increases the convenience of online searching and again is more efficient in both time and cost.

Although the older-style printed index can be touched, picked up and perused, it takes up physical space. Print indexes have fixed entries listed under a set of pre-established headings and subheadings and you can see the whole thing at once. When conducting a search in a printed index, you need to first know the precise terms (known in library lingo as 'controlled vocabulary') used in the index. If multiple terms describe your topic, you then have to look up each term separately and read all the entries listed in an attempt to eliminate non-applicable articles. This elimination process is based largely on the title. For large topics, index entries have the potential to be endless, and the process of elimination is time consuming and confusing.

If you do have access to both the printed and electronic versions of CINAHL or *Index Medicus* (MEDLINE), try the following Student Challenge.

Student Challenge

Comparing Printed and Electronic Indexes

Do a search of the nursing literature in the year 2001 for articles that give information about nursing care of persons with Alzheimer's disease.

1. Use the print index first.
2. Time each search.
3. What difficulties did you encounter with each search method?
4. What did you like about each method?
5. Compare your results. Are they similar? Which method produced the best materials?

How Do You Successfully Search for Information?

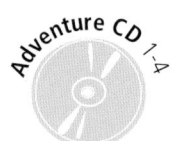

A **search** is conducted using indexes, abstracts and catalogues to find information about specific subjects. As you have probably discovered, searching for a known book or article by title or by author is fairly easy. Searching for unknown materials on a subject you're interested in is a little more complicated. If you have ever done a search and received a message that says, 'there are 2346 matches' or 'there are no matches meeting your search parameters', you know what we mean. This section is designed to help make your searches smoother and more productive.

Clearly define your mission

What is it that you expect to find from your trip to the library? What is your subject area? What are the key concepts and subconcepts for that subject? Which concepts are most important? What information do you already have? Reading your own textbooks or reference books for background information before you go to the library can help focus and direct your search. Look at the references listed in these books. You might find sources on your topic that you can look up in the library.

> **HINT** It helps to read your own textbooks or reference books for background information before you go to the library.

Choose appropriate resources

Books tend to give you standard accepted information and practices. They provide good baseline data on a subject, particularly if the subject area is new to you. If you already have a working baseline and are looking for current information, then skip the books and go straight to the journals. Journals provide more current information than books. They report changing trends and practices. Research journals provide the results of the latest research studies. Do you need definitions, statistics, trends, or professional or government standards about a topic? These are usually found in reference materials or the special documents sections of the library. Dictionaries and encyclopaedias can give you quick definitions and overviews of your subject matter.

Choose appropriate indexes

You will save a lot of time if you choose the appropriate index. When skimming the list of available periodical indexes, some choices are obvious. You don't look in the literature or philosophy indexes for a nursing topic. But there are several indexes for nursing journals, including CINAHL and *Index Medicus* (MEDLINE). There are also indexes from other disciplines that might have information about a related topic in nursing. For example, you might locate articles for case management in the *Social Work Abstracts*. Each index has a primary area of focus, and advantages and limits. A description of the purpose of a particular index and a list of the journals included is usually readily available in the library. These descriptions may be available in print and/or on computer. Reading these descriptions can help you decide which database to use. Another useful database is EBMR *Full Text*, a specialised database for locating full-text evidence-based publications.

Define your search parameters

Electronic databases operate with a special vocabulary. However, the computer helps you define the preferred terms to use in a search. If you enter a term, it will supply alternative terms for use. It will also let you view the entire directory if you want to see how it is organised. Different databases use different listings of terms. MEDLINE uses a medical subject-heading (MeSH®) directory. CINAHL uses its own specialised thesaurus. Many other databases use Library of Congress headings or their own specialised subject directories.

Place limits on your search

You want to make your search as precise as possible. If you have several key terms, use them. Set other limits such as gender, age and/or time factors if you know them. You can always lift some of the limits if you don't find what you want. Let's say, for example, that we want to find out the latest information on the effects of menopause on individuals with diabetes mellitus. If we enter the word 'diabetes' to search MEDLINE, for example, we would get more than 147,000 different citations. If we use the words 'diabetes mellitus' we come up with around 134,000 citations. The words 'diabetes mellitus AND menopause' narrow it down to fewer than 500 citations. If we narrow the search to include only adult females, we get around 300 citations. If we further limit the search to articles written in English and published from 2000 to 2001, we get a manageable number of citations.

All computerised search databases have rules for use. The more you know about these rules and how to use them, the more successful your search will be. Most databases use something called Boolean operators. These operators are just words (e.g. AND, OR, NEAR, NOT) that help you link key terms together to get certain results. Look at the diabetes–menopause example in Table 1-1. As you can see, OR is the least restrictive link and NOT is the most restrictive link. Other operators may be used to place limits on such things as age, gender, type of journal, years of publication and so on.

A few databases use a technique called *probabilistic searching*, which gives you a list of articles ranked from most to least likely to be relevant, based on a set of supplied search terms (e.g. diabetes mellitus, menopause, female, adult). Articles containing all the terms would be high on the list, and those containing one term would be at the bottom of the list. You can even weight the terms to indicate which are more important in the search (e.g. the terms *diabetes mellitus* and *menopause* could be more heavily weighted than female or adult).

TABLE 1-1 Example of a Boolean Search

Connector	Example	What Happens
or	Diabetes mellitus *or* menopause	Retrieves all citations containing the words 'diabetes mellitus' or the word 'menopause' in an article.
and	Diabetes mellitus *and* menopause	Retrieves all citations containing both the words 'diabetes mellitus' and the word 'menopause' in an article.
near	Diabetes mellitus *near* menopause	Retrieves all citations containing both the words 'diabetes mellitus' and the word 'menopause' in the same sentence of the article.
not	Diabetes mellitus *not* menopause	Eliminates any citations containing the words 'diabetes mellitus' that also contain the word 'menopause'.

The best way to become proficient at using search operators is through informed practice. Many students do not make full use of electronic system capabilities, but you should remember that these systems are expensive and universities invest a great deal of money in them because they are so crucial to your learning. Read the materials available on conducting a search. Ask for assistance if you aren't finding anything or if you're finding too much. Explore various search options and see what happens. Most importantly, practise, practise, practise. (Hint: Make sure you correctly spell all the terms that you enter for a computerised search.)

View your search results

Once you have defined and run your search, you'll want to view the results. The first viewing screen usually contains each citation with the option to view an abstract or full text if available. Simply looking at article titles or journal names helps you eliminate more articles from your search. If a citation looks promising, you may want to look at the abstract.

In the example about menopause and its effects on diabetes, a preview of the final citations led to about 20 articles that looked like useful possibilities. We asked the computer for the abstracts on these articles and found that around five of the articles looked promising. We then went to the shelves and skimmed the full texts of those articles. Three were useful, so we made copies of them.

Looking at the citations may also give you clues about making a search narrower. For example, when we did the search using just the word 'diabetes', the very first citation was about diabetes insipidus, leading us to add 'mellitus' to the term 'diabetes' to be more specific.

Now that you have had a little practice, try the following Student Challenge and do another search, using the computer and whichever electronic resources you deem most appropriate. Use the information from the successful search section and the knowledge gained from the previous Student Challenges to assist you.

Student Challenge

Putting It All Together

Search for updated information on a basic nursing skill (such as handwashing, blood pressure readings or temperature taking).

1. Define what you are looking for.
2. What resources will you use? Why did you choose them?
3. Describe how you conducted your search. What parameters did you use? How did you limit the search?
4. How many different searches did you do? What guided your decision-making processes during the search process? What aspects of your search approach worked and what didn't work?
5. Print the end results of your search. Locate the articles you think are most pertinent to your selected topic. Do they contain the information you need?

Resource Kit

Library help guides: Many libraries offer printed help guides designed to make library use easier. Collect them, read them, use them.

HELP! Button: Electronic databases all come with a Help button. It is designed to help you make the best use of that database. Click on it whenever you are stuck in an electronic search process and need guidance.

Librarians: Don't forget to use these helpful resources. Don't be shy. They field all kinds of seemingly dumb questions.

> 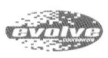 Visit this book's Evolve website at http://evolve.elsevier.com/AU/Borbasi/maze for further information.
>
> Check out the puzzles, mazes and games on your CD-ROM.

Acknowledgment

The authors wish to acknowledge the assistance of Ms Raechel Damarell, Subject Librarian, School of Nursing and Midwifery, Flinders University in the adaptation of this chapter.

References

American Library Association (ALA) (1986). *ALA World Encyclopedia of Library and Information Services*, 2nd edn. ALA, Chicago.

Australian Library and Information Association (ALIA) (2002). Statement on information literacy for all Australians. Online. Available: http://www.alia.org.au/policies/information.literacy.html 12 Mar 2003.

CINAHL Information Systems. About CINAHL. Online. Available: http://www.cinahl.com 12 Mar 2003.

Feather J, Sturges P (1997). *International Encyclopedia of Information and Library Science*. Rutledge, New York.

National Library of Medicine PubMed (1999). The NLM PubMed Project Overview. Online. Available: http://www.ncbi.nlm.nih.gov/pubmed/overview 12 Mar 2003.

http://evolve.elsevier.com/AU/Borbasi/maze

Learning Objectives

After reading this chapter and following critical reflection the student will be able to:

1. Describe the internet and relevant internet components and services.
2. Use three different approaches to web navigation.
3. Send and receive electronic mail with attachments.
4. Explore listservers, newsgroups and/or chat rooms.
5. Discuss possible applications of FTP and Telnet.
6. Access library filing systems (indexes, catalogues) over the internet.
7. Use professional databases available on the net.
8. Locate print and electronic journals available on the net.
9. Discuss professional communication and education opportunities available via the internet.

Chapter Outline

What Is This Chapter All About?
What Is the Internet?
What Does the Internet Offer?
World wide web
Communication tools
Traditional services
How Do You Use the Internet?
Navigating the web
   Uniform resource locator
   Hypertext links
   Search engines
Communicating on the net
   Email and listservs
   Newsgroups and chat rooms
   Audio and video possibilities
Trying traditional tools
How Do You Use the Net for Professional Purposes?
Information access
Communication possibilities
Ongoing educational opportunities

Chapter 2
Surfing the Internet

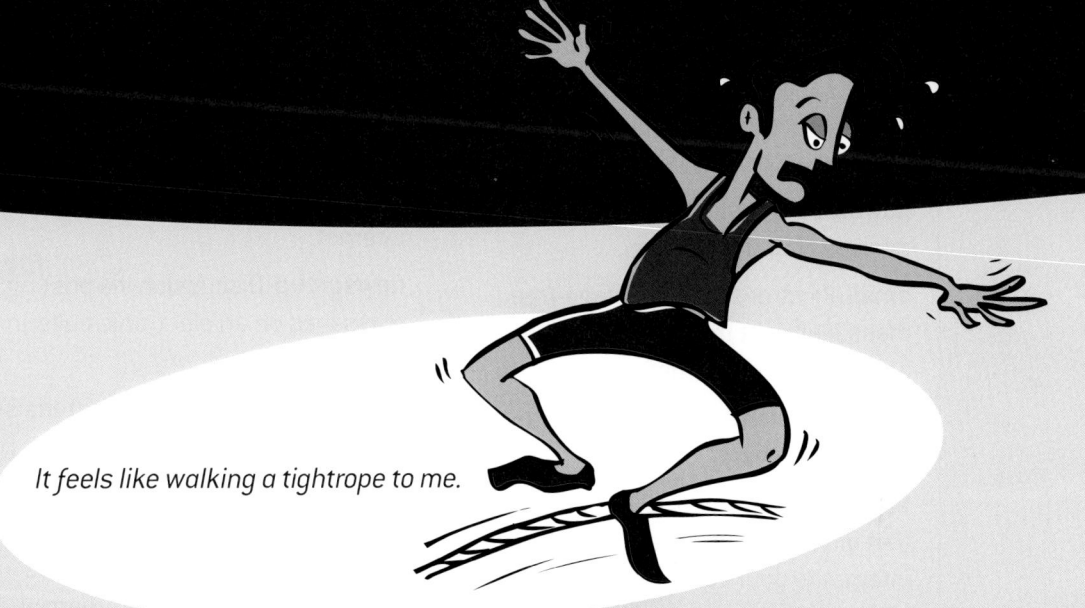

It feels like walking a tightrope to me.

Student Quote

'I feel like an explorer setting out in uncharted territory … It's exciting and scary at the same time.'

Abstract

Technology and the internet are changing the way we find, use and share information. The internet is a worldwide, interconnected network of computers. You can tap into stored information and databases and send and receive communications from individuals or groups. To use the internet you need a computer, a connection source and a service provider. All internet locations are identified by an address (i.e. the uniform resource locator, or URL). Navigating the net is enhanced by the use of web browsers and search engines. Library catalogues, indexes and other resources are available on the internet, including various health-related databases such as MEDLINE and CINAHL. Full-text print journals and electronic journals are increasingly available. The internet provides instant communication to professional colleagues from across the globe. You can take a course, search for a job or hold a meeting over the internet. It holds new hope in the quest for information literacy.

Key Terms

Net Nomenclature

bookmark A way to mark and easily access a favourite or frequently used website in Netscape Navigator (referred to as 'Favorites' in Internet Explorer).

browser Program that opens and displays pages on the world wide web.

download Transfer a file from the internet to your computer.

email Electronic mail; postage-free messages sent from one computer to another via the internet.

file attachment File that is added to an email message.

file transfer protocol (FTP) Program that allows you to transfer files from the internet to your computer.

home page The first or base page for a website. It often serves as a map, directing you to places of interest on the site.

hypertext Electronic document format that permits links to other web pages or other related websites. The link is underlined and can be accessed by a mouse click on the link.

hypertext markup language (HTML) The codes and instructions used to control the appearance and function of a website. It inserts links, graphics and other multimedia objects on the web page.

hypertext transfer protocol (HTTP) The language used to transfer web pages over an internet connection. The first letters in a URL for a site on the world wide web.

internet service provider (ISP) Company that provides a connection to the internet (e.g. Telstra BigPond, Ozemail).

listserver (listserv) Electronic mailing list.

log off Disconnect from the internet.

log on Connect to the internet.

navigate Move from site to site on the internet.

newsgroup Discussion via posting messages on an electronic bulletin board.

online (1) Computerised materials that are accessed by other computers (e.g. a computer network). (2) Having an active connection to the internet.

online service Range of services provided by an online commercial network (such as CompuServe, AOL, Prodigy). Examples of services include access to the internet, news, games, travel information and so on.

search engine Tool for finding and retrieving specific information on the web (e.g. Yahoo!, Lycos, Go.com, Altavista, Excite).

server (host) Computer that offers an information service over the internet.

Telnet Software that lets users log on to another computer from a remote site. It shows text only, no graphics or pictures.

uniform resource locator (URL) The address system used by the internet to assist in locating a web page or file.

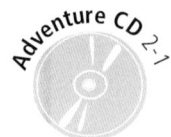

upload Transfer a file from your computer to another computer, using the internet.

user Client that communicates via computer and uses internet services offered by servers or hosts.

user name The name you use to identify your computer to another computer or computer system.

web page One screen on a website.

website Sequence of web pages created by an individual or organisation for conveying information.

world wide web (www) Collection of computers on the internet that are interconnected by hypertext and store websites.

Easy access to ever more affordable, powerful and user-friendly microcomputers has forever changed the way we interact with the world around us. The computer revolution is in full bloom and has spawned the internet. This information highway can instantly link us to people and resources around the world. It is changing the way we work and play. We can buy a car or shop for groceries without leaving the house. We can meet and chat with new friends in Canada, Japan or Brazil. We can send or receive reams of material at the push of a button. We can tap into the latest information available about almost any subject imaginable. The internet is erasing boundaries of time and distance. It allows us to explore new worlds and ideas, to sail into uncharted waters and to become players in an exciting adventure.

What Is This Chapter All About?

You have explored the library as a resource that can help you become and remain information literate. This chapter introduces you to another way to keep up with the rapid information growth of our times. We take you on a tour of the internet and explore its potential, investigating what it is, what it can offer and how to use it. We focus on the internet as a tool for locating and accessing information resources. The ability to use the internet can extend and enhance your library skills and make finding needed professional information easier, less time consuming and more convenient. Picture this: it's 11 pm and you're all ready for bed. In a panic, you realise that you have an assignment due in two days and you haven't even started on it. The library is closed so you can't even do a literature search. Now imagine conducting a search from your bed, in your pyjamas, on your laptop, at midnight. Fantasy? No, thanks to the internet. If this sounds like a tool you would like to exploit, read on.

HINT If you are already an accomplished internet user, you might want to skim the first part of this chapter and concentrate on the section that addresses use of the internet for professional purposes.

What Is the Internet?

The internet is, in the broadest sense, a microcosm of our world. It reflects a vast variety of cultural and societal views and allows people across the planet to share ideas on a personal level never before possible. In a more literal sense, the internet is a huge network of interconnected computers located all over the world. These computers are linked by a series of networks. Some of the computers in the network are known as hosts or servers, because they 'serve' information in various ways to computer owners known as clients or users.

> The internet is a huge network of interconnected server and user computers located all over the world.

Anyone with a computer, a modem and an account can access the internet and communicate with all the other participating computers. This means that you, as an internet user, can interact with people from around the world. You also have access to a vast array of information and resources stored on those computers. The internet currently connects millions of computers and is more than doubling in size every year.

> Anyone with a computer, a modem and an account can access the internet.

The internet, or 'net' for short, began as a highly specialised network of computers designed by the United States military in the 1960s. Other governmental agencies, universities and research institutions began to use it in the 1970s to exchange scientific and technical information. In the 1980s, libraries and other professional associations began using the internet to exchange scholarly information. Then an explosion occurred in the personal computer industry, and the ready availability of personal computers allowed individuals access to the net.

The 1990s marked a rapid evolution of the internet. It has become a personal communication exchange and commercial marketplace, as well as an information resource. Local, state and national governing bodies; professional and community associations; educational and research institutions; and businesses and individuals use the net. It is used for learning, research, business and pleasure, and remains relatively lacking in structure and control. There are few rules and no central organising concept. Even the 'experts' struggle to keep up with the changes.

The potential of the internet seems limitless, but that very potential also presents challenges (Box 2-1). The biggest challenge when using the internet is learning to

navigate the net efficiently and effectively. Think of it as an adventure because the net can be a powerful tool for communication, information retrieval and learning.

> **BOX 2-1** Some Issues Encountered When Using the Internet
>
> **Confusion and chaos:** The internet operates in a freewheeling culture with few rules, limits or boundaries. No entity exercises control over net offerings and there is little regulatory control over net transactions.
> **Needle in a haystack:** The number of internet websites is growing at an incredibly fast pace. No single search device has been devised that allows efficient access to everything on the net. Sometimes you have to wade through a haystack of useless and irrelevant junk to find the needle that you need.
> **Time drain:** Although touted for its instant access and speed, it is easy to spend hours moving and scrolling through various web pages on the internet, with little to show for the effort.
> **Questionable reliability of information:** Anyone is free to post information, and this leads to a dilemma about the accuracy and reliability of such information. The exact source and that source's credibility are often hard to determine on the internet.

What Does the Internet Offer?

There are many services on the internet. The world wide web (www) and electronic mail (email) are probably the best known. Other applications include listservs, newsgroups, chat rooms, audio and interactive video, file transfer protocols (FTP) and Telnet. Each of these is described in the following sections.

World wide web

The **world wide web (www)** or 'the web' is the most rapidly growing portion of the internet. Although the terms 'internet' and 'world wide web' are often used interchangeably, the web is in fact a subset of the internet. The web is a huge, loosely organised collection of documents on thousands of topics stored on various computers worldwide. The collection is located on various **websites**, each containing numerous **web pages** of material. These web pages use a variety of multimedia resources with a mixture of text, sound, graphics, colour and sometimes videos.

The pages are linked by **hypertext**, which allows you to move from one page to another or from one website to another by clicking on a highlighted word with your computer mouse. This is often termed 'surfing'. For example, you might be on a website about the care of diabetes mellitus and discover links to a diabetic diet, insulin or foot care. (More about navigating the web later.)

Communication tools

There are a number of ways to communicate with others over the internet. These range from email to chat rooms, newsgroups and videoconferencing. A discussion of communication tools follows.

Electronic mail (**email**) allows you to send and receive messages over the internet. You can even attach and send computer files, called **file attachments**, with your message. The message travels postage-free and arrives at its destination in a matter of seconds. As a student, you can send and receive messages to and from faculty members or you can send a term paper or care plan by attaching it to a message. You can converse with nursing students in other universities around the world. Email also allows you to send a message to multiple people simultaneously. A *listserv* is an email list that is organised around a particular area of interest. To use a listserv, simply send an email message to the owner of the list, who then distributes the message to all the members of a particular interest group who have subscribed to the list.

Newsgroups are electronic message boards that allow you to post and receive messages to and from participants in that newsgroup.

Chat rooms are similar to newsgroups, except that you can carry on typed conversations with people who are currently logged on to their computers and are tuned into a particular chat room. So feedback in a chat room is immediate, whereas feedback in a newsgroup is delayed. Some schools of nursing have chat rooms to allow students to interact with the faculty as well as one another. This is particularly so with distance programs.

If you have the right hardware and software, you can use the internet as a telephone and actually speak to people through an internet connection. If you add special video equipment, you can hold video conversations and actually see the person as you talk. You can even hold videoconferences. As technology continues to improve, this use of the internet will become more common.

Traditional services

Two older or more traditional systems on the internet that you may still see in action are **Telnet** and **file transfer protocols (FTP)**. Telnet connects a text-only computer to one or more remote locations via the internet. It requires special software to establish a connection. Some universities and libraries still use Telnet systems.

File transfer protocol is a particular process used to transfer files across the internet. Typical files include public domain software, lesson plans, electronic books, research reports and graphics.

How Do You Use the Internet?

To use the internet you need access. This requires a computer, an internet connection and an **online service** or **internet service provider (ISP)**. The most common connection is through a modem. Satellite dishes, cable television and digital subscriber lines (DSL) also offer internet access in some locations. The modem is used to dial up a commercial online service such as AOL or Telstra.com, or to connect to an ISP such as BigPond or Ozemail. These services typically charge a subscription rate. Some ISPs provide free connections, but you are likely to be subject to a barrage of advertisements. (The Resource Kit at the end of the chapter lists several online services and ISPs.)

Once you have a connection, you are ready to **log on** to the net. However, you need a program that will let you take advantage of the resources on the internet. Two popular programs, Internet Explorer and Netscape Navigator, enable you to browse the web, send and receive email, access newsgroups and chat rooms, use an electronic telephone and edit web pages. Even though they allow you to access multiple internet resources, they are often called **web browsers**. One of these programs may have come with the purchase of your computer, or your ISP or online service may have provided it to you. Both systems look similar and operate very similarly (Fig 2-1) and both are available for Macintosh and Windows computer operating systems.

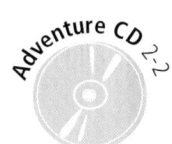

Navigating the web

The browser that is built into the Internet Explorer or Netscape Navigator program serves as your guide to the world wide web. As you will discover, it is easy to lose track of where you are on the web. A browser allows you to track the websites you visit, to revisit previous sites and to save favourite sites so that you can find and visit them easily.

When you first connect to the internet, you will automatically connect to the front page of your online or internet service provider and to your web browser program. Your screen will display a home page from your service provider with the browser toolbar and menu at the top (Fig 2-1).

a

![Internet Explorer toolbar]

b

![Netscape Navigator toolbar]

Figure 2-1 a *Internet Explorer toolbar* ***b*** *Netscape Navigator toolbar*

Uniform resource locator

There are three major ways to move around the web from that initial page. The first is by entering the address of a particular site you wish to visit. Each place on the internet has a **uniform resource locator (URL)**, which is an address for a specific location on the internet. For example, http://collingwoodfc.com.au/ is the URL for the Collingwood Football Club website.

If you know an address, you can enter it on the location line of your web browser and it will take you directly to that site. Various print, CD-ROM and online directories list website addresses. They often resemble telephone directories. There is even a website yellow pages. You will also notice that an increasing number of businesses, newspapers and television programs are posting their URLs.

> **HINT** You must type the URL exactly as it appears. If you add a space, omit a dot or misspell a word, the site can't be located. However, you can omit the 'http://' at the beginning of a web address. The web browser will automatically insert it for you.

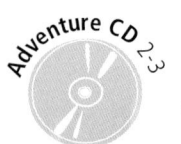

Examining a URL can tell you something about the site. Figure 2-2 presents the elements of a URL. To see how URLs work, try the following Student Challenge.

Student Challenge

Using URLs

If you have internet access, try the following:

1. Collect three or four URLs you have seen mentioned in a newspaper, magazine, on television or in another source.
2. Connect to your ISP and web browser.
3. Enter one of the URLs in the address or location text box on the browser. (Hint: On most browsers, the text box to type in the URL is located right below the toolbar and above the page viewing area.) You may have to erase an existing URL before entering the new URL.
4. Highlight the URL you have entered and click on it or click the 'Go' button to the right of the text box, or press 'Enter' on your keyboard.
5. You should now be looking at the first page of the site that you entered the address for.
6. Now enter another URL and repeat the procedure described above. You have now moved to another specified site.

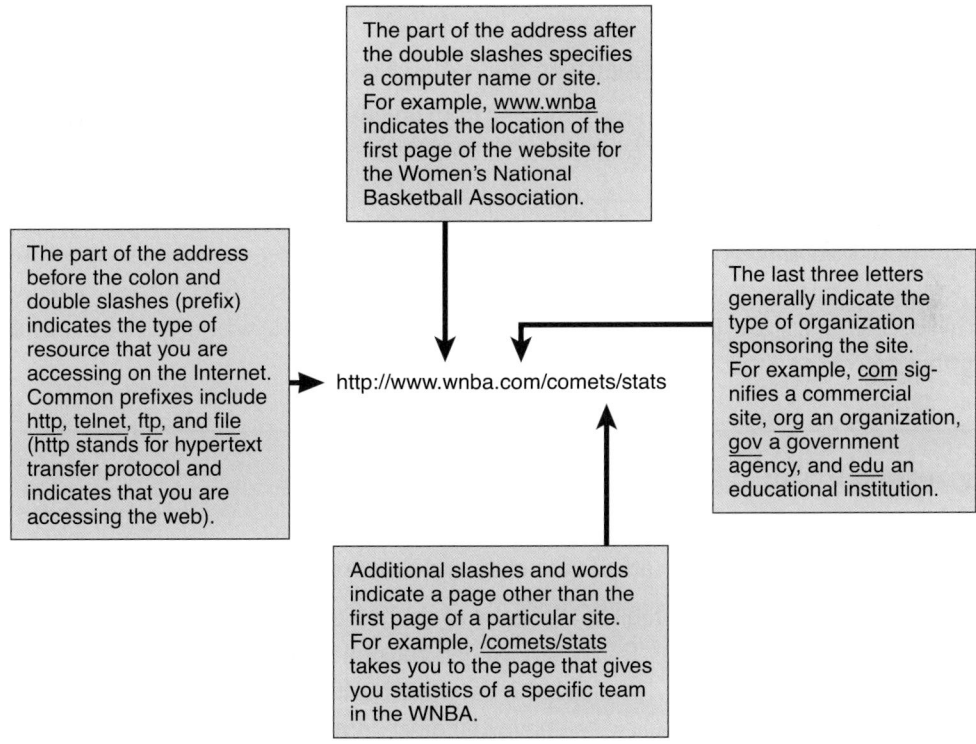

Figure 2-2 *Elements of a uniform resource locator (URL)*

Hypertext links

A second way to move around the web is by clicking on the highlighted web links or icons (little pictures) found on each web page. These are known as *hypertext links*. When your mouse pointer moves over a link, the pointer will change form (e.g. the pointer may change from an arrow to a hand). This alerts you to the presence of a link. These send you instantly to other pages within that site or to other related sites.

> **Student Challenge**
>
> Leafing Through Links
>
> Using one of the sites that you found by entering a URL, try the following:
>
> 1. Look at the web page. Note that some of the text is highlighted and underlined. These are hypertext links. Click on one of these links. You have just moved to another web page.
> 2. Check the address window on your web browser. Note how the URL has changed. If the address has been added to, you have moved to another page. If the information right after 'www' has changed, you have accessed a new site.
> 3. Explore the pages for this website by clicking on various links and viewing several web pages.
> 4. Try clicking on icons and boxed text. These may also be links.
> 5. Play around, enjoy the feeling of moving from link to link and page to page. When you are done, don't log off (disconnect). Do the next challenge first.

By now you have probably discovered that you can become lost in the forest, so to speak, rather quickly. This is why a web browser is a useful tool. The web browser can help you leave a trail of bread crumbs to mark where you have been. Try the following Student Challenge.

> **Student Challenge**
>
> Trailblazing or Trial Browsing
>
> You should be using the results of your click-and-link exercise.
>
> 1. Locate the web browser toolbar at the top of your screen. Click the 'Back' button on your web browser toolbar. This will move you back one web page. Click the 'Back' button again. Do it again. Now click the 'Forward' button. This will move you forward one web page with each click. You have just discovered a basic way to retrace your path when you want to revisit a previous page or advance to the next page.

2 If you have Internet Explorer, click the 'down' arrow located to the right of the 'Back' button on your browser toolbar. A list of the pages you just visited will appear. Click on one of these pages. You will go right to it. This can save you multiple clicks on the 'Back' button.

3 Click the 'down' arrow to the right of the address or location window. It lists the URLs for the sites you have visited most recently. Note that it lists only the site, not the various pages in the site. Click on one of these sites.

4 Do you want a comprehensive record of where you have been on the web? If you have the Internet Explorer browser, click the 'History' button. Click on the week and the day you are interested in. Click on the site you are interested in. You will see a trail of all the pages you visited in that site. If you have Netscape Navigator, open the 'Communicator' menu and choose 'History' to produce the history list.

5 Do you want to save a site or a page you really like and want to visit again? To bookmark a website, bring the site or page up on your screen. If you have Internet Explorer, open the 'Favorites' menu and click on 'Add to Favorites'. Your page is permanently saved for you. Anytime you want to access it, just click the 'Favorites' button on the toolbar and then click on the saved web page of your choice.

If you have Netscape Navigator, open the 'Bookmarks' menu located to the left of the location box and click 'Add Bookmark'. To get a bookmarked page just click the 'Bookmarks' menu and select the web page of your choice.

6 Explore the other buttons on your web browser toolbar. Can you figure out what they do? Open up the various drop-down menus for your browser. Check out the help menu. Don't be afraid to try out buttons and menu options. Have fun, explore and play.

Search engines

A third way to navigate the web is by using a search engine. **Search engines** are tools that allow you to search for information by using key words. You will find that they resemble the search tools you used in Chapter 1 when doing index searches. Various search engines are available to help you do a search of websites. Some of the most commonly available engines are described in Box 2-2.

Navigating the Web

Navigate the web by:
1 *Entering the URL of the website*
2 *Clicking on hypertext links*
3 *Using search engines.*

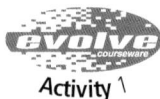
Activity 1

BOX 2-2 Sample Search Engines

The website for each of the following search engines is accessible through this book's Evolve website at http://evolve.elsevier.com/AU/Borbasi/maze.

- **AltaVista** is a very comprehensive search engine with a large and reliable index. It has basic and advanced search capabilities. You need to have fairly narrow search parameters or you will get an overwhelming response to your search query.
- **Excite** may be helpful when you are not quite sure what term or terms to use in a search. It uses a method known as *concept searching*. This means it will not only look for the key words entered, but will also look for materials based on the idea the terms convey. It will also suggest related terms to use. If you find a source you like, Excite also has a feature that lets you search for similar sources by clicking on the 'more like this' option.
- **Go.com** allows you to search other internet sites in addition to websites, such as news stories from the newswire services. It also has a special feature called 'imageseek' that lets you look for pictures or graphics.
- **Google** allows you to search the entire web or just Australian sources. You can also search specific sites (e.g. universities). Google also suggests alternative spellings if it appears that you have made a typo when keying in your key words for a search.
- **HotBot** is a comprehensive search engine that is very user friendly. It will guide you through the process and allows you to search by date or by domain type (e.g. you can limit your search to educational sites or delete commercial sites).
- **Lycos** uses probabilistic searching and lists search results in rank order of relevance to your search. It also has a browseable index.
- **Magellan** not only does a search, but also rates and reviews many of the sites located. You can search the entire Magellan database or limit your search to the reviewed and/or top quality sites.
- **Northern Light** is one of the latest 'in' search engines because it will directly link you to full text resources and a way to order them online.
- **Yahoo!** allows you to use a subject index or key word search approach. You can even conduct a key word search within a selected index category. Yahoo! also has hypertext links to other search engines. For these reasons, many people consider Yahoo! to be the best overall search engine available.

Many other search engines also exist. Some are very specialised and search only certain segments of the web. These may be helpful for narrowing a technical or specialised search. For example, some search engines search only news or health sources or reference resources. Others, known as 'metasearch' tools, allow you to use a number of different search engines at once for a more global search. Although metasearch tools permit a wide search, they seldom offer you the ability to refine a search. Box 2-3 presents examples of specialty and metasearch tools. We will explore professional health care search indexes later in this chapter.

> **BOX 2-3** Specialised Search Engines
>
> The website for each of these search engines is accessible through the book's Evolve website at http://evolve.elsevier.com/AU/Borbasi/maze.
>
> **Specialty Search Engines**
> *My Virtual Reference Desk* is an electronic source for locating many of the same materials you would find in the reference section of a library, including dictionaries, encyclopaedias and quick facts.
> *Internet Public Library* permits you to search for many resources that you might find in a public library. It leads you to many full-text references and sources.
> *News Index* lets you search for current news stories worldwide.
> *Achoo* helps web browsers look for medically related topics for consumers.
> *Health A to Z* is a search tool for heath-related topics for consumers.
>
> **Metasearch Tools**
> *Cyber411* searches 16 search engines simultaneously with one set of terms and removes duplicate entries. It allows use of Boolean operators.
> *Dogpile* allows you to use up to 25 different search engines in any sequence you designate for one set of key search terms. It also has a link to Metafind.
> *Metafind* allows you to search several engines sequentially and sort your results while the search engine remains running in the background.
> *Inference Find* lets you do parallel searching. It filters out duplications in your search efforts and clusters your results for you.

Activity 2

You have access to all these engines through your ISP or by using the URL address of the particular engine. Each of these search engines uses slightly different search methods and indexing systems. This means you need to rely on the Help feature when first using a particular search system. This allows you to get a feel for how that system operates. A perfect search system would help you find all the relevant information about your topic that is available on the web. Such a search engine does not exist. If you use several different search engines for the same topic, you will get differing results. Some engines use Boolean search logic and others use probabilistic methods. Each has a unique indexing system. Some allow you to search only by key words. Others allow you to search by key words or to use a subject index.

If you want further information on search engines and how they work, log on to the book's Evolve website at http://evolve.elsevier.com/AU/Borbasi/maze and link to the Spider's Apprentice website. This site explains how search engines work,

Activity 3

gives you tips on conducting and refining a search, provides ratings for several popular search engines and even lets you try out several search engines.

Ultimately, the best way to view the way that search engines work and to see the difference in results is to use and explore a few of them. Try the following Student Challenge.

> **Student Challenge**
>
> Sampling Search Engines
>
> Decide on a specific subject area you're interested in. Get adventurous and have fun. Explore the art of making bread, caring for your cat, or old movies. Use your imagination. Once you have an area of interest, log on to your ISP and web browser. Then do the same search using three or four different general search engines.
>
> 1 Note the rules for searching for each search engine that you try.
> 2 Note the different special features available.
> 3 Compare the results from the various searches.
> 4 Which search engine was the easiest to use? Which gave you the best results?
> 5 Try a specialty topic and use a specialty search engine.
> 6 Try one of the metasearch tools.

Communicating on the net

A number of communication opportunities await you on the internet. You can send and receive electronic mail with individuals and groups. You can post messages, chat online, use the telephone or hold videoconferences. With a little basic information, you will be a confident communicator in no time.

Email and listservs

To send email over the internet, you need an internet mailing address and electronic mail software. Several internet sources provide free email accounts and email software. Chances are, however, you already have email access, since it is one of the services included when you subscribe to an online service or an ISP. An email feature is also included with the Netscape Navigator and Internet Explorer web browser packages. All these services provide help to use the email program feature. You will get guidance in setting up an email account and obtaining an email address.

An email address consists of two basic parts: the **user name** and the host name. These two parts are connected by an '@' symbol. You determine the first part of the address. The second part of the address is dictated by the service that supplies your internet account. Examining an email address reveals information about the location of the account (Fig 2-3).

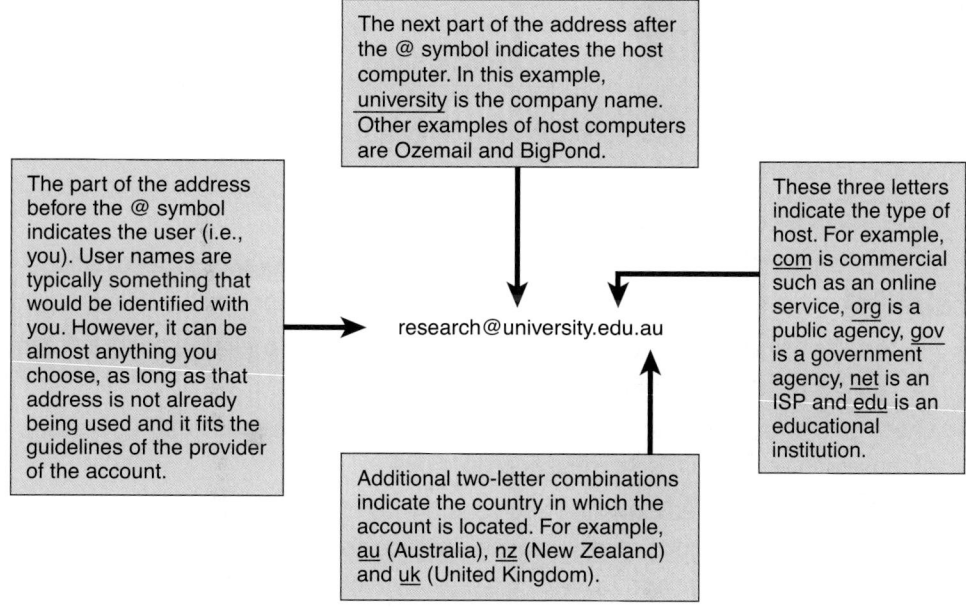

Figure 2-3 *Elements of a sample email address*

Once you have a functioning email account, you are ready to send and receive mail. This is easy. First you connect to the internet. Then you call up your email software program. If you subscribe to an ISP or online service, you can connect by using the icon or link that appears on the opening page immediately after you connect to the internet. It will be labelled something like 'message centre' or 'mail centre'. If you are using your web browser's email capabilities, the Netscape email program is called 'Netscape Messenger' and the Internet Explorer email program is called 'Outlook Express'.

All email programs look slightly different and have slightly different menu systems, but they all have common features. They allow you to compose and send messages to anyone with an email account (provided you know their email address) and to read and save or print messages sent to you by others. They also let you keep an email address book. All these features are easily accessible through various menu options or toolbar buttons. Many programs offer several features that enhance sending and receiving mail.

- You can attach and **upload** one or more files when sending a message.
- You can **download** files sent to you by others.
- You can add graphics and special formatting to your messages.
- If you get a special digital certificate and key, you can even send and receive messages that are in code and unreadable by anyone except authorised users.

> **Student Challenge**
>
> Email Explorations
>
> If you have access to an email account and are not yet familiar or comfortable with using it, try the following:
>
> 1 Have the email address of one or more friends or fellow students handy.
> 2 Get on the internet and access your mail centre. Explore the various menu options and toolbar buttons. If you are unsure about what they are for, use the Help feature.
> 3 Try to compose and send a message to your friends. In the message, instruct them to reply by email to your message.
> 4 Check your email address book. It should automatically have the email addresses of those people you just sent messages to.
> 5 When you have finished exploring and sending, log off. Come back later and check for messages. When you have messages, practise opening them and reading them. Try printing them out. Try saving a message to a file. Try deleting a message.
> 6 If you are having difficulty with sending or receiving and the 'help' function is no help, try asking a friend who is an email user to demonstrate for you. Or purchase a basic book on internet use (see the Resource Kit at the end of this chapter for suggestions).
> 7 If you are feeling comfortable with your email prowess, try attaching and sending files. Have someone attach and send a file to you. Try downloading the file to your computer and opening it.

Activity 4

As an internet user, you have access to listservs, which allow you to send email to an entire group of people who share a common interest. To do this you simply subscribe to that particular listserv (subscriptions are free) and send an email message to the listserv address. This message is then sent to the other subscribers of that listserv. You also receive email messages from other subscribers. If you want to receive lots of email, just join a listserv. Thousands of listservs are available. If you're interested, you can access a listserv directory on the web such as Liszt Select. (This site is accessible through the Evolve site.) Over 250 health-related listservs are listed in this particular directory. This site also contains links to other listserv directories.

Newsgroups and chat rooms

Newsgroups and chat rooms also allow you to communicate over the net. Over 20,000 newsgroups or bulletin board sites are available on the internet. On this type of site you can post messages for any subscriber to read and respond to. Messages and replies are clustered together to establish a conversational flow. Like listservs, newsgroups revolve around particular interest areas. Some of these newsgroups have a moderator or manager who sorts through messages and makes decisions about what is posted. Others are totally uncontrolled and all messages are posted. If you're interested in newsgroups, most search engines allow you to search for them. You can also tap into a website specifically devoted to newsgroups. They have search mechanisms and category links. One such site is Google, which you can access through the Evolve site. If you find a newsgroup of interest, you can subscribe to it at no charge. You can even post messages and ask people to reply privately via your email address rather than responding on the bulletin board.

Activity 5

You can also communicate with one or more people by typing back and forth to each other in a chat room. The main difference between chat rooms and listservs or newsgroups is that you are holding a running conversation with others who are online at the same time you are. If you're interested, you might want to visit Yahoo! (remember this search engine?), because it also offers a number of chat rooms. It will also allow you to search for other chat rooms. Chat rooms are also available from your online service or ISP.

Audio and video possibilities

With the right equipment and an internet phone program you can talk to anyone else who also has the right equipment and software program. You can also place conference calls. Technology that even allows for videophone calls and video-conferencing is available. These relatively recent technological innovations are not yet in common use, but prices are falling and their use is expected to expand rapidly.

Trying traditional tools

File transfer protocol is still a very useful process for transferring files from one computer to another over the net. It has now been incorporated into use of the web and you can perform this procedure with the help of your web browser. However, it is not a web application. File transfer protocol is often used to obtain updated versions of software programs and internet tools that you are already using. You can also use FTP to transfer *shareware* (free or nominally priced software programs).

To perform a file transfer procedure you need a web browser and the URL of the file you want to receive. You simply connect to your web browser, type the URL in the address or location box and click on the URL. A file directory will appear. You scroll through the directory and click on the file you want and it will appear on your screen. You can then save the file to whatever location on your computer you choose.

If the file you are transferring is a compressed or *zipped* file (a large file that has been condensed for easier storage and transfer), you will need a special piece of software to decompress or unzip the file to read or use it. Your web browser or ISP usually provides you with information that allows you to directly download such a program for use. Winzip is a common unzipping program that can be purchased for a nominal fee.

Telnet allows you to log on to a specific computer on the internet from a computer at another site. You may wonder why this is important in light of all you have just learned about the web. Some computer information and services are not currently available on a website, and access is only possible through a Telnet connection. To log on to another computer site, you must have some type of Telnet software and the Telnet URL for the computer you wish to access. Telnet URLs start with telnet://. Some libraries have Telnet connections that allow you to log on to their library computer and use their catalogue and indexes. You could check and see whether your library uses Telnet—if so, you may want to investigate how you can use it.

How Do You Use the Net for Professional Purposes?

Many professional uses have already been alluded to in this chapter. You may already be using some of the ideas we are about to cover. If so, good for you. This section examines some of the ways that you can make the internet work for you to enhance your professional life. Our focus is on the information and communication capabilities of the internet.

Information access

Many professional information sources are available on the internet. You have access to a wide variety of databases, patient and nursing education resources, as well as some full-text and virtual nursing journals. One of the most helpful things to be discovered is how to conduct a library search from your own personal computer at any time you choose. Your university will have facilities for online off-campus searches or remote access. Explore this possibility with the following student challenge.

> **Student Challenge**
>
> ### Making the Most of Library Resources
> Check with your library to see what kind of remote access you have to their electronic resources. Explore the requirements for use of remote library access.
>
> 1. Is such access possible?
> 2. Is it available to you?
> 3. What are the procedures for requesting access?
> 4. What equipment and software are needed?
> 5. Is a special password required?

If you don't have remote capabilities through your local academic or health sciences library, don't despair. You can also conduct index searches by accessing MEDLINE or CINAHL through other websites. MEDLINE is produced by the National Library of Medicine (NLM®) and is available free of charge through a number of websites or through commercial vendors for a fee.

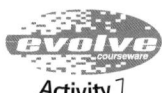

Activity 6

One of the better known access sites is PubMed. PubMed is the NLM search mechanism that allows you to search the MEDLINE and PREMEDLINE® databases. PREMEDLINE is a fairly new service that allows you to search basic citation information and abstracts before the full citation record is generated and added to MEDLINE. This means you can find the most current material available. New records are added to PREMEDLINE every day.

CINAHL is also accessible from a website. (This site is available through Evolve.) However, because CINAHL is a commercially maintained index, an access fee is charged for use of the search mechanism. They do offer student discounts. Membership gives you online full-text access to approximately 17 print nursing journals, as well as the CINAHL database (CINAHL 2003). Most of the current full-text offerings for these journals begin with 1997 or 1998 issues and are available for published articles at least six months to one year old. A listing of these journals and their tables of contents is accessible on the website free of charge. You may wish to locate the website and explore it to determine whether a subscription would be helpful to you.

Activity 7

Electronic journals and online versions of print journals are beginning to appear in nursing. CINAHL offers access to an electronic journal entitled *Online Journal of Clinical Innovations*. This journal focuses on research reports and clinical innovations. There is an annual subscription fee and the journal is produced quarterly. Articles from this journal can be downloaded and printed out for no additional fee.

Another electronic nursing journal, *Online Journal of Knowledge Synthesis for Nursing,* is sponsored by Sigma Theta Tau (Sigma Theta Tau 2003). (This site is accessible through Evolve.) This journal provides full-text critical reviews of current research as it pertains to clinical nursing practice. Check to see whether your library carries subscriptions to one or both of these electronic journals. If so, you may have remote online access through connection with your library internet site.

Activity 8

Other electronic nursing journals include the *Online Journal of Issues in Nursing,* sponsored by Kent State University. This is a peer-reviewed journal with an interactive format. You can view and download all articles at no charge. Southern Cross University also has an online journal called the *Australian Electronic Journal of Nursing Education.*

A wide range of healthcare-related databases and professional sites are available to you via your computer and an internet account. A brief sample of such websites and databases is provided in Box 2-4.

Activity 9

> **BOX 2-4** Selected Professional Websites and Databases
>
> The website for each of these is accessible through this book's Evolve website at http://evolve.elsevier.com/AU/Borbasi/maze.
>
> - **Nursing Society**—the website for Sigma Theta Tau. It contains information about the society, grants and research activities, online publications and eligibility requirements, among other topics.
> - **Australian Nursing Federation (ANF)**—the website for the ANF provides access to policies and reports as well as tables of contents and information about the *Australian Nurses Journal* (ANJ) and the *Australian Journal of Advanced Nursing* (AJAN).
> - **College of Nursing**—the website provides information about the College library and online services as well as information about research and publications.
> - **Royal College of Nursing, Australia (RCNA)**—this website offers conference information, online forums, publication information and information about scholarships.
> - **Hardin Meta Directory of Internet Health Sources**—a metalisting with links to indexes that index healthcare sites. A huge listing of nursing indexes is found here.
> - **Nursing Net**—just one of the indexes from the Hardin site. This is a good electronic guide for nursing journals and other publications and references as well as continuing education sites and employment postings. It even links you to an online discount bookstore.
> - **Nursing World**—the website for the American Nurses Association (ANA). You can link to state nursing association sites, check nursing and healthcare policy, read up on credentialing issues and do much more.
> - **Online Books**—an index with links to over 9000 full-text books available for online reading free of charge. It has a large medical and healthcare section.
> - **Journals**—an index for journals, magazines and newspapers.
> - **US Library of Congress**—the online catalogue for this government organisation. Links to other library catalogues, search mechanisms and resource help are available at this site.
> - **US Centers for Disease Control**—provides access to thousands of health-related statistics, including morbidity and mortality statistics from the National Center for Health Statistics and government information on hundreds of health-related topics.
> - **US National Institutes of Health**—the home base for several government agencies of interest, including the National Institute for Nursing Research (NINR) and the National Library of Medicine (NLM).
> - **Australian Institute of Health and Welfare**—provides access to a wealth of health- and welfare-related statistics and information. Lists of publications and online data are included here.

Evolve will link you to a special website set up just for this learning package. It contains hypertext links to related areas of interest, content updates, author information and more. If you have not already done so, take a minute to use Evolve and log on to explore the website. Try the following Student Challenge.

Student Challenge

Evolve Magic

1. Log on to the Evolve website at http://evolve.elsevier.com/AU/Borbasi/maze.
2. Add the website to your Favorites or Bookmarks list.
3. Explore the site and see what is offered.
4. Find out a little about us (your textbook authors).
5. Read up on some frequently asked questions.
6. Check out available links, then log off and insert your CD-ROM for this text.
7. Note the Evolve button located at the bottom of the main menu and submenus. It allows you to go directly to the Evolve site from the CD. Try it out.

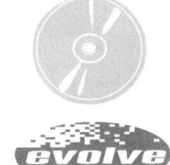

Communication possibilities

Communication capabilities on the net provide a wide range of professional possibilities, including interaction with fellow students and faculty at your university via email. Some universities allow you to submit assignments using email attachments—you will need to check the policy of your institution before doing this. You can send and receive messages to and from other professional colleagues worldwide. You can hold discussions with colleagues about patient care issues, brainstorm about solutions to clinical problems and more by using listservs, newsgroups or chat rooms. A number of professionally related discussion groups are available already on the net. You could even start your own.

Student Challenge

Communication Contingencies

1. Explore professional listservs and newsgroups on the net. (Hint: Remember Liszt Select, Google and your search engines.)
2. See if your school or university is on the web. If so, check to see what discussion groups they have available.

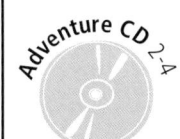

Ongoing educational opportunities

The ease of access to the internet and the web has also opened up new avenues in education and learning opportunities. It is now possible to take courses over the net. Many of these feature interactive classrooms where you can talk with lecturers and fellow classmates online through audio or videoconferencing capabilities. The concept is known as *distance learning*. Many universities are starting remote-site campuses to offer classes in areas with little access to university settings. Continuing education opportunities abound on the internet. Although these opportunities are relatively new, they are growing rapidly. It may be possible someday to earn a degree by completing most or all of your coursework requirements online. We are entering a new era that is filled with possibilities and promise for taming the information revolution.

Resource Kit

Finding Internet Service Providers

If you have a computer with Microsoft Windows, you can find out about major ISPs by using the Internet Connection Wizard located in your Internet Explorer program (look under Tools, Internet options). The wizard can also help you download the software required to set up your chosen ISP and then make the connections to run the ISP.

You can also find local ISPs in the *Yellow Pages* telephone directory under the heading 'Internet Services'.

Easy-to-Use Guides to Help You Log on to and Use the Internet

Eager B (1999). *Internet quick reference*. Indianapolis, Que. *A quick reference, visually oriented, economical.*

Levine JR, Baroudi C, Young ML (2000). *Internet for Dummies*. IDG Books. *A more comprehensive reference, easy to follow, economical.*

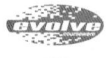 Visit the book's Evolve website at http://evolve.elsevier.com/AU/Borbasi/maze for further information.

 Check out the puzzles, mazes and games on your CD-ROM.

References

CINAHL Online. Available: http://www.cinahl.com 12 Mar 2003.
Honor Society of Nursing, Sigma Theta Tau International. Online. Available: http://www.nursingsociety.org 12 Mar 2003.

http://evolve.elsevier.com/AU/Borbasi/maze

Learning Objectives

After reading this chapter and following critical reflection the student will be able to:

1. Describe the components of effective reading.
2. Discuss factors that influence reading rate and comprehension.
3. Examine personal reading skills.
4. Explore strategies to increase reading effectiveness.
5. Define summarisation/abstraction.
6. Describe the steps necessary for competent summarisation.
7. Apply abstraction skills to selected materials.
8. Describe the factors that influence the quality of information.
9. Discuss ways to evaluate the quality of information.

Chapter Outline

What Is This Chapter About?
What Is Effective Reading?
Reading rate and comprehension
Reading more effectively
What Is Summarisation/Abstraction?
How Do You Evaluate Information?
Factors affecting information quality
Evaluation skills

Chapter 3
Reading Faster, Reading Smarter: Managing Information Wisely

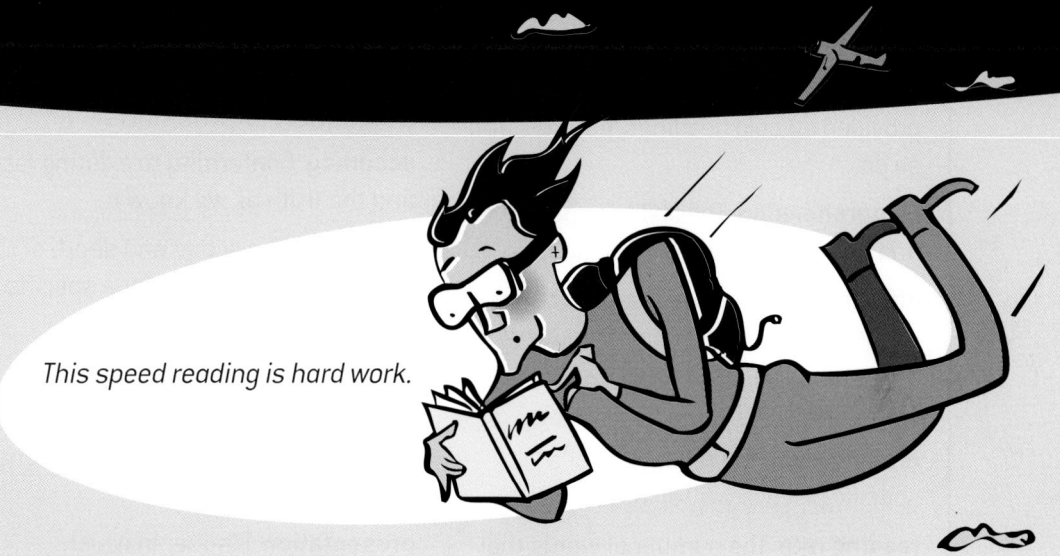

This speed reading is hard work.

Student Quote
'Breaking the highlighter habit has made me focus more when I read.'

Abstract
Efficient use of information requires the ability to effectively read, to competently summarise, and to critically evaluate the various sources we locate. Speed and comprehension—the cornerstones of effective reading—are affected by factors such as difficulty level, reading level, subject familiarity, mechanical skill, and various internal and external environmental factors. A consistently used and organised reading strategy can increase reading effectiveness. The ability to summarise and restate what has been read ensures a greater understanding and grasp of the subject matter. As the quantity of available information increases, we must be able to quickly evaluate the quality of such information. Several factors help determine quality of information: these include accuracy, adequacy, balance, currency, presentation and reliability.

Key Terms

Reading Rhetoric

abstract Summary of the essential characteristics of something more extensive (e.g. a summary of a research article).

advance organisers Preselected mental landmarks that serve to organise materials as you read. They are often provided by bold headings, outlines and so on.

comprehension The ability to perceive and understand concepts or ideas.

effective reading rate The number of words that can be read in a minute while maintaining a high level of comprehension.

reading level The readability of a specific piece of written material.

reading rate The number of words that can be read in a minute.

reading strategy (method) System that breaks a reading assignment down into manageable parts that are more readily processed.

speed reading Reading at an increased rate through techniques that encourage fewer eye fixations on the page.

summary Concise recapitulation of previously stated information that captures the main ideas.

Evaluation Expressions

accuracy Conformity to existing facts and the truth as we know it.

adequacy The scope and depth of information presented for a specific audience.

balance Presentation of competing points of view.

currency The immediacy of presented information.

presentation Manner in which information is displayed.

reliability Dependability and trustworthiness of information.

What Is This Chapter About?

Now you have learned how to gather information effectively, the next step is to dissect and use that information efficiently. This includes the ability to effectively read, competently summarise and critically evaluate the information at hand. Some of you are probably good readers and may view reading as enjoyable. Others of you may see reading as a necessary chore. Still others may find reading a frustrating experience. Whatever your feelings, there are ways to improve your abilities and make the time you spend reading more productive. This chapter discusses effective reading, competent summarisation and critical evaluation issues, and examines ways to improve your skills in each area. You can practise these skills through doing the Student Challenges and the CD-ROM games and puzzles.

What Is Effective Reading?

Reading can be broken down into two basic types: fun reading and learning-related reading. Each type requires differing levels of focus. Fun reading is reading for pleasure and may include browsing the latest *Who* magazine, scanning the morning newspaper, or curling up with a good mystery novel. Reading for fun does not require the same level of preparation, attention or thought as reading to learn. This chapter focuses on reading to learn.

Effective reading is the ability to read quickly and comprehend the materials at hand. Your reading rate and comprehension are key factors in reading effectively. These two components are closely related. Your ability to grasp relevant ideas as you read increases your reading speed. Speed without comprehension is of little value. However, a slow, plodding, laborious approach to reading can lead to frustration and loss of your train of thought.

Reading rate and comprehension

Reading rate is defined as the number of words that can be read in a minute. An effective reading rate is defined as the number of words that can be read per minute while maintaining a high level of comprehension. **Comprehension** is defined as the ability to grasp ideas and to understand the concepts being presented.

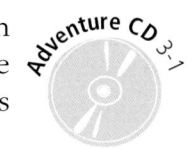

Reading rates and comprehension are affected by a number of factors that emanate from the material, the reader or the environment. These include the difficulty level of the material, the reading level at which the material is presented, the reader's familiarity with the subject area and mechanical reading skills, and internal and external environmental distractions.

Factors Affecting Speed and Comprehension

Source factors:
- *difficulty level*
- *reading level*

Reader factors:
- *familiarity with subject*
- *language skills*
- *mechanical skills*

Environmental factors:
- *internal distractions (fatigue, hunger, illness)*
- *external distractions (noise, temperature, light)*

Information comes in varying degrees of difficulty or complexity. Complex and abstract concepts require more thought and more careful reading. This slows the rate at which they are read. Some subjects that are more complex are harder to grasp and apply than others. Materials that contain highly specialised and/or technical information have a higher level of difficulty. This is true even if the reader is familiar with the subject being presented. For example, an article about the anatomy and physiology of pain is harder to read than an article about the nursing care of a person experiencing pain.

Reading level refers to the readability of a given piece of written material. It is affected by the number of syllables in words and the number of words in sentences. The higher the average number of syllables per word and words per sentence, the greater the reading level. As reading level rises, comprehension requires more effort and reading rate slows. When material is loaded with three-syllable words and 22-word sentences, the brain tends to struggle. However, very low reading levels result in a dull and monotonous presentation. A succession of six-word sentences full of monosyllables can be mind numbing. Do not confuse readability with difficulty. Difficulty refers to the idea being presented, whereas readability refers to the presentation of the idea. Even simple ideas can be made hard to read, and difficult ideas can be presented in reader-friendly form.

> Do not confuse readability with difficulty. Difficulty refers to the idea being presented, whereas readability refers to the presentation of the idea.

Reading level is usually calculated and expressed as some form of index. These indexes typically report a value that can be matched to the educational level required to read a particular document with ease (e.g. year 6 versus year 12 reading). Generally, the higher the number of the index, the harder the material is to read. If you use the Microsoft Word (version 95, 97 or 2000) word processing package on your computer, you can calculate a readability score on any document you write. It is located under the Tools menu under grammar options. One of the most popular readability indexes is the Gunning Fog Index, which is fairly easy to calculate by hand. The steps are presented in Box 3-1.

BOX 3-1 Calculating the Gunning Fog Index

Step 1. Select a sample.
Choose a 100-word (to the nearest sentence) sample from the material to be analysed.

Step 2. Determine the average number of words per sentence.
Divide the total number of words in the sample by the total number of sentences in the sample.

Step 3. Determine the percentage of words with three or more syllables. Divide the number of three-plus syllable words by the total number of words. (Do not count the following as three-syllable words: capitalised words, hyphenated words, or words for which the addition of an 'es' or 'ed' makes the third syllable.)

Step 4. Calculate the grade level index: add the result of step 2 to step 3 and multiply by 0.4.

Example:
Step 1: 110-word passage
Step 2: 110 words in 11 sentences 110/11 = 10
Step 3: 21 three + syllable words out of 110 words 21/110 = 19%
Step 4: Add average words (10) to percentage of polysyllable words (19) and multiply by 0.4 (10 + 19 = 29 x 0.4 = 11.6).
Result: Reading level is year 11–12.

Sources: Gunning Fog Index 2003; Doell 2003.

If you're having trouble reading a particular piece of information, you might want to check the reading level at which it is written. Try the following Student Challenge.

Student Challenge

Reading Readability

1 Using selected samples (a paragraph or two) from each of the following sources, calculate a reading level.
   a this textbook
   b one of your other textbooks
   c an article from a popular magazine
   d a source you considered very difficult to read and understand
   e a student paper or assignment you have written
2 Compare the results from the various samples. How do they compare? What did you learn?

Familiarity with the subject and the vocabulary used greatly affects reading rate and comprehension. If you have insufficient background in a particular subject, you are handicapped when you try to read about it. The unfamiliar concepts and ideas require additional thought. Words may be foreign or used in specialised ways for various topics. Vocabulary is particularly important to reading because the words on the page are actually tools for building thoughts. It is difficult to formulate or extract ideas from your reading if you are unfamiliar with several of the words being used to present those ideas.

Lack of familiarity with the words on the page also greatly slows your reading rate. A nurse researcher can read most nursing research articles with relative speed and high-level understanding. As a nursing student, you might arrive at a lower level of understanding after a much greater time investment. As a nurse, to read effectively you need to be equipped with a good general vocabulary and specialised vocabularies from several fields, including chemistry, biology, physiology, pharmacology, medicine and nursing.

This means you need to develop quite sophisticated language skills. Even people who have a wide general vocabulary can struggle with the specialised vocabulary needed to study and practise nursing. Some students, particularly those who have English as a second language, might face even more challenges. You will find that your university has support available for students who need to develop study and reading skills. These services are provided by Student Learning Centres. When you are starting out with your study, medical terminology can be difficult to understand, but strategies like learning prefixes and suffixes will help you understand the meanings of many of these new words. Lists of medical prefixes and suffixes can be found in most medical/surgical fundamentals nursing textbooks.

Reading requires certain mechanical skills. If the reader is lacking some of these skills, both reading rate and comprehension can be affected. These skills include the way the eyes focus when reading, the way words are viewed on the page, the way the eyes fix on and sweep a page, and the smoothness or flow of the process. Focus in reading means you read for ideas rather than words. You are tuned into the meaning behind the words. You have a purpose for reading such as understanding a key point or looking for an answer to a question or a solution to a problem. Words are viewed as thought clusters rather than as single entities. The eyes sweep the page with few fixations (pauses as the eyes move across the page). You take in groups of words at a time. The lips are still, and reading is silent. If reading mechanics are lacking, then the reading rate slows. A sufficiently slow rate affects comprehension. It is difficult to pick out key ideas if you are concentrating on seeing and reading each word.

There are courses that teach you to increase your rate and comprehension by improving your reading mechanics. These are often known as **speed-reading** courses. They teach you techniques that allow you to take in large groups of words on a page while controlling your eye movements. These techniques force you to see and consider several words as a single unit. Although you will never read technical material at a high rate of speed, it is a valuable skill to be able to view words in groups rather than as single entities.

Internal and external environmental factors can also affect your reading speed and comprehension. If you are tired, anxious, sick, hungry, or otherwise distracted, your ability to focus and read effectively is affected. Likewise, if the room is too noisy, too hot, too cold, too dark, or the site of other activities, your ability to concentrate and read is affected. You may have discovered that there are times when you are more alert and better able to concentrate. If so, take advantage of these times.

Reading more effectively

An organised approach to reading can help you read more actively and understand what you are reading. A good **reading strategy** breaks the reading assignment down into manageable parts and helps you process one part before moving on to the next. A number of reading strategies have been advocated to increase reading effectiveness. Several of these are listed and described in Box 3-2. If you do not already have a proven reading strategy, you may wish to read further about some of the described strategies and try out one or more of them—see the Resource Kit at the end of this chapter for references. Having a reading strategy is more important than the particular strategy you choose. The reason a systematic approach is effective is because it allows you to organise and focus your reading.

> **BOX 3-2** Effective Reading Strategies
>
> **SQ3R**—Survey, Question, Read, Recite, Review. Devised in the 1940s by Francis Robinson for students at Ohio State University, this system has been used for years, and a number of variations have come from this original work.
> **SQ4R**—A variation of the above method, SQ4R adds a record step to the process, in which the user records key ideas on paper or note cards.
> **OK5R**—Overview, Key ideas, Read, Record, Recite, Review, Reflect. This strategy offers yet another twist on the basic strategic formula.
> **SSS**—Skim, Scrutinise, Sweep up. By now you should be seeing a pattern.
> **PRR**—Preview, Read actively, Recall. This reading strategy is endorsed by several university study skills programs.

As you look at Box 3-2, note that all the strategies have common tactics. They all advocate that you first survey or preview the material to get an overview of what you are about to read. This means paying attention to advance organisers. Advance organisers are things such as the table of contents, preface, chapter outlines, learning objectives, titles, subject headings, abstracts, introductions and summaries. These are placed in material specifically to help you organise your thoughts. They prepare you to read by providing a road map to the presented material. They tell you in advance what points are important and help to establish ties between major information segments.

These reading strategies also ask the reader to examine or scrutinise what they are reading. This means identifying main ideas and key points and asking how they relate to other key points. It means getting a firm understanding of what you are reading and addressing points that are confusing or unclear. It means looking for signs that indicate how the information is organised or what is important. These signs include information emphasised by highlighting or boxes. Words such as 'first' or 'second', 'for example', 'in summary' or 'finally' also serve as signals.

Finally, these strategies ask the reader to review what has been read. When you finish reading the material, you need to gather all the key ideas and summarise what you have gleaned from the material. Check your summary of key points against the author's by rereading the summary, key points, or abstract of the material. Now is the time to note and clear up points of confusion. It is also a good time to physically make notes of the key ideas and points you have pulled from the material.

Do not use a highlighter or underline phrases in the material. Highlighting does not require you to pull out and examine relationships between key ideas. Many people also use highlighting as an escape tactic to delay the hard work of thinking about what they are reading. They highlight anything that looks important, with the promise that they will read and make sense of it later. It isn't unusual to see student texts with entire pages highlighted. Something about having to write down your thoughts encourages you to more clearly refine your understanding. The physical act of writing also serves to lodge the idea more firmly in your memory.

HINT Do not use a highlighter when reading.

Try the following Student Challenge and see if you have some system in place for effective reading.

Student Challenge

Strategic Strategies

Respond to the following questions and directions using this textbook as your example.

1. Did you examine and survey the general text layout before beginning your first reading assignment (e.g. preface, table of contents, glossary, appendices, special supplements)?
2. Do you know what general layout and features are included in each chapter?
3. Did you preview the outline and learning objectives for this chapter before you began reading it?

4 If not, take some time to do that survey now. What did you learn from your examination of the text?

5 When you read, do you ask yourself what the central point is in each paragraph? Do you make use of the abstract provided with each chapter?

6 Do you pay attention to the boxed materials? Figures? Tables? Charts? Diagrams?

7 Did you make note of the defined terms?

8 Are you doing the student challenges? CD-ROM exercises?

9 When you finished the first two chapters, were you clear about the key points? Did you have any questions? If so, did you actively seek and find answers?

10 If your reading skills need refining, then find a reading strategy and incorporate it in your reading sessions. (Hint: Your library probably has a number of resources filed under 'effective reading' or 'effective study'.)

There are other tactics you can employ to read more effectively. These are listed in Box 3-3.

BOX 3-3 Tips on Effective Reading

1 **Prepare your environment.** Banish as many distractions as possible. Find a quiet, comfortable, well-lit place to read. Have all the necessary supplies such as pens, note paper and other resources ready before you begin.

2 **Prepare yourself.** Select times of the day when you are alert and at a mental peak. Schedule reading times in advance and keep the appointment. Read in manageable chunks. Remember, concentration requires energy. If you find your mind wandering or you are having trouble seizing on the key ideas, take a five-minute break.

3 **Read actively.** Think about what you are reading. Read with a purpose. Actively search for key points and ideas. Look for examples or illustrations of those ideas. See if you can think of other examples. Make connections between the ideas being presented. Get a picture of the whole idea in each paragraph, each section and each chapter.

4 **Use tools to increase understanding.** If you are unfamiliar with the subject, you may want material that provides background before tackling material that addresses specific issues on a subject. If you are unfamiliar with the vocabulary, use a dictionary as you read and apply what you find back to the materials you're reading.

5 **Increase your mechanical skills.** (1) Read phrases rather than individual words. Very few ideas are expressed in single words. Reading in phrases allows you to

better follow the meaning of the material. (2) Eliminate reading out loud, word pronunciation and lip movements. These are indications that you are reading words rather than phrases, which means you are focusing on the words themselves rather than the ideas they represent. (3) Reduce rereading to a minimum. Often the next phrase or sentence will offer an explanation, making rereading unnecessary. Reread only if the point is still unclear after you complete a section.

What Is Summarisation/Abstraction?

The ability to understand and condense what you have read into a few well-chosen words is an important skill. Summarisation is the ability to capture the key ideas or main points in a clear, concise form. A **summary** briefly states the essence of what has been previously presented. An **abstract** is a synonym for 'summary'. It is often placed at the beginning of a chapter or article, while a summary is most frequently placed at the end. We are using the word 'abstract' in this text because it is the term you will see most frequently when reading research articles. You will also find an abstract at the beginning of each chapter in this text.

The ability to competently summarise any material requires that you have a fundamental understanding of the concepts being presented in that material. You can use the following questions to test your understanding of the material you are reading.

1 Can you grasp the ideas being expressed and distinguish key ideas from secondary points?
2 Can you express key ideas in words different from those used by the author?
3 Can you identify supporting evidence for a particular point?
4 Can you give examples to illustrate that point?

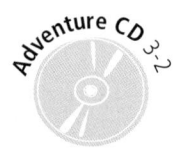

If you are having difficulty separating out the main or key points as you read, remember to use the cues presented by the material. Check for advance organisers. Look for bold topical or section headings. Search for signal words. If you cannot express the author's ideas in your own words, then you are having trouble comprehending what is being said. You may need to reexamine the paragraph. Is the concept foreign to you? If so, seek additional resources. Are some of the words unfamiliar? If so, consult a dictionary. Are you tired, distracted, or not thinking clearly? If so, take a break and reread it when you have a clearer focus.

To provide supporting evidence, you must see the relationships between and among the points being presented. The same mechanisms you use to pull key ideas also help in visualising secondary and supporting ideas. When you think the concept is clear, test yourself by coming up with a specific example of the concept.

If you have difficulty with this, scan the material and see if a sample example was provided.

Let's use a paragraph from this chapter as an example of the art of summarising.

> *Effective reading is the ability to quickly read and comprehend the materials at hand. Your reading rate and comprehension are key factors in reading effectively. These two components are closely related. Your ability to grasp relevant ideas as you read increases your reading speed. Speed without comprehension is of little value. However, a slow, plodding, laborious approach to reading can lead to frustration and loss of your train of thought.*

The paragraph's main idea is that good reading has two interconnected elements—speed and understanding. Its first sentence tells you what the two elements are. Note that the second sentence repeats this same idea using different words. The authors then tell you that the elements are related and use supporting examples to expand on the relationship of the two elements. This paragraph also sets up the following paragraphs, which discuss reading rate and comprehension in more depth.

Let's look at another example.

> *Now that you have learned how to effectively gather information, the next step is to efficiently dissect and use that information. This includes the ability to effectively read, competently summarise and critically evaluate the information at hand. Some of you are probably good readers and may view reading as enjoyable. Others of you may see reading as a necessary chore. Still others may find reading a frustrating experience. Whatever your feelings, there are ways to improve your abilities and make the time you spend reading more productive. This chapter discusses effective reading, competent summarisation and critical evaluation issues, and examines ways to improve your skills in each area. You can practise these skills through doing the Student Challenges and the CD-ROM games and puzzles.*

This is the first paragraph in this chapter. The main idea is to inform the reader that this chapter addresses ways to use information by examining abilities to read, summarise and evaluate. This paragraph not only provides a link with the previous two chapters, it also serves as an advance organiser. It tells you what general topics to expect in this chapter. It also reminds you that student learning activities are available to help you master the content.

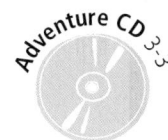

Now put your summary skills to the test with the following Student Challenge.

> **Student Challenge**
>
> Summary Skills
>
> Select several (at least five) paragraphs from this chapter. Summarise each paragraph in one sentence.
>
> 1. How did you decide what the main idea was? Did you make use of advance organisers? Signal words?
> 2. Do your summary sentences use your own words? If not, try restating the summary again.
> 3. Can you think of a way to illustrate the main idea? Cite examples from two or three of your summaries.
> 4. Did you have any trouble understanding what was being said? If so, what did you do to help you understand?

How Do You Evaluate Information?

As greater amounts of information become more easily accessible, it becomes increasingly difficult to judge its quality. Your excursions on the internet should have already alerted you to this problem. So one of the critical issues facing us in this 'age of the information explosion' is how to assess the quality of the information to which we are exposed. Chapters 1 and 2 addressed the issue of finding information. Now we are going to talk about how to decide whether the information we locate is adequate.

Factors affecting information quality

Several factors—accuracy, adequacy, balance, currency, presentation and reliability—affect the quality of information. **Accuracy** is associated with the content of the material. Accurate information is the result of an active effort to confirm or verify and shows conformity to existing facts (can be verified through other sources). **Adequacy** refers to the scope and depth of information presented. Adequate information provides the reader with materials that are sufficient in scope and depth for the specific purposes of that reader. **Balance** deals with acknowledgment and presentation of competing points of view. Lack of balance leads to bias. **Currency** addresses the immediacy of the material and whether it accurately reflects ongoing changes in a particular field of study. **Presentation** has to do with whether the content is presented in a well-organised manner. **Reliability** is often connected with the source of the material. Reliable information is consistently dependable and comes from a generally proven and trustworthy source.

> Factors affecting the quality of information:
> - *accuracy*
> - *adequacy*
> - *balance*
> - *currency*
> - *presentation*
> - *reliability*
> - *evaluation skills.*

Evaluation skills

Several considerations can help you make judgments about the quality of the information you are using. The first consideration is the source of the material. If you have tapped into materials from published textbooks, reference books or recognised journals, there is a reasonable expectation that the material has been reviewed and edited by authorities in the area. You may wish to check this out. Many text and reference books list contributing authors and/or reviewers and their credentials in the front of the book. Journals may be refereed or peer reviewed (i.e. the article is sent for critique by one or more experts in the field before being accepted for publication). This is an additional sign of quality. This means that most traditional sources (textbooks and journals) have been adequately reviewed and evaluated by a reputable publisher and are generally trustworthy.

However, if you have pulled the information from the internet, evaluating the source requires more effort. Look first at the three letters in the URL, which tell you what type of organisation is sponsoring the site. (Note: some sites don't use this identifier.) If it is a commercial organisation (.com), ask yourself what they are selling and whether this might bias their presentation of data. In other words, treat the information like you treat advertisements. If the address is for a nonprofit organisation (.org), ask yourself what their purpose and agenda is and what audience the materials are geared for. Government (.gov) and educational (.edu) sites are generally good sources of reliable information.

Whenever possible, check the author's credentials and affiliations. Although this is often difficult on the internet, the more reliable sources usually provide this information on the site. Because there are no editors or quality checkpoints for much of the material on the internet, you need to exercise greater caution and scepticism about the information you find. (Note: some sites, particularly professional sites, have editorial or peer review. When this is the case, it is clearly stated on the site.)

The second thing you can do is evaluate the types of materials you are using. Is the information from a primary or a secondary source? A primary source is the original source of the data. A secondary source secures the data from the primary source. The secondary source should cite the primary source when securing such data. This allows you, the reader, to access the primary source, if you wish, for more information about a specific point. (Note: footnotes or cited references tell us when data is from another source.) Is the material intended for a professional or lay audience or the general public? This often changes the presentation manner, breadth and depth of coverage. You need to decide whether the material contains enough information for your purposes.

Third, evaluate the timely nature of the information. Check the publication date and see how current the information is. If you are seeking information in a rapidly changing field or subject, this step is crucial. Remember that information in a book is probably already three to five years old when it is first published, so sometimes data in textbooks is dated. It can be a worthwhile exercise to check the reference list of textbooks to see just how current the information is that the authors drew on when the book was published. On the other hand, information in journals tends to be from six months to two years old when published. However, this is not always the case. Close reading of research papers can sometimes reveal a long lapse in time between collection of data and publication. The internet, with posted conference proceedings and electronic journals, has the potential to provide the most current resources available. Of course, again, this is not always the case, as some web pages are not updated regularly. When you are looking at internet sites, check to see when the information was last updated. This is usually posted on the site home page. (Hint: Page info on Netscape Navigator also provides this information.)

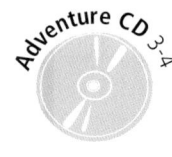

Finally, look at the content of the material itself. Is it presented in a well-organised and straightforward manner? Are major points adequately illustrated and explained? Are arguments backed up with supporting material such as referenced citations? Is the presentation balanced, and does it include alternative points of view? Does the material make sense? Is the material logical? Is the material adequate, or does it leave the reader with partially answered or unanswered questions? Compare the content with other sources. Look for similarities and differences. How do various sources agree or disagree? What common ground can you find?

Try the following Student Challenge and see what you discover.

> **Student Challenge**
>
> Checking Sources
>
> 1. Check the front of this book for a list of authors and reviewers and their credentials.
> 2. Look at two or three nursing journals and locate their policies for manuscript acceptance. Did you find any that were peer reviewed? If not, check the *Journal of Nursing Scholarship* or *Journal of Advanced Nursing*. How could you tell they are peer reviewed? How do peer-reviewed journals look compared to a journal like the *Australian Nurses Journal*? What are the most noticeable differences between them?
> 3. Check out some of the health-related websites on the internet. What information was available about the source of the information? Could you distinguish professional and academic sites from general sites? Could you tell how current the data were?
> 4. Check out one of the internet sites that posts professional conference proceedings. Find a newsgroup or other forum on the web that is for healthcare professionals. Explore it and see what it has to offer. Did you find any ground-breaking information?

Much of the evaluation process requires you to think critically about your resources. That means not taking material at face value. Just because information is published or appears on the internet in electronic form does not necessarily mean it is correct or current. Now that you are studying nursing you need to develop critical thinking skills. This means you need to ask questions, cross-check resources against one another, and bring a healthy degree of scepticism to your reading. For example, it is quite possible that segments of material in your current nursing textbooks are no longer valid because they are outdated.

This is particularly true of information that is time sensitive. When a text cites statistics, make a habit of looking at the date of the reference material. Consider too when data collection took place. When the text describes certain procedures or tests, ask yourself whether that material is the most current or if other technology has replaced that which is described. Ultimately you must make a judgment about whether a particular resource can be trusted to provide the quality information that you need.

Activity 10

> **Resource Kit**
>
> Reading Strategy References
>
> Robinson F (1970). *Effective study*, 4th edn. Harper & Row, New York. *This book is out of print but can still be found in many academic libraries and can be located at used bookstores through the Amazon.com website. A link to Amazon.com can be found on this book's Evolve site.*
>
> Wahlstrom C, Williams B, Dansby C (1999). *The practical student*. Wadsworth, Boston. *This book has several good study skills in addition to a chapter on effective reading that examines the SQ3R system.*
>
> Johnson D, Johnson C (1998). *Learning power*. Simon and Schuster, New York. *Another general study reference with a chapter on the SSS reading strategy.*
>
> Grammar Checkers, Reading Ease and other Faery Tales 2003. Online. A link to Grammar Checkers can be found on this book's Evolve site.
>
> 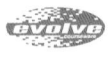 Visit the book's Evolve website at http://evolve.elsevier.com/AU/Borbasi/maze for further information.
>
> Check out the puzzles, mazes and games on your CD-ROM.

References

Doell D (2003). Gunning Fog Index. Online. Available: http://www.pima.edu/~ddoell/tw/gfiex.html 12 Mar 2003.

Gunning Fog Index 2003. Online. Available: http://isu.indstate.edu/nelsons/asbe336/PowerPoint/fog-index.htm 12 Mar 2003.

Microsoft Word (1997). Readability scores, Microsoft Word 97 Help menu.

Section 2

Talking the Talk

Learning the Language, Defining Research, and Exploring Quantitative and Qualitative Perspectives … Jump In

Health care and healthcare technology are becoming increasingly complex and expanding at a rapid rate. The practice of nursing changes on a daily basis. How do we cope? How can we keep our knowledge base and our practice current? Research is the key. It provides a solid foundation on which to base our practice. This means that as nurses we need to incorporate nursing research findings into our practice settings. This is commonly referred to as evidence-based practice. To do this we must be able to read, understand and apply the available research literature. This section defines research, explores quantitative and qualitative research methodologies, and provides you with the vocabulary and tools to read and understand research articles.

http://evolve.elsevier.com/AU/Borbasi/maze

Learning Objectives

After reading this chapter and following critical reflection the student will be able to:

1. Explore preconceived self-notions about research.
2. Define the terms 'research' and 'nursing research'.
3. Describe ways to acquire knowledge.
4. Discuss why nursing research is important.
5. Describe the historical development of nursing research.
6. Discuss nursing research priorities.
7. Delineate future directions for nursing research.

Chapter Outline

How Do You Feel About Research?
What Is Research?
What is knowledge?
    Tradition and custom
    Authority
    Trial and error
    Personal experience
    Intuition
    Reasoning
    Research

What is nursing research?
Why Is Research Important?
Why is nursing research important?
A Historical Look at Nursing Research
Nursing research in Australia
The Future of Nursing Research
Who Is Involved in Nursing Research?
ANC competencies and how they relate to research

Chapter 4

Research: What, Why, Where and Who?

Now class, 'research is the systematic, controlled, empirical and critical investigation of hypothetical propositions about presumed relations among natural phenomena' (Kerlinger 1973).

Student Quote

'At first I thought this learning about research was going to be a total waste of time. Now I'm excited because I'll be giving the very latest in nursing care to my patients.'

Abstract

Research is one way we acquire knowledge. Others include tradition, authority, trial and error, personal experience, intuition and reasoning. All these methods provide viable options to make sense of the world. Research offers us a systematic way to confirm existing knowledge and to build new knowledge. Nursing research explores issues important to nursing, to refine and expand the body of nursing knowledge. Although research in nursing was slow to develop, it has become an institutionalised force and now has an increasingly vital role in the practice of nursing in this complex and rapidly changing society. Nursing continues to grapple with ways to better facilitate the use of nursing research findings in the clinical practice setting.

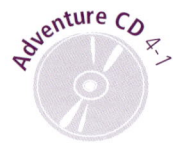

> **Key Terms**
>
> ### Knowledge Nomenclature
>
> **authority** Knowledge gleaned from the expertise of others.
>
> **epistemology** The philosophical theory of knowledge.
>
> **intuition** Insight into the whole of a situation without possessing readily supportable or confirming data.
>
> **knowledge** Essential information about the world around us that allows us to function more effectively.
>
> **personal/lived experience** Knowledge derived from the cumulative experiences of living.
>
> **tradition** The handing down of knowledge from one generation to the next.
>
> **trial and error** The process of trying a succession of alternative solutions until one solves the problem at hand.
>
> ### Research Nomenclature
>
> **bias** Any influence that may alter the outcomes of a research study.
>
> **clinical nursing research** Nursing research that has a direct impact on nursing interventions with clients.
>
> **deductive reasoning** Logical system of thinking that starts with the whole and breaks it down into its component parts.
>
> **dichotomy** Division into two parts.
>
> **empirical** Data generation through objective means.
>
> **hegemony** Dominance, usually of one group over another.
>
> **inductive reasoning** Logical system of thinking that begins with the component parts and builds them into a whole.
>
> **nursing research** Research usually conducted by nurses to generate knowledge that informs and develops the discipline and practice of nursing.
>
> **paradigm** Set of philosophical assumptions that underpin one's approach to inquiry.
>
> **reasoning** Use of logical thought patterns to solve problems. May be inductive or deductive in nature.
>
> **research** Systematic process using both inductive and deductive reasoning to confirm and refine existing knowledge and to build new knowledge.

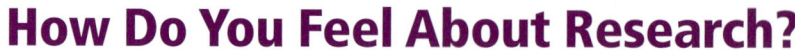

How Do You Feel About Research?

The first thing we do when facing a new class of research students is to pose a series of questions, such as: What image comes to mind when we say the word 'research'? What are your feelings about studying research? Is research important to nursing? Who should do or use research?

Just about now, many of you are probably wondering why you are studying research. You may have a vague notion of what research is but be unsure about what it has to do with the day-to-day practice of nursing. You may think only intellectual types are attracted to research, and you may worry about whether you'll be able to understand and make sense of it all. Although you probably agree that research has a place in nursing, you may think someone else should be doing or using it and that your time could be better spent on other pursuits. Or you may be excited and curious about this course but somewhat anxious about getting started.

Let's begin with the premise that research is an important tool in the rapidly changing practice of nursing. It can be used by all nurses at all educational levels and at all stages in their careers to do their jobs more effectively. This means you can use research right now to improve the care you give to patients in the clinical area. With that premise in mind, this chapter seeks to introduce the concept of research in a general context and within the specific context of nursing. It explores the ways we come to know about the world. It also looks at the importance of research in nursing, and the history and future of nursing research. Finally, it defines research roles and discusses obstacles to the use of research findings.

> Research is an important tool in the rapidly changing practice of nursing.

Student Challenge

Preconceived Notions

Consider each of these questions one at a time and record your answers.

1. What image comes to mind for the word 'research'? Paint a word picture or draw an image. For example, you might think of a little eggheaded bald man with glasses, bent over a microscope in a tiny, cluttered back room.
2. What characteristics does a researcher possess? List traits you think it takes to be a researcher.
3. How do you feel about research? About your study of research? Use feeling words like happy, sad, scared or anxious. Then try to examine why you might be feeling that way.
4. Do you think research is important to nursing? Why or why not?
5. Who do you think should do nursing research? Use nursing research? Do you picture yourself involved with research? Compare your answers with two or three of your peers. Discuss similarities and differences. What do your answers tell you? Did you learn anything that might be useful as you begin your study?

What Is Research?

Research literally means to search again or to examine carefully. It employs a systematic process to ask and answer questions that generate knowledge. The research process is often compared to the problem-solving process because they are similar—both employ a systematic approach in an attempt to answer a question. However, there are several important differences. The research method is much more formal and has identified standards and conditions that guide the process. Problem solving is concerned with an immediate solution for a particular situation. Research seeks answers that can be applied to other situations. Finally, problem solving seeks to find a solution within the boundaries of what we already know, whereas research seeks to confirm or refine what we think we know or to discover new knowledge. In fact, research often occurs because existing knowledge is inadequate to solve a particular problem that has been raised.

What is knowledge?

Knowledge is the comprehension and understanding of facts, truths or principles. It is the information we use to conduct our personal and professional lives. The study of (theorising) knowledge is called **epistemology**. We acquire knowledge in several ways.

We may use more than one method at a time in working on a solution to a problem or the answer to a question that is troubling us. All the methods are viable options and valid at various times. Each offers us a way to deal with the world. All possess strengths and weaknesses. The ultimate task is to recognise and use them all to our best advantage. The following sections discuss each in a little more depth.

Student Challenge

Thinking About Thinking

1. Either alone or with a small group of friends, brainstorm how you come to know what you know.
2. When you are finished, compare your list to the list in Box 4-1.
3. Any surprises? Did you come up with ways that are not listed?
4. Can you think of examples of how you use each of these sources of knowledge in your daily life?

> **BOX 4-1** Sources of Knowledge
>
> Tradition and custom
> Authority and role models
> Trial and error
> Personal experience
> Intuition
> Reasoning
> Research

Tradition and custom

Knowledge derived from **tradition** is 'truth' that is passed to us from previous generations. It is often a reflection of our culture or heritage. It involves those things we know or do because 'this is the way it has always been'. We usually accept these truths as given, with little questioning. This can be advantageous because it offers a common cultural ground from which to communicate and make decisions. Many practices that evolve from this kind of knowledge are ritualistic in nature. The reason or rationale for such practice may have been lost or may have disappeared over the years.

An example of this is provided in the following story. Two friends were preparing dinner together. One of them took the roast, cut off each end, and then placed it in the oven to brown. The other asked, 'Why did you cut off the ends first?'. 'I don't know,' said the first, 'It's the way my mother taught me.' However, being curious, she called her mother and asked for an explanation. Her mother didn't know either, having learned to cook a roast by watching her mother. So the woman called her grandmother in search of an answer. 'Well,' the grandmother said, 'I used to cut the ends off the roast because the dish I cooked it in was too small to hold the whole thing.'

Large segments of information and several practices in nursing are based largely on tradition. For example, we routinely take patients' vital signs each shift and provide daily baths and linen changes. Can you think of other examples? Many of these practices were originally instituted for good reasons. However, much like cutting off the end of the roast, the reason for the practice may no longer be viable. So it might be to our advantage to more critically examine those things in nursing that we 'know' by tradition or things that we do because that's the way it is customarily done. However, some of these practices persist even when we have evidence that the practice is unnecessary or not effective.

Authority

We rely heavily on individuals who are 'experts' in certain areas to provide us with information about various topics so we can make better informed decisions and better learn how to perform certain functions. The first **authority** figures we encounter are our parents. When we go to school, we begin to rely on teachers and textbooks for expanding our knowledge base. We also rely on the opinions of authorities that have expertise in areas we do not. This is a natural evolution and to be expected because it would be impossible for us to be knowledgeable about everything. As we choose a profession, we look to authorities in the field to teach us what they know. When we imitate the example set by authority figures, they serve as role models. Student and novice nurses can gain confidence and competence by selecting and using nursing academics or expert clinicians as role models.

The caution when using knowledge gleaned from authorities or in imitating their behaviours is to pick your authorities and role models carefully. Ask yourself questions such as: What makes this person an expert? What is their educational background and experience? How did they come to know? Do I accept the word of my lecturers and tutors or practising nurses without question? How well read and current are my nursing academics? Are they involved in scholarly activity and research? Are their clinical skills current? What about the nurses I see in the clinical area? Do they keep up with the latest discoveries in their specialty area? Do they show evidence of critical thinking in their clinical decision making, or do they justify actions with 'that's the way we do it here'?

Textbooks and other information sources often assume an authority role in the life of a nursing student. We tend to assign a lot of credibility to the written word. Do you take every piece of information you read at face value? Do you know if you are learning the best information available? Do you regularly use nursing journals as information sources? As you learned in the previous chapter, the information in most textbooks is at least three to five years old by the time it is published. One academic we know co-authored a quick reference handbook on diseases. Within one month of sending her work to the publisher, six major developments occurred that affected the content of that book. The book itself was not available until a year after she finished writing. She doesn't even want to count the number of changes that occurred in that one-year period. So, view the information critically. Is it in line with other authorities in the same area? Is it backed with sound rationale? Is it presented clearly and logically? Is it current? This is particularly timely advice in the age of an information explosion in which material is readily available on every topic imaginable.

Trial and error

The process of **trial and error** uses a successive number of alternative solutions to a problem until one works, to solve the problem at hand. It is often used when we have little frame of reference to draw on, when seemingly equal options are easily accessible and/or when we have exhausted standard approaches. This approach tends to be haphazard and results often cannot be reproduced a second time. Did you ever try to reproduce a meal that you just sort of threw together with a little of this and a little of that and have it actually turn out as tasty as the first time around?

We may also wind up using one option when another would work better. This occurs because the selected option adequately solves our problem, leaving the better option unexplored. For example, have you ever played around in a trial-and-error fashion to produce a certain result with your computer, and then proudly shown the results of your handiwork to a more computer-literate friend, who shows you how to get the same result in one or two key strokes or mouse manoeuvres? Of course this then renders your solution laughable and needlessly convoluted.

Using a system of trial and error may also entail a certain amount of risk. Using trial and error to learn to play 'Commando' on the computer is acceptable. If your character gets blown up, you just start over. Using trial and error to find the correct dose of medication for a patient could spell disaster. However, trial and error can bring about surprising results. When you approach an obstacle from a 'let's try this and see what happens' perspective, you are not bound by the restraints of logic. This type of exploration may provide solutions that might never have been attempted with a more 'logical' approach.

Personal experience

Knowledge derived from the cumulative experiences of living is familiar and powerful. It comes from seeing, hearing, touching, tasting, feeling and doing it ourselves. It is first-hand knowledge. We know it because we were there. We know it because we have been there before. We are intimately acquainted with this form of knowing. We trust it and value it highly in our decision-making process. It is personal. We witnessed it while it was happening. The more experience we gain in a situation, the greater our comfort and skill in that situation. As the number and variety of our experiences increase, we transfer, adapt and extend knowledge learned from previous situations to fit new situations. As the depth and breadth of our experience grows, our operating knowledge base becomes increasingly complex. **Personal experience** is individual and is often hard to translate or explain to others, particularly those who have no similar experience.

Personal or first-hand experience is also a useful tool in the professional arena. Patricia Benner (1984) describes five levels that a nurse goes through in developing clinical expertise: novice, advanced beginner, competent, proficient and expert.

Movement from one level to the next occurs with experience. Experience is only gained when previous knowledge is refined or challenged by actual clinical evidence. The novice nurse begins with knowledge gained in large part from authoritative sources and from the ability to reason and solve problems based on that body of knowledge. Experience is then added to the equation. Expertise develops over time when the nurse tests and refines her body of knowledge in real-world situations. Thus, according to Benner, experience is a necessary prerequisite for developing expertise.

Intuition

Intuition is a 'hunch' or 'gut feeling' about a situation that is not readily explained or easily backed up by logic or facts. It is an insight or understanding of the whole seen apart from its component parts. Intuition is closely tied to personal experience. Extensive personal experience allows an ingraining of knowledge so that it becomes second nature. Acting on this deeply embedded knowledge often occurs automatically and quickly as a flash of insight, an immediate recognition of the whole. It is often difficult to even recall or recount what produces this insight. Intuition has long been discounted because it is not easily examined or readily categorised. It also appears to occur apart from consideration of available facts and use of a reasoning process. So, in a society that holds logic at a premium, intuition is labelled as unreliable or as a lucky guess.

Benner (1984) describes intuition as perceptual awareness. Intuition in her estimation is not a lack of knowledge or a lucky guess. Rather it is deep knowledge derived from long hours of clinical observation and experience. It is being attuned to very subtle shifts that may be important only in the case of a specific patient. Benner (1984) documents several instances where expert nurses recognised impending warning signs of a life-threatening situation long before the so-called 'objective signs' revealed that something was going wrong. This type of clinical knowledge needs greater study so it can be more clearly understood and taught.

Reasoning

Reasoning is the use of logical thought patterns to solve problems. It can be broken into two broad subcategories: inductive and deductive reasoning. **Inductive reasoning** begins with several specifics or facts and builds a larger picture or whole that incorporates the smaller pieces. The accuracy of such reasoning rests with which pieces of information are chosen to build the larger whole. **Deductive reasoning** starts with the big picture or the whole and tries to break it down into its smaller parts. Reasoning allows us to try out alternatives in our mind and to select the one that seems to fit the situation best. It can, however, stifle creativity and overlook viable alternatives that may appear logically inadequate. No evaluation mechanism is built into the reasoning process. Much of the utility of our reasoning process is tested through experience in real-world situations.

Research

Research is a combination of deductive and inductive reasoning processes. It is a systematic process used to confirm and refine existing knowledge and to build new knowledge. Inductive reasoning allows us to generate new concepts and theories; deductive reasoning allows us to test out those concepts and theories. Quantitative research is used to describe, explore, explain or predict observable or measureable conditions. Qualitative research allows us to identify, examine and explain the experiences of an individual or group. We talk in depth about these two types of research in later chapters.

> Research is a systematic reasoning process used to confirm existing knowledge and build new knowledge.

Research has built-in checks and balances as well as evaluation mechanisms. It seeks to acknowledge and reduce bias. However, all sources of knowing are influenced by personal bias. All that we learn is filtered by our own set of views, and we have a tendency to use incoming knowledge to confirm those already held views. Thus, when filtering information, we tend to note and remember those things that support our views and ignore or deny those that are contrary.

Is research then a magic bullet, an answer to all questions, a solution to all human problems? Of course not. It is a very specific set of processes designed to examine only those problems that can be directly or indirectly seen, touched, heard, tasted or smelt. Research cannot be used to produce answers about fundamental moral or ethical issues such as whether abortion is good or evil or whether cloning is right or wrong. It cannot take the place of philosophical debate about the meaning of life or the existence of a 'higher power'. The research we conduct is only as good as the limits of the study and the way the study is designed, and all studies have limits or flaws. Some explorations using the research process are even out of reach because we haven't yet invented the instruments that would allow us to measure what we want to study. Results obtained from the research process provide us with reasonable or plausible answers. The knowledge gained is never final or absolute. It is, in fact, always subject to ongoing investigation and scrutiny. Research is a tool, albeit a very powerful one, to explore the world around us.

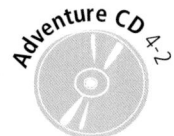

> Research is a tool to explore the world around us.

What is nursing research?

Nursing research is simply research that addresses issues important to nurses and the nursing profession. Nursing research uses the research process as a tool to search for, develop, refine and expand a body of knowledge that shapes and enhances the practice of nursing. Research can be classified as nursing research when the research endeavour produces knowledge relevant to nursing. This includes the areas of clinical practice, education and administration, as well as various professional issues. The focus in this text is on nursing research that has a direct impact on nursing interventions with clients. This is often referred to as **clinical nursing research**.

> Nursing research uses the research process as a tool to search for, develop, refine and expand a body of knowledge that shapes and enhances the practice of nursing.

Why Is Research Important?

The ultimate importance of research is found in its definition. It generates knowledge. This in turn allows us to make better informed decisions and choices. It may validate existing practices built through tradition, intuition and personal experience. It may examine tried and true practices and make them more efficient, less expensive or less complicated. It may explore ways to tackle newly evolving problems in an increasingly complex world. Most importantly, research contributes to better healthcare outcomes for consumers.

Why is nursing research important?

Nursing research serves several purposes for nursing as a profession and for nurses as individuals. It provides a standard and reliable knowledge base upon which to build the practice of nursing. This in turn ensures that the care given to clients is the best possible at the time. So nursing research plays an important role in guiding and improving the delivery of nursing care to clients. Research-based practice ensures the delivery of up-to-date nursing care and the implementation of new ways of nursing.

Professions are commonly judged by the body of knowledge they generate. A clearly defined knowledge base built on a strong research foundation lends credibility to nursing as a distinct profession. The more defined this knowledge base, the clearer the role of the nurse in the delivery of health care. If nurses can more clearly define their role, then they can more clearly articulate distinctions and similarities between their own roles and those of other healthcare professionals. This in turn allows consumers of health care and potential clients to better see and value the contributions of nurses and nursing as a profession.

The practice of nursing in today's litigious society demands increasing accountability for one's actions. Consumers demand reasons for nursing interventions. Thus nurses need sound rationales for their decisions and actions. A knowledge base grounded in the findings of sound research provides such rationales. Individual nurses need a current knowledge base in order to be responsible and accountable to the consumer. This is the nub of evidence-based practice and is written into the Australian Nursing Council (ANC, formerly Australian Nursing Council Inc, or ANCI) competencies.

Nurses are increasingly called on to document the cost effectiveness of the nursing care that is given. Many healthcare facilities have tried to reduce costs by substituting untrained personnel for nurses. In part this is because nursing services consume such a large part of an institution's budget. Research can demonstrate that effective nursing care leads to fewer patient complications, shorter hospital stays or fewer readmissions, and that nursing cutbacks actually increase overall institutional costs (Joint Commission on Accreditation of Health Care Organisations 2001; *New York Times* 2002).

A Historical Look at Nursing Research

Research is a relatively new addition to nursing's toolbag of knowledge sources. While the first research efforts can be traced back to Florence Nightingale, little formal research was carried out by nurses until the late 1940s. The progress of nursing research is closely tied to the development of nursing and nursing education.

Research was slow to develop in nursing. Schools evolved from military and religious roots and stressed order and obedience. Inquiring minds had little place in this system of education. Instead, dedication to hard work and submission to authority were valued. Training was viewed as an apprenticeship, with long hours and rote repetition the order of the day. Nurses had little free time and little say in their own training or work. The traditional subservient role of women in society reinforced the values promoted by hospitals and hospital schools of nursing.

Only when nursing began to move toward advanced education and affiliation with university settings did nursing research begin to emerge. This move began in the United States. Ironically, it was research by investigators in other disciplines that exposed the deficiencies in the preparation of nurses and urged better educational opportunities and a move to university settings. Sociologists found the study of nurses and nursing as a work culture particularly fascinating. As a female-dominated occupation, nursing held special appeal for sociological investigation. Nursing work, habits, roles and attitudes were dissected and reported for decades in sociological literature.

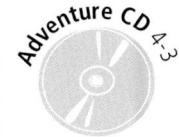

World War II increased the demand for nurses and sparked interest in nursing as a profession. Nurses and nursing were in the spotlight. In the US, funds for development were suddenly available from government and private sources. US nurses began to push for basic and advanced education in university settings. Nursing research got a major boost in that country with a nursing research centre and a nursing foundation established to promote nursing research. A journal was created to publish the results of that research. More nurses were receiving advanced degrees and had expertise in research. Unfortunately, most of these degrees were in fields other than nursing. Thus, early research efforts by nurses tended to ask questions about the education, psychology or sociology of nurses.

In the 1960s and 1970s and still in the US, the number of nurses with advanced degrees and research skills continued to increase and the push for doctoral preparation in nursing began. Formal support mechanisms for research and research funding in nursing increased and stabilised. Nursing practice was becoming more standardised, complex and specialised. Nursing education at the master's level became more common and emphasised specialisation in rapidly emerging specialty areas. Research was carried out to establish standards for specialty practice. Nurses began to turn to nursing care and clinical practice to provide questions for research. The focus of study shifted from nurses to the practice of nursing. Nursing theories evolved that attempted to describe and explain the practice of nursing. These theories began to be tested by nurse researchers. Practice-related research flourished and by the end of the 1970s, two new research journals were launched in the US to handle the nursing research explosion. In 1988 the US National Center for Nursing Research was federally mandated and funded under the National Institute of Health (NIH). In 1993 it was named an institute in its own right.

Nursing research in Australia

In Australia such developments took longer. The move to tertiary education only began in earnest in the mid-1980s. In the US, however, by the 1980s there was already a critical mass of nurses with doctoral degrees and research skills, and many Australian nurses went to the US to study for higher degrees. The Dawkins reforms in the late 1980s saw the merger of colleges of advanced education and universities, and resulted in the basic entry for nursing in Australia becoming an undergraduate degree, with nursing research identified as a crucial component. The inception of postgraduate degrees led to further growth in nursing research, although in the early stages much of this research was about nursing education and nurses themselves (Roberts & Taylor 1998).

As increasing numbers of nurses (mostly academics at this stage) conducted research, the Royal Australian Nursing Federation (RANF, now known as the ANF) launched the *Australian Journal of Advanced Nursing* in 1983, to create an outlet for research publication. Since that time, other key nursing bodies have also committed to encouraging research activity. The Royal College of Nursing Australia (RCNA) has developed a position statement on nursing research that can be accessed through its web page (http://www.rcna.org.au/content/nursing_research .doc) and has funding available nationally for research and scholarships. The ANF is committed to increasing the research capacity of the organisation. For example, the South Australian branch of the ANF has recently employed a joint appointee with the tertiary sector for the explicit purpose of informing strategic nursing research and development. Its website provides details of organisations that offer national research funding opportunities (try http://www.anf.org.au/nno/default.htm) for nurses. The incorporation of a competency statement about nursing research into the ANC competencies for beginning practitioners confirms the profession's commitment to research (Roberts & Taylor 1998; ANC 2000). The New Zealand Nurses Organisation (NZNO) has a well-developed nursing research section (NRS).

In the early stages of their research endeavours, US nurses leaned heavily towards empirico-analytical research, while nurses in Australia, influenced by the feminist movement, favoured qualitative research methodologies, although in both quarters there are now moves to eclecticism. In much the same way as in the US, nursing research in Australia has been through a process of evolution. Much work has been done in refining and expanding nursing research efforts. Through such international and national efforts, nursing today has established a firm foundation for its practice through research. Most Australian undergraduate students now study research as part of their degree, and honours programs are available for talented students to develop research skills early in their careers. In Australia and New Zealand there are numerous doctoral programs in nursing. Centres for nursing research are beginning to proliferate in many hospital and university settings and Clinical Professors of Nursing have been established through university/industry partnerships. The quality and volume of nursing research continues to grow, and an increasing number of research journals have been launched to help disseminate nursing research findings. Clinical practice specialty groups progressively fund, promote and publish research in their respective specialty areas.

In 2002 the focus of nursing research in the Western world shifted to the exploration of nursing practice. While research remains predominately initiated and conducted by people affiliated in some way to the university sector (i.e. academics and students), research questions (the substance of research) to a much larger extent are being generated by clinicians, and more and more clinicians are joining with academics to form research teams. Moreover, research teams are expected to be multidisciplinary and cross-institutional. Traditionally, Australian researchers have relied on the Australian Research Council (ARC) and the National Health and Medical Research Council (NH&MRC) to support research but must now look increasingly to nontraditional sources. As national research funding becomes increasingly competitive, collaborative cross-disciplinary research that clearly demonstrates health outcomes is more likely to get funded. It is an exciting and optimistic time for nursing research. Box 4-2 presents some highlights in the development of nursing and ultimately nursing research in Australia. In New Zealand the Health Research Council provides funding for health research, and the New Zealand Nurses Organisation and the Nursing Education and Research Foundation (NERF) offer a range of grants and scholarships for nurses. The NERF has an excellent online index of New Zealand nursing research that can be accessed free of charge.

> **BOX 4-2** Nursing Highlights in Australia
>
> | | |
> |---|---|
> | 1868 | Lucy Osborne arrives at the Sydney Infirmary to establish the first hospital-based school of nursing based on the Nightingale system |
> | 1899 | Formation of the NSW Trained Nurses Association, which later became the Australasian Trained Nurses Association |
> | 1903–51 | *Australasian Nurses' Journal* published; later *Australian Nurse's Journal* |
> | 1923 | The Australian Nursing Federation becomes the first national nursing organisation |
> | 1924 | Nurses Registration Act passed through parliament |
> | 1931 | NSW Nurses' Association founded |
> | 1943 | The Kelly Report (NSW) published. First major investigation of modern nursing in Australia |
> | 1949 | The NSW College of Nursing is established |
> | 1950 | The College of Nursing Australia, established in Victoria, begins offering postgraduate courses |
> | 1967–74 | Nine reports published on the issue of the education preparation of nurses and nursing in NSW |
> | 1967 | First combined degree and nursing course offered at UNE |
> | 1969 | Truskett Interim and Matron's Reports released |
> | 1972 | Nurses Education Board (NEB) established in NSW |
> | 1973 | Nurses Education Board Act passed through parliament in NSW |
> | 1975 | Goals in Nursing Education Report Parts 1 & 2: 'Nurse education: what future?' First national approach to transferring nursing education to the higher education sector |
> | 1978 | Six colleges of advanced education offer undergraduate courses in nursing |
> | 1978 | Sax Report on Nurse Education and Training: Report of the Committee of Inquiry into Nurse Education and Training to the Tertiary Education Commission, released |
> | 1983 | *Australian Journal of Advanced Nursing* first published |
> | 1985 | Nurse education and training moved to the tertiary sector in NSW—diploma of applied science (nursing) offered at colleges of advanced education |

1993	Full transfer of nursing education across Australia to the tertiary sector
1990	Amalgamation of colleges of advanced education with universities—bachelor degree in nursing becomes requisite for registration
1990	ANRAC (Australian Nurse Registering Authorities Conference) developed national competencies for registered nurses
1992	*Contemporary Nurse* first published
1992	Australian Nursing Council (ANC) established. First peak body concerned with regulation of nursing
1993	*Australian Nursing Journal* (ANJ) published by Australian Nursing Federation (previously *Australian Nurse's Journal*)
1993	Full transfer of nursing education across Australia to the higher education sector
1993	Code of Ethics for Nurses in Australia first developed
1994	Nursing Education in Australian Universities: Report of the National Review of Nurse Education in the Higher Education Sector 1994 and Beyond (Reid Review). Review found the transfer to be successful
1994	*Collegian, Journal of Royal College of Nursing, Australia* first published
1994	*Nursing Inquiry* first published
1995	Nurse Practitioner Project Stage 3—Final Report of the Steering Committee (NSW Health)
1995	*International Journal of Nursing Practice* first published
1996	Joanna Briggs Institute for Evidenced Based Nursing and Midwifery established at Royal Adelaide Hospital
1997	National Review of Specialist Nursing Education (Russell, Gething & Convery)
1999	'Rethinking Nursing': report of a national nursing workforce forum held in Canberra to identify future challenges in Australian nursing
1999	First national scoping study of the mental health nursing workforce in Australia
2001	Nurse supply and demand to 2006: projections and issues. A project carried out for the Australian Council of Deans of Nursing (Preston)
2002	Revised Code of Ethics for Nurses in Australia 2002
2002	Senate Inquiry into Nursing Report 'The patient profession: time for action'
2002	National Review of Nursing Education Report: 'Our duty of care'

Activity 11

> **Student Challenge**
>
> Netting Nursing Organisations
>
> 1. Log on to the internet and check out the RCNA website. Explore the history of the RCNA and discover its central mission.
> 2. Can you find out who the Executive Director of the RCNA is? Do you think she/he is qualified for the job? What did you base your evaluation on?
> 3. Do you think it is important for nurses to have their own national professional organisation? Why or why not?
> 4. Click on Policy, then Policy development, then Position statements and guidelines, and read the Position Statement on Nursing Research.
> 5. Go to the International Council of Nurses home page.
> 6. Explore the history of the ICN and discover its central mission.
> 7. Click on ICN Policies, go to Nursing Profession, scroll down to Nursing Research and read the ICN Position Statement.
> 8. Do you think it is important for nursing to have its own international governmental institute? Why or why not?
> 9. Access the following websites:
>   - The National Institute of Nursing Research
>   - Sigma Theta Tau
>   - Nursing Research Section, NZ Nurses Organisation.
> 10. Explore what they have to say about their organisations and the emphasis they place on nursing research.
> 11. On the Sigma Theta Tau website search for Xi Omicron, which is the chapter in Australia. Do they encourage student membership? If so, what are the criteria for students to join?

The Future of Nursing Research

In Australia a national nursing research agenda has not been clearly defined, although the establishment of a National Institute of Nursing Research much like the one in the US to develop broad research priority areas for the profession cannot be far off. In Australia research priorities in health are set by federal agencies such as the NH&MRC (http://www.health.gov.au/nhmrc/) and these are generally very broad. Research priorities are also established at State level through Departments of Health or Human Services (see Department of Human Services South Australia http://www.dhs.sa.gov.au, NSW Health http://www.health.nsw.gov.au, Department of Human Services Victoria http://www.dhs.vic.gov.au/). The Priority-Driven Research Program (State/Commonwealth Research Issues Forum) provides competitive funding for conducting health service research identified as a priority by the States/Territories and approved by the Australian Health Ministers Advisory Council (AHMAC). National research priorities are also set through the Commonwealth Department of Education, Science and Training (DEST; http://www.dest.gov.au), who have a link to National Research Priorities on their home page. In New Zealand the Ministry of Health (together with the Health Research Council) identifies areas for health promotion and research interest (http://www.moh.govt.nz/moh.nsf).

> **BOX 4-3** National Research Priorities for Australia's Future Prosperity
>
> An environmentally sustainable Australia
> Promoting and maintaining good health
> Frontier technologies for building and transforming Australian industries
> Safeguarding Australia
>
> Source: Prime Minister of Australia media releases. Online. Available:
> http://www.pm.gov.au/news/media_releases/2002/media_release2018.htm 6 Jan 2003.

Many health organisations publish research priorities including, for example, the World Health Organization (WHO) and the State Government Departments of Health or Human Services. Descriptions of these can be accessed on the world wide web.

The future for nursing research in the twenty-first century promises to be bright and challenging. With the development of a national organisation for nursing research, research priorities are likely to be directed at nursing practice. There will also be an increased emphasis on building on the results of completed studies. This includes repeating studies using various subjects in a variety of settings (replication). There will also be an ever-greater push to find ways to ensure that nurses use the results of all this nursing research in the course of their day-to-day practice (discussed in more depth in Chapter 12).

> **Student Challenge**
>
> Foraging for Future Research
>
> 1 Log on to the internet and check out the US National Institute for Nursing Research (NINR) strategic plans for the twenty-first century (http://www.nih.gov/ninr/research/diversity/mission.html).
>
> 2 Check out the NINR Areas of Research Opportunity for the years 2002 and 2003. Compare them with those for 2001, cited in Box 4-4. How have they changed?

3 Discuss the delineated areas. What relevance do they have to what you see in the clinical area?

> **BOX 4-4** NINR Areas of Research Opportunity for 2001
>
> Chronic illnesses or conditions
> Enhancing adherence to self-management of chronic illness
> Managing diabetes in minority groups
> Behavioural changes and interventions
> Using telehealth as a mode of intervention to improve clinical nursing care
> Collaborating with clinical trials supplements
> Compelling public health concerns
> Enhancing end of life/palliative care
> Promoting health disparities centres and career development
> Provision of training opportunities in clinical genetics research
>
> Source: NINR 2001 NINR areas of research opportunity, Online. Available: http://www.nih.gov/ninr/research/dea/2001AoRO.html 6 Dec 2003.

Who Is Involved in Nursing Research?

Nurses at all levels have a role to play as either consumers or producers of nursing research. Consumers of nursing research are responsible for reading current research and adapting useful findings to their practice. Producers design and implement research studies and disseminate the study results for consumers to use. While some countries delineate levels of research participation by educational level for nurses, in Australia under the aegis of the ANC competencies, all registered nurses are required to be at least consumers of research. The priority is to read and use research results in the clinical setting.

ANC competencies and how they relate to research

The ANC National Nursing Competency Standards are core standards that are expected to be exhibited by all nurses for registration. In developing the competencies the ANC has taken account of the contemporary role of the registered nurse and provided a benchmark for nurses in daily practice. Aspects covered include clinical practice, management of care, counselling, health promotion, client advocacy, facilitation of change, clinical teaching, supervising, mentoring and research. The ANC has recently developed principles for the assessment of national competency standards to guide their use in determining competency.

The Domain 'Critical Thinking and Analysis' incorporates research as follows:

Competency Unit 6
Values research in contributing to developments in nursing and improved standards of care.
Element 6.1: Acknowledges the importance of research in improving nursing outcomes.
Element 6.2: Incorporates research findings into nursing practice.
Element 6.3: Contributes to the process of nursing research.

Source: Australian Nursing Council (2000). ANC National Nursing Competency Standards for the Registered Nurse and Enrolled Nurse. Online. Available: http://www.anci.org.au/competencystandards.htm. Last updated 7 Nov 2002.

Resource Kit

Nursing Research Journals

Australian Journal of Advanced Nursing

Journal of Advanced Nursing

Nursing Research

Research in Nursing and Health

Applied Nursing Research

Nursing Science Quarterly

Journal of Nursing Scholarship

Useful Websites

Australian Nursing Federation (http://www.anf.org.au/)

Royal College of Nursing Australia (http://www.rcna.org.au/)

Australian Nursing Council (http://www.anc.org.au/)

National Institute of Nursing Research (NINR) (http://www.nih.gov/ninr/about.html)

New Zealand Nursing Council (http://www.nursingcouncil.org.nz)

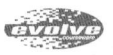 Visit the book's Evolve website at http://evolve.elsevier.com/AU/Borbasi/maze for further information.

 Check out the puzzles, mazes and games on your CD-ROM.

References

ANC (2000). *National competencies for the registered nurse*, 3rd edn. Australian Nursing Council, Canberra.

Benner P (1984). *From novice to expert: excellence and power in clinical nursing practice.* Addison-Wesley, Menlo Park, Calif.

Joint Commission on Accreditation of Healthcare Organisations (2001). Health care at the crossroads: strategies for addressing the evolving nursing crisis. Online. Available: http://www.jcaho.org/news+room/press+kits/nursing+shortage+press+kit.htm 12 Mar 2003.

Kerlinger FN (1973). *Foundations of behavioral research*, 2nd edn. Holt Rinehart & Winston, New York.

New York Times (2002). Patient deaths tied to lack of nurses. Online. Available: http://www.nytimes.com Last updated 8 Aug 2002.

NINR (2000). NINR Areas of research opportunity. Online. Available: http://www.nih.gov/ninr/research/dea/2000AoRO.html 10 Mar 2003.

NINR (2001). NINR areas of research opportunity. Online. Available: http://www.nih.gov/ninr/research/dea/2001AoRO.html 6 Jan 2003.

Roberts K, Taylor B (1998). *Nursing research processes: an Australian perspective.* Nelson, Melbourne.

Russell RL (1990). *From Nightingale to now: nurse education in Australia.* WB Saunders, Sydney.

http://evolve.elsevier.com/AU/Borbasi/maze

Learning Objectives

After reading this chapter and following critical reflection the student will be able to:

1. Define quantitative research.
2. Describe quantitative research classifications.
3. Discuss the phases of the research process.
4. Describe the steps involved in conceptualising a study.
5. Describe the steps involved in designing a study.
6. Describe the steps involved in conducting a study.
7. Describe the steps involved in analysing a study.
8. Describe the steps involved in using study results.
9. Discuss the relationships among phases of the research process.
10. Cite examples of steps and phases of the research process.

Chapter Outline

What Is Quantitative Research?
Quantitative Research Classifications
Reasons quantitative research is conducted
Time span and point of data collection
Purpose
Research design
What Is the Research Process?
Phase 1: Conceive the study
    Identify the problem
    Review the literature
    Define a theoretical framework
    Formulate variables
Phase 2: Design the study
    Select research design
    Identify sample and setting
    Select data collection methods
    Evaluate instrument quality
Phase 3: Conduct the study
    Get approval to use human subjects
    Recruit subjects
    Collect data
Phase 4: Analyse the study
    Describe the sample
    Answer the research questions
    Interpret the results
Phase 5: Use the study
    Recommend further research
    State implications for practice
    Disseminate results

Chapter 5

Quantitative Research: Summing It Up

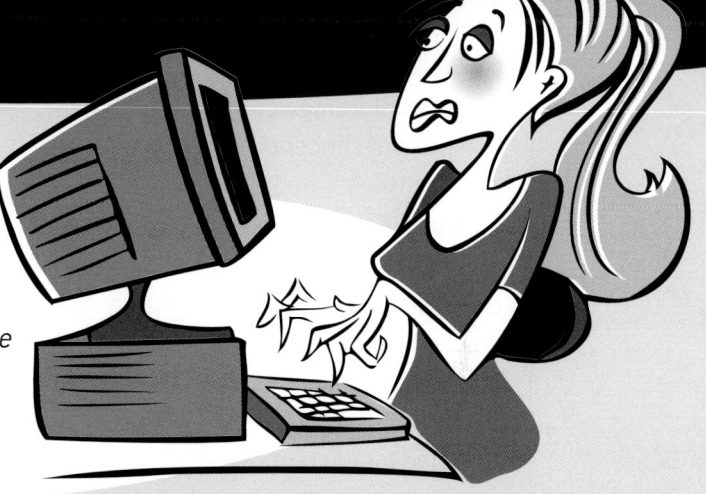

Hmmm! There has to be a statistic here somewhere that will make my results come out with the right answer.

Student Quote

> 'Once you understand what all those terms mean, and learn that there is a set structure and defined process for doing a (quantitative) research study, it's not so hard to follow what's happening.'

Abstract

Quantitative research is a systematic logical process used to answer questions about measurable concepts. It can be classified in numerous ways, including via the stated goals of the research or by the choice of research design. The research process is a circular one comprising an orderly series of five phases that move the researcher from formulation of researchable problems to discovery of probable answers. The phases begin with conceptualisation and crystallisation of the problem. This problem is grounded in a literature base of previous research and theory. A study plan is then developed that specifies a research design, the subjects to be studied, and the instruments to be used for measurement. The study is implemented and data are collected using a set of ethical guidelines. Data are analysed statistically, and research questions are answered and placed in a theoretical context. The findings are examined for their relevance to nursing practice and future research. Results are communicated to research consumers.

Key Terms

Quantitative Connections

concept Mental picture of an object or phenomenon. Concepts may be concrete or abstract.

conceptual definition Statement attaching a specified meaning to a word (e.g. what the word means for a particular research study).

conceptual framework Loosely related collection of concepts that have not yet been tested.

constant Characteristic that does not vary for a particular research study.

control Mechanisms used by the researcher to reduce the influence of extraneous variables.

data Measurable bits of information collected for the purpose of analysis.

data collection The gathering of information necessary to address the research problem.

dependent variable Variable that is affected by the action of the independent variable.

descriptive statistics Statistics used to describe and summarise data.

ethics committee Committee responsible for review of research proposals to ensure that human subjects are protected from harm.

experimental research Quantitative research in which one concept (independent variable) is manipulated to determine whether another concept (dependent variable) is affected.

extraneous variable Variable that interferes with the relationship of the independent and dependent variables in a specified study.

findings Results of the statistical analysis of study data.

generalisation The ability to apply study results from the sample to the population.

hypothesis Statement of predicted relationship or difference between two or more variables. A hypothesis contains at least one independent and one dependent variable.

implication Inference drawn about the results of a research study.

independent variable Variable that causes a change in the dependent variable.

inferential statistics Statistics that are used to study relationships or differences among variables in a sample and infer the results back to the population.

informed consent An agreement by a research subject to participate voluntarily in a study after being fully informed about the study and the inherent risks and benefits of participation.

instrument Device or technique used to collect data in a research study (e.g. biophysical instruments such as glucometers, psychological instruments such as questionnaires or interviews, behavioural instruments such as observation).

literature review Critical summary of available theoretical and research literature on the selected research topic. It places the research problem for a particular study in the context of what is currently known about the topic.

manipulation Intervention or treatment introduced by the researcher in an experimental study.

measurement Set of rules used to assign numbers to variables.

nonexperimental research Quantitative research in which concepts are not manipulated, but are examined as they occur naturally.

nonprobability sample Sample selected using nonrandom techniques.

operational definition Specifies how a variable is to be measured.

population All known subjects that possess a common characteristic of interest to a researcher.

probability (random) sample Sample selected using techniques to ensure that each subject in the population has an equal chance of being selected.

problem statement Interrogative or declarative statement that describes the purpose of a research study, identifies key concepts and sets study limits.

quantitative research Systematic process used to gather and statistically analyse information that has been measured by an instrument and converted to numerical data.

recommendation Statement derived from a research study to guide future research about a specified topic.

reliability Characteristic of a good instrument; the assessed degree of consistency and dependability.

research design The overall plan for collecting data in a research study.

research process Orderly series of phases and steps that allow the researcher to move from asking a question to finding an answer.

research question Use of an interrogative format to identify the variables to be studied and possible relationships or differences between those variables.

sample Subset of a population selected to participate in a research study.

sampling The process used to select the sample.

setting The physical location and conditions under which a research study takes place.

systematic review Review or scientific study that seeks to answer a clear question by locating and appraising all published and unpublished works on the subject.

theoretical framework The theoretical foundation or frame of reference for a research study.

theory Integrated and interrelated set of concepts used to explain some phenomenon.

validity Characteristic of a good instrument; the extent of an instrument's ability to measure what it purports to measure.

variable Concept, characteristic or trait that varies (e.g. takes on measurably different values) within an identified population in a research study.

Within research there are several paradigms that are grounded in different philosophical approaches. For the purposes of this book we are going to concentrate on introducing you to the main ones you will encounter as beginning readers of research, and beginning students of nursing. These major paradigms are called quantitative and qualitative. However, as you develop a wider range of reading you will encounter research and scholarship grounded in other approaches, such as postmodernity or critical social theory.

This chapter addresses quantitative research, and Chapter 6 addresses qualitative research. The intent of these two chapters is to provide you with working knowledge of both research approaches. This will give you the necessary background and vocabulary to recognise, read and use the findings from the nursing research literature. This chapter defines quantitative research, explores various ways in which quantitative research can be classified, and identifies and discusses the specific steps of the quantitative research process.

You may find the next two chapters difficult to read and comprehend. That is to be expected, because you are learning a new vocabulary. Don't panic. Remember what you learned in Chapter 3, and use your reading strategy. Take the time to thoroughly read and summarise the material. These two chapters provide the foundation you need to enable you to read and apply research results. Take a deep breath and attack this chapter one paragraph at a time. You can do it.

HINT The Glossary contains many of the terms used in this chapter even though they are not located in your Key Terms list. So take advantage of the Glossary. It is located at the back of the book, and it is on the CD-ROM.

What Is Quantitative Research?

Quantitative research is a systematic, objective process used to gather and analyse information that has been measured by some kind of instrument. Instruments are used to convert information into numbers. Quantitative research uses statistics to manage those numbers. The statistics may describe the numbers or analyse the numbers. This allows the researcher to draw a numerical picture of the information collected, to look at how the things being measured are alike or different, and to make decisions about whether things are related or different, or to determine whether one thing causes another to react in a certain way.

> Quantitative research is a systematic process used to gather and statistically analyse information that has been measured by an instrument and converted to numerical data.

Quantitative research uses a logical approach that emphasises deductive reasoning. It has several identifiable characteristics. It begins either with an educated guess (hypothesis) about how the **concepts** to be researched might be related, or with a question (research question) about what is to be explored or described. It studies only quantifiable concepts (concepts that can be measured and turned into numbers). The process is very structured. It seeks to be objective and tries to limit or control the effects of things not being studied. This approach yields results or **findings** that are clearly defined and easily interpreted.

However, this approach has limitations. It is not readily used to study complex issues in which a large number of factors are at play. It cannot study concepts that cannot be numerically measured. Also, although objectivity is prized and strict controls are imposed to ensure this objectivity, bias is inevitable and begins with the researcher's interest in a particular area of study. It continues when the researcher makes predictions or hypotheses about the expected results. The researcher often becomes highly invested in ensuring that those predictions are supported by the study's outcomes. There have been numerous reports about researchers who resort to various conscious and unconscious means to ensure certain results. An example of this was reported in a newspaper story that told of a scientist who faked data to try to prove that there was a relationship between electric power lines and an increased incidence of cancer (Seyfer 1999).

Quantitative Research Classifications

Several different terms are used to describe or classify quantitative research. We explore some of the more common classifications and terms so they will be familiar to you when you encounter them in the literature. Quantitative research may be classified in the following ways: the reasons for conducting the research, the span of time in which data collection occurs, the point at which data are collected, the number of subjects sampled, the purpose or aim of the research, and the research design or statistical method used (Box 5-1). Studies may fall under several of these classification schemes. Thus, you might see a particular study described as a cross-sectional, descriptive, nonexperimental study.

BOX 5-1 Classification Systems for Quantitative Research

Reasons conducted:
- Basic (pure)
- Applied

Time span:
- Cross-sectional
- Longitudinal

> Point of data collection:
> - Retrospective (*ex post facto* or after the fact)
> - Prospective
>
> Purpose or aim:
> - Descriptive
> - Exploratory
> - Explanatory
> - Predictive
>
> Research design:
> - Experimental
> - Nonexperimental (correlational)

Reasons quantitative research is conducted

Pure or basic research is done to establish or extend fundamental concepts and theories. It is a search for 'knowledge for knowledge's sake'. The findings may have no immediate practical application or benefit. Applied research is conducted for practical purposes and is directed at solving an immediate problem. Applied research is often based on a foundation of basic research, and its results often suggest further areas for basic research study. Because nursing is a practice discipline, most of the research in various nursing research journals is applied research. As a consumer of nursing research who desires to improve clinical practice, you will likely be most interested in applied research.

> Applied research is used to find solutions to clinical problems in nursing.

Time span and point of data collection

Research is sometimes described by the span of time used to collect the data for the study or to indicate when data were collected. Cross-sectional studies use data collected at one point in time. Longitudinal studies use data collected at several points over a longer time period. Measurements of the identified concepts may be taken many times over several months or years. Prospective studies analyse data collected on factors or events as they occur. Retrospective studies analyse data on factors or events that occurred before the onset of the research study.

Purpose

The two categories most helpful in describing a quantitative study are classification by purpose, and classification by design. You may recall that in Chapter 4 we said, 'quantitative research is used to describe, explore, explain or predict observable measurable conditions'. Thus this particular classification scheme informs us about the general purpose of the research study.

A descriptive study does as its name implies; it *describes* the concepts under study. It commonly looks at the prevalence, magnitude and/or characteristics of the concept. It may classify various factors in the study. A recent example of a descriptive nursing research study can be found in Lengacher et al's study (2002) to establish the frequency of complementary therapy use in women diagnosed with breast cancer. The survey was also used to determine demographic and clinical factors associated with the use of complementary therapy. Another example can be found in a study by Mimnaugh et al (1999), which described the types and intensity of sensations experienced by postoperative patients during the removal of tubes.

Exploratory studies *explore*. They are used to investigate a particular concept about which little is known. They go beyond describing concepts and begin to examine the relationships or differences between the concepts and other factors. For example, Gallinagh et al (2002, p 147) explored 'the use of physical restraints as a safety measure in the care of older people in four rehabilitation wards'. Their study examined the prevalence and type of physical restraint used with older persons and looked at relationships between restraint use and variables such as age and gender, staffing and time of day.

Explanatory studies *explain*. These studies try to discover why a certain concept or phenomenon occurs. They search for cause and effect or interactive relationships between concepts. They are often linked with theory and represent a way to organise or integrate the relationships among various concepts or factors. For example, in an explanatory study Pryor et al (2002) looked at the effect of supervision on the injury experience of children unintentionally hurt in agricultural accidents. The research was underpinned by a recognised Injury Model.

Predictive studies *predict*. Once events are explainable, the next step is to try to predict what will occur with one factor if a change happens in related factors. Studies that try to predict what will occur are called predictive studies. For example, Jennings-Dozier (1999) studied whether certain factors would predict which women would get a Pap smear.

Research design

There are two major research design categories: experimental and nonexperimental. These descriptions tell us how the research study has been designed. In **experimental research**, the researcher manipulates one concept under study to see how that manipulation will change or affect another concept under study. For example, an experimental study by Gawlinski & Dracup (1998) looked at whether positioning affected oxygen saturation in critically ill patients. The position of patients was manipulated to see if oxygen saturation changed (e.g. the patients' positions were changed and then their saturation levels were measured).

In **nonexperimental research**, there is no manipulation. The concepts are just studied as they occur naturally. For example, in a study about pregnant and nonpregnant adolescents and self-esteem (Connelly 1998), the researcher did not manipulate the concept of pregnancy (i.e. she did not decide who got pregnant and who did not). She simply chose teens who were already pregnant and teens who were not. She then measured the self-esteem of both groups. Nonexperimental studies are sometimes referred to as correlational studies or nonintervention studies. Correlational is really a descriptor used to describe the type of statistic used to analyse the data.

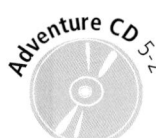

> There are two major research design categories: experimental and nonexperimental.

Student Challenge

Scrutinising Study Classifications

Go to the library and look up the research studies cited as examples in the previous paragraphs. Don't worry about being able to decipher them at this point.

1. Can you tell why they are classified as they are? Choose several other nursing research articles.
2. Can you pick out the studies that are quantitative? (Hint: Look for studies that have numbers and symbols and talk about various types of statistical analysis.)
3. Could you determine any further classification of the quantitative studies you looked at? This can be more difficult. Some will tell you in the title or the abstract. Others give some clues but fail to identify the study classification. For example, an experimental study might talk about an intervention or use of experimental and control groups (e.g. randomised control trial).

What Is the Research Process?

The **research process** is an orderly series of phases and steps that allow the researcher to move from asking a question to finding an answer. The answer, in turn, suggests new questions. Thus research (the act of re-searching) can be envisioned as a circular process with attendant phases and steps, as illustrated in Figure 5-1. These phases and steps guide the research process. Although they occur in the general order indicated by Figure 5-1, the order may vary, steps may overlap, and the researcher may shift back and forth between various steps or phases. In some studies, certain steps are unnecessary and are omitted. However, we can use these phases and steps as a guide to paint a picture of the research process. This will help you understand what the researcher goes through when conducting a study.

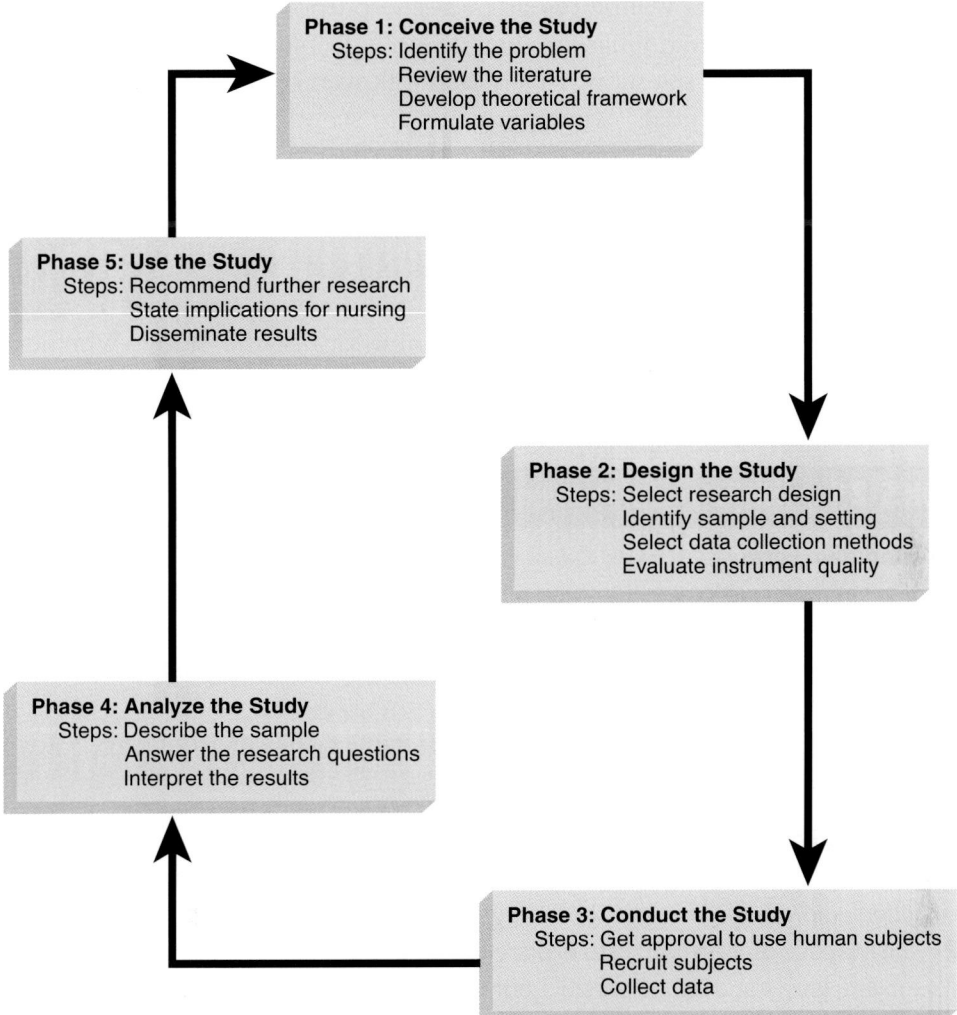

Figure 5-1 The phases and steps of the research process

Phase 1: Conceive the study

The first task at hand for any researcher is to make a decision about what to study. The activities in this phase involve reading, theorising and thinking about the area of interest. Thus the steps of problem identification, literature review and theoretical framework development often occur simultaneously and lead to the formulation of research hypotheses or research questions. In the following sections, we examine each step individually.

Identify the problem

The **problem statement** describes the focus or intent of the research study. It identifies what concepts will be researched. The purpose of the study (i.e. intent, goal) is also described and limits are drawn. Some problems are stated directly and simply in the form of a question. This is then followed by a broader description of the study's purpose or goals. Some problems are stated in a declarative form and labelled as a statement of purpose. The declarative form contains the aim (to describe, explore, explain or predict) of the research as well as the concepts to be studied. It may also contain information about the research design (e.g. is it experimental or nonexperimental?). Examples of both forms can be seen in Box 5-2. Many research studies include more than one problem statement or statement of purpose. This may indicate increased complexity of the study. Whether the researcher uses a problem statement or a statement of purpose or both, the intent is the same. These statements guide and focus the research.

> **BOX 5-2** Sample Forms of Problem Statements
>
> **Interrogative Form**
> 1. What characteristics are common among elderly individuals who seek care in an emergency department?
> 2. Does parental presence affect anxiety and behaviour of young children undergoing suture repair of a laceration?
> 3. Can oxygenation be improved in premature infants by use of extratactile stimulation?
>
> **Declarative Form**
> 1. The purpose of this nonexperimental study is to describe the characteristics of elderly individuals who use the emergency department.
> 2. The purpose of the study is to explore the influence of parental presence on anxiety levels and behaviours of young children who get sutures for a laceration.
> 3. The purpose of this experimental study is to determine whether a stimulation protocol will improve the oxygenation of premature infants.
>
> *Examples are taken from student theses.

Review the literature

The **literature review** involves a search for information that is relevant to the identified problem area. It tells us what is currently known about the area under study and places what is known in context. This allows the researcher to see how their particular study fits into a larger picture. It is much like looking at the picture on the box when trying to put a jigsaw puzzle together. The literature review also helps develop the theoretical frame of reference for the study. Finally, it may also serve to better refine and define the problem being studied. It may even provide information about the best way to design the study or the best way to measure the concepts being examined.

This sounds straightforward enough. You are already familiar with the procedures used to conduct a literature review. Electronic databases of catalogues and periodical indexes are used for the search, and the identified concepts and related terms form the core focus of the search. Several information sources, as shown in Box 5-3, are of interest to the nurse researcher. These should look familiar to you. Research studies that have examined some of the same or similar concepts are the most helpful and form the backbone of the literature review.

BOX 5-3 Information Types and Sources

Research studies:
- Nursing research journals (e.g. *Australian Journal of Advanced Nursing, Contemporary Nurse, Journal of Nursing Scholarship, International Journal of Nursing Practice, International Journal of Nursing Studies, Journal of Advanced Nursing, Nursing Science Quarterly, Nursing Research, Research in Nursing and Health*)
- Research findings in other nursing journals (*Online Journal of Knowledge Synthesis, Evidence-Based Nursing, Evidence-Based Mental Health,* various nursing specialty journals)
- Research journals in related fields
- Systematic reviews
- Dissertations and theses
- Research conference proceedings or paper presentations

Theoretical and conceptual discussions:
- Nursing books
- Nursing journals such as *Advances in Nursing Science, Nursing Inquiry*
- Books in related fields

Facts and statistics:
- Government documents
- Professional documents (published by RCNA, ANC, ANF etc)

Opinions and anecdotes on nursing and health-related issues:
- General nursing journals and broadsheets (*ANF Journal, The Lamp, Nursing Standard, Nursing Outlook, Nursing Review* (RCNA), *Connections* (RCNA), *Kai Tiaki,* specialty journals)
- Journals in related fields
- Newspapers, internet websites, television

The literature review should be comprehensive, balanced and relevant. In other words, it should cover all the current theoretical and research content on the defined concepts in the problem statement. Information should be included whether or not it supports the researcher's line of thinking. The review should draw the core of information from other research efforts. It should rely heavily on primary sources of information (articles written by the person who actually conducted the research being reviewed). Secondary sources (descriptions of research studies by authors other than the researcher) should be used only to provide information about additional primary sources.

Define a theoretical framework

A **theoretical framework** uses a theory or theories to form a theoretical foundation or frame of reference for the research study. A **theory** consists of several concepts that are well integrated and interrelated and are used to explain some phenomenon. The concepts and many of the relationships have been previously tested and researched. You have probably studied many theories in the course of your nursing education. Nursing uses several theories from related disciplines (e.g. Selye's (1956) theory of stress, Maslow's (1943) theory of human motivation, Erikson's (1950) theory of development).

Nurses have also developed several theories to explain nursing practice (e.g. Orem's (1971) theory of self-care, King's (1971) theory of system transaction and goal attainment, Rogers' (1970) unitary man theory). Theories help us pull complex concepts together. They demonstrate how these concepts interact and function as a larger whole. This allows us to more effectively order our own knowledge and increase our understanding of the bigger picture.

A theoretical framework helps the researcher explain or predict study outcomes and to link those outcomes to the existing body of knowledge. Not all research studies use a theoretical framework. Sometimes a theory is not yet available because the area of research is new. Descriptive and exploratory studies often lack a theoretical frame of reference.

In these instances, some researchers use a conceptual framework. A **conceptual framework** is a loosely related collection of concepts that have not yet been tested. However, as nursing science grows, the use of theoretical frameworks grows in nursing research. The relationship of theory and research is a circular one (Fig 5-2). Theory supports and suggests research problems. Research findings confirm or refute theory explanations. This allows theories to be revised and provides additional avenues for research.

A researcher who is doing pure or basic research may be devising numerous research studies for the express purpose of testing and refining a particular theory. Researchers who are doing applied research can increase the usability of their research findings by relating them to theory. For example, a researcher might be

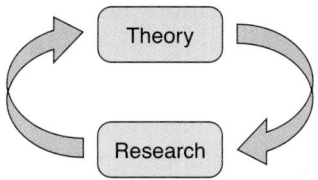

Figure 5-2 *Relation of theory and research*

interested in investigating the characteristics of individuals who consistently take their antihypertensive medications and those who do not. If the researcher conducts the study without a theoretical framework, the findings might identify whether any characteristics distinguish medication takers from nontakers.

However, suppose the researcher decides to use Orem's self-care theory as a theoretical framework. Now the researcher can relate the characteristics of medication takers to the concept of self-care. Those individuals with sufficient self-care agency would be expected to engage in self-care practice (e.g. taking medication). Those with self-care deficits would be expected to need nursing assistance. Thus research findings that identified characteristics of medication takers versus nontakers could be seen as factors that promote self-care agency (takers) or self-care deficit (nontakers). Nurses could then apply those characteristics to other situations in which the patient is expected to carry out prescribed healthcare regimens. This might allow the nurse to anticipate when individuals need nursing assistance to overcome a self-care deficit. This example illustrates how use of a theoretical framework can help researchers and research consumers expand the applicability of research findings.

Formulate variables

Variables are identified concepts or traits that are measured, manipulated or controlled in a research study. A **variable** is a concept or trait that varies. These traits may be associated with organisms or with the environment. For example, gender is an organism variable because some organisms are male and some are female. Weather (rain, sun, snow, hail and so on) is an example of an environmental variable. Almost any concept, characteristic or trait that can be observed and/or measured can be considered a variable. When a characteristic or trait does not vary within a given research study context, it is called a **constant**. For example, if researchers wanted gender to be a constant, they might select only females as subjects for their study. Researchers often use constants to exert control over variables they don't want to study but that might otherwise interfere with the study results.

Variables may take different forms. They may be classified by quality or quantity. Qualitative (categorical) variables change in terms of the presence or absence of a specified trait (e.g. male or not male, married or not married, blue-eyed or not blue-eyed). Quantitative (continuous) variables change in terms of amount or degree (e.g. income, height, weight). These variables can be described in numbers and fractions of numbers. Classifying variables as qualitative or quantitative becomes more important in a later phase of the research study because researchers choose certain analytical tools based on this variable classification.

Another way to classify variables is to determine whether a particular variable is acting as an independent variable, a dependent variable or an extraneous variable in a research study. These distinctions in variables are usually used when the purpose of the study is explanatory or predictive, but they may be seen in exploratory studies in which relationships or differences are being researched.

The **independent variable** is used to explain or predict the change or variation in the **dependent variable**. For example, in a study that is researching whether a 'low-fat diet' will decrease 'cholesterol levels', the 'type of diet' is the independent variable, and the 'level of blood cholesterol' is the dependent variable. The independent variable can be considered the cause, while the dependent variable is the effect.

An **extraneous variable** can also affect the dependent variable and interfere with the relationship of the independent and dependent variables. In the previous example, the extraneous variables 'exercise' and 'menstrual cycle' might also affect 'cholesterol levels'. Can you think of other extraneous variables that might affect 'cholesterol levels'? Researchers try to identify all potential extraneous variables so they can **control** them and keep them from interfering with the variables under study. The literature review helps them identify these extraneous factors. We discussed one form of control the researcher uses by turning an extraneous variable into a constant. Sampling and statistical techniques are also used to help the researcher exert control over extraneous variables.

Once variables are identified, they must be defined. Variables are defined in two ways. The first is a **conceptual definition**. This is the type of definition you are familiar with, the kind you look up in the dictionary. It tells what the word means in the given context of a particular study. The second definition is an **operational definition**. This definition spells out how the variable will be measured. For example, the variable 'anxiety' might be conceptually defined as 'uneasiness or apprehension about an impending event'. The operational definition might state that 'anxiety will be measured using the Clinical Anxiety Rating Scale'. Operational definitions are often decided on in phase 2 of the study.

In a specific research study, variables come from the concepts identified in the problem statement and are specified in the form of research questions or hypotheses. The population to be studied is also specified in the research questions or hypotheses. (We discuss populations in the next phase of the research process.) Box 5-4 provides examples of research questions and hypotheses as derived from the problem statement.

When research questions are used, the purpose of the study is descriptive or exploratory, and a theoretical framework is rarely identified. **Research questions** use an interrogative format to identify the variables to be studied and possible

> **BOX 5-4** Sample Research Questions and Hypotheses
>
> **Problem Statement**
> 1. What common characteristics are possessed by elderly individuals who seek care in an emergency department?
> 2. Does parental presence affect anxiety and behaviour of young children undergoing suture repair of a laceration?
> 3. The purpose of this experimental study is to determine whether a stimulation protocol will improve the oxygenation of premature infants.
>
> **Questions/Hypotheses**
> 1. What percentage of total emergency department visits are by elderly persons? What are the presenting chief complaints of the elderly? Is use affected by time of day, season of year, availability of GP, public or private status, gender or age of the elderly?
> 2. Will there be a difference between the anxiety levels and disruptive behaviours of young children whose parents are present during laceration repair versus those with no parental presence?
> 3. Premature infants who receive extratactile stimulation will have higher P_{O_2} levels than those who do not.
>
> *Examples are taken from student theses.

relationships or differences between those variables. Example 1 in Box 5-4 is from a descriptive study and shows questions used to identify and describe the variables (number of ED visits, chief complaints, time of day, season of year, ED category, payment method, gender and age) and the population (elderly persons using the ED). In the second example from an exploratory study, a question asks about differences on two dependent variables (anxiety levels, disruptive behaviours) for two different groups of individuals (children with and without parental presence). Parental presence or absence is the independent variable and young children with lacerations are the population. Research questions serve as queries about variables and how they might interact with one another. Research questions are used when no concrete information is available to predict an answer.

A **hypothesis** is an 'educated guess' about the relationships between variables and the expected outcomes of the study. It tries to predict the nature of the relationship between variables. The researcher makes these 'educated guesses' based on the review of literature and the theoretical framework. The results of the research study will either support or refute the hypotheses established in the first phase of the study. Research studies that use hypotheses are usually either explanatory or predictive in nature.

All hypotheses contain at least one identifiable independent variable and at least one dependent variable. Some hypotheses are labelled as simple. They contain one independent and one dependent variable. Other hypotheses are labelled as complex hypotheses because they contain more than one independent and/or dependent variable. Example 3 in Box 5-4 is from an explanatory study and shows a hypothesis that predicts one group of infants will be better oxygenated than another group. The independent variable in this hypothesis is the presence or absence of extratactile stimulation, and the dependent variable is Po_2 level. The population is premature infants.

Phase 1 can be thought of as the conceptualisation phase. It lays the foundation for the research study. When done well, the foundation is firm. When this phase is not well thought out, the study rests on a slippery slope, which makes the findings of the study suspect. Now you have read about phase 1, try the next Student Challenge.

> **Student Challenge**
>
> ### Perusing Phase 1
>
> Select several quantitative nursing research studies from your library. Use the nursing research journals or student theses or dissertations if they are available.
>
> Scan these studies and see if you can identify each of the elements we have discussed in phase 1. Remember, the studies may not contain all elements.
>
> 1. Find the problem statement. Can you find examples of the interrogative form and the declarative form? Did the studies label it as a problem statement? If not, look for a statement such as 'the purpose of the study was …' or examine the title or the abstract.
> 2. Was a literature review present? Did it help you better understand the context of the study?
> 3. Was a theoretical framework identified?
> 4. Can you identify the variables being studied? Can you find the research hypotheses or research questions? Can you identify independent and dependent variables? What about extraneous variables? (Hint: Look for phrases such as … was controlled using …). Did the researcher state how the variables were defined?
>
> Were different elements easier to spot in some studies than in others? Were some elements obvious in all the studies? Were any elements missing in all the studies you looked at?

Phase 2: Design the study

In phase 2 of a research study, the researcher makes decisions about how to conduct the study. The researcher designs the study and plans methods for conducting the study. The sample is chosen, a setting is determined, variables are operationally defined, instruments are selected and evaluated, and procedures for data collection are outlined. These decisions have implications for the credibility of the results of the study. If the research design is flawed, then the findings are suspect. Let's examine each step involved in making decisions about the study design. The order of the steps may vary slightly when making decisions, but all the steps are crucial in the design process.

Select research design

The **research design** is the overall plan that guides the way the study is conducted and analysed. As we stated earlier when discussing classifications of research studies, there are two major categories of quantitative research design: experimental and nonexperimental. There is one important distinction between experimental and nonexperimental designs. The researcher is an active agent in an experimental study, deliberately manipulating the independent variable in an attempt to change the dependent variable. This manipulation is often labelled a treatment or an intervention. In a nonexperimental study, the researcher is an observer and recorder, and there is no manipulation or treatment.

Experimental designs

Experimental designs are characterised by three factors: (1) manipulation, (2) use of a control group, and (3) random assignment. All these factors allow the researcher greater overall control of the experiment and are used to ensure that changes in the dependent variable are not caused by extraneous variables. As previously discussed, **manipulation** is the treatment or intervention the researcher carries out on the independent variable to try to get the dependent variable to change.

> Experimental designs use (1) manipulation, (2) control groups, and (3) random assignment to make sure changes in the dependent variable are not caused by extraneous variables.

To make sure the change in the dependent variable is because of the treatment (manipulation) and not some other factor (extraneous variable), the researcher puts some of the subjects into a control group and some subjects into a treatment group. The control group does not get the experimental treatment (manipulation). The treatment group does get the experimental treatment (manipulation). If the dependent variable changes for the treatment group and does not change for the control group, then the treatment is probably causing the change. Look at Example 3 in Box 5-4. This is an experimental study. The researcher had two groups of premature infants. The treatment group got the extratactile stimulation treatment (manipulation). The control group got the usual care given by the nurses in the neonatal intensive care unit (NICU). Po_2 levels (dependent variable) were measured for both groups. The researcher was looking for an increase in Po_2 for the treatment group and no increase in Po_2 for the control group.

Random assignment is the third characteristic of experimental designs. To guard against bias, the researcher randomly assigns subjects to a treatment or control group and randomly decides which group will get the treatment and which group will not. Random assignment means every subject has an equal chance of being in either group and each group has an equal chance of being designated as the treatment group. In Example 3 in Box 5-4, the infants were randomly assigned to Group 1 and Group 2 using a table of random numbers (Box 5-5). The treatment group was then selected by placing two pieces of paper with the words 'Group 1' and 'Group 2' in a hat. One piece of paper was drawn, and that group was designated as the treatment group.

BOX 5-5 Sample of a Section of a Table of Random Numbers

77	51	30	38	20	19	50	23	71	74
21	81	85	93	13	51	47	46	64	99
99	55	96	83	31	86	83	42	99	01
69	97	92	02	88	93	27	88	17	57
68	10	72	36	21	62	53	52	41	70

All experimental designs use manipulation. Some, however, fail either to use a control group or to use random assignment because it is not always possible to have a control group or to decide who should go into one group or the other. When one of these two factors is missing, it is called a quasi-experimental design. A quasi-experimental design must then use other ways to ensure that the study results are valid. One way to do this is to take extra measurements of the dependent variable, or to measure the dependent variable before and after the treatment.

Nonexperimental designs

Nonexperimental designs do not use treatments or attempt to manipulate the independent variable. These designs use what is already occurring in a particular setting with a particular group of subjects to describe or explore relationships between certain variables. Descriptive nonexperimental designs do not even have an identified independent variable to manipulate. Example 1 in Box 5-4 is a descriptive, nonexperimental design. The researcher is simply collecting data on several variables and describing the results. Example 2 in Box 5-4 is an exploratory, nonexperimental design with an independent variable—parental presence or absence. The researcher is looking to see if parental presence affects anxiety and behaviour (dependent variables). However, the researcher did not decide when the parents would be present or absent. She simply noted whether the parents were present or absent during the suturing procedure, and measured anxiety and behaviour in the child.

When a study contains independent and dependent variables and the researcher chooses not to manipulate the independent variable, it is usually for one of three major reasons: (1) all events have already occurred, (2) the variable cannot be manipulated, or (3) it would be morally or ethically wrong to manipulate the variable. In a retrospective nonexperimental study the researcher simply collects data on the variables after they have already occurred. Take the example of the infant stimulation study. Suppose that the researcher located two different hospitals—one offered extratactile stimulation as a part of routine care for all premature infants and the other offered no extratactile stimulation. Further suppose that the researcher collected charts of premature infants in both hospitals, looked up recorded P_{O_2} levels, and compared the P_{O_2} levels of a group of stimulated infants with a group of nonstimulated infants. This is a nonexperimental research design in which the researcher is looking at variables that have already occurred.

> When a researcher chooses not to manipulate the independent variable, it is usually for one of three major reasons: (1) all events have already occurred, (2) the variable cannot be manipulated, or (3) it would be morally or ethically wrong to manipulate the variable.

Many variables cannot be manipulated. If researchers are interested in whether gender affects longevity, for example, they cannot manipulate the gender variable. They cannot make males become females to see if that change will make them live longer. If researchers are interested in whether ageing affects calcium levels in the blood, they cannot manipulate the age variable (i.e. they cannot make someone get older). In these instances, the researcher must examine the variables as they naturally occur.

Other variables can be manipulated, but to do so would present an ethical dilemma. When researchers were studying the effects of smoking on health, they did not manipulate the variable of smoking. They did not decide who would smoke and who would not smoke because it would not be ethical to force someone to smoke. So, smoking is a variable that can be manipulated, but for ethical reasons it is not. We discuss how subjects are protected against possible unethical treatments in phase 3.

When a variable cannot be manipulated or when manipulation would cause an ethical dilemma, nonexperimental research designs must be used. This does not mean that nonexperimental designs cannot be used to explain or predict. We can use sophisticated statistical techniques to examine relationships among variables and to predict how they should function under various circumstances.

Identify sample and setting

Once the research design has been established, the subjects and setting for the study must be considered. The **setting** is the physical location for and the conditions under which the study takes place. For example, the study involving children and suture repair took place in the suture room of a Level 2 ED in one children's hospital. The study involving premature infants and stimulation took place in a NICU of a large teaching hospital. Premature infants from around the city are transferred to this unit, which has computerised equipment capable of continuously monitoring Po_2 levels on all infants.

The subjects of interest for a research study are known as a **population**. These subjects possess certain common characteristics or traits that identify them as a part of the population. For example, 'young children with lacerations that require sutures' are the subjects of interest in Example 2 in Box 5-4. Study subjects need not be human; they might be animals such as white mice, bacterial colonies in petri dishes, data such as vital signs, or objects such as charts. A **sample** is a portion or subset of a population (Fig 5-3). Populations are usually large, so the researcher chooses a part of the population to make the study more feasible. Subjects are selected using a process known as **sampling**.

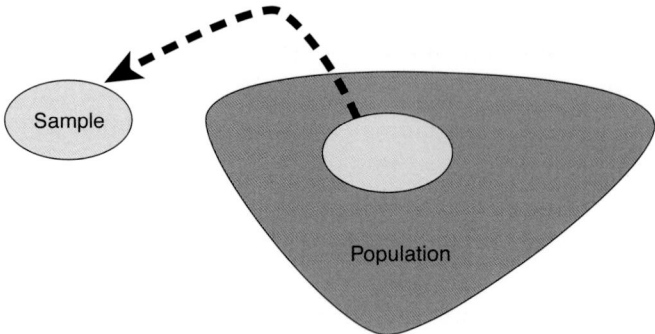

Figure 5-3 *Sampling*

When the researcher selects the sample, he or she tries to make sure the sample characteristics resemble the population characteristics as closely as possible so the sample represents the population. If a sample is representative of the population, the study results can be applied to the whole population. For example, if the children in the laceration study were less anxious during the suturing process when a parent was present, it is helpful if that finding can be applied to all children with lacerations. The ability to apply study results from the sample to the population is known as **generalisation**. The type of sampling process chosen determines whether study results can be generalised from the sample to the population.

There are two major categories of samples: (1) probability and (2) nonprobability. Box 5-6 presents and defines sample categories and subcategories. Review these so you can recognise the vocabulary used to describe sampling in a research article and can distinguish between probability and nonprobability types of samples.

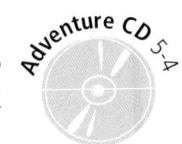

BOX 5-6 Categories of Samples

Probability Sampling—Random Selection
1. A **simple random sample** is the most basic form of probability sampling in which all subjects in a population are numbered, and a sample is selected randomly using a lottery or table of random numbers.
2. A **stratified random sample** is subdivided into groups according to some characteristic (e.g. gender—males and females; or ethnicity—those from an English-speaking background, those from a non-English-speaking background, Torres Strait Islander or Aborigine). The subsets are then randomly sampled.
3. A **cluster sample** is a multistage sampling in which larger clusters (groups) are randomly selected first (e.g. hospitals) and then smaller clusters are randomly chosen (e.g. patients).
4. A **systematic sample** selects every *kth* (e.g. every fifth or seventh or twentieth) subject from a randomised list.

Nonprobability Sampling—No Random Selection
1. A **convenience (accidental) sample** selects the most convenient subjects at hand.
2. A **quota sample** is conveniently selected according to prespecified characteristic(s) (e.g. gender or ethnicity).
3. A **purposive sample** uses subjects that are handpicked by the researcher, based on a set of defined criteria.
4. A **nonrandom systematic sample** selects every *kth* (e.g. every fifth or seventh or twentieth) subject from a nonrandomised list or every *kth* subject as they become available (e.g. every third patient admitted to the unit).

In a **probability sample**, the subjects are chosen at random. Each subject in the population has an equal chance of being in the sample. Probability samples ensure mathematical representation of the population. Therefore when researchers choose probability sampling techniques, they ensure that the results of the study can be generalised to the population. Subjects in a **nonprobability sample** are not chosen at random. There is no way to assess whether they are representative of the population. Therefore the results can only be applied to the sample and cannot be generalised to the population. The sampling method used is a very important thing for you to note when you read research studies, because it tells you whether you can apply the study results to your situation. If a nonprobability sample was used, the results may or may not be applicable to your clinical situation.

> The sampling technique tells you whether you can apply the results in your clinical situation with confidence.

At this point you may be asking, 'If probability samples are so much better than nonprobability samples, why would a researcher ever use a nonprobability sample?' Good question! Nonprobability sampling may be preferable for several reasons—it is less expensive and requires less time and fewer resources and, sometimes, generating a probability sample is not possible. For example, it may not be possible to generate a list of every subject in the population because no comprehensive source exists. At other times, generating such a list can be prohibitive in terms of time and expense. Think about compiling and numbering a list of 1000 or 10,000 or 100,000 subjects in a population. Access to certain subjects in a population may also be cost prohibitive (e.g. subjects in another city, state or country). Access to certain subjects may be denied by the institutions or by the subjects themselves. Some populations are hidden and/or hard to access (e.g. stigmatised populations such as sex workers). You will find that many nursing research studies use nonprobability sampling techniques. As computers generate ever-growing databases, as research funding and support increases for nursing research, and as the research studies and researchers grow in sophistication and complexity, this situation is beginning to change.

The size of the sample is also important in making the sample representative of the population. As a general rule of thumb, the larger the sample, the more representative it is of the population. The researcher considers several factors when selecting a sample size. These include the size of the population, the availability of the population, the characteristics of the population, and the cost and time expended per subject, and the power analysis required to ensure that findings are significant. The size of the sample also affects the statistical techniques that can be used. Statistics used to analyse several variables simultaneously (multivariate statistics) require larger sample sizes. When you read a research study, check the sample size. If a sample is small (under 30 subjects), particularly if it is a nonprobability sample, use the study results with caution.

> Use study results with caution when the sample is small and sampling is nonprobable.

Select data collection methods

To examine the proposed research questions or hypotheses, the researcher must be able to collect measurable information on the variables. These measurable bits of information are known as **data**. Data are collected using an **instrument**. Instruments that collect quantitative data can be classified by the type of data they are designed to collect. Data are generally physiological, behavioural or psychological in nature. Physical measurements generally require specialised biophysical instruments and specialised expertise on the part of the user. You are familiar with several of the biophysical measurements used in healthcare and healthcare research. Examples include sphygmomanometers, thermometers, manometers, pulse oximeters, glucometers, ECG machines, EEG machines, transducers and so on. We regularly use these instruments in clinical practice. Researchers also use them to measure physiological variables.

Behavioural data (observable actions of the subject) are generally collected through observation. In quantitative research these observations are evaluated and assigned numeric values. For example, degree of uncooperative behaviour was observed and rated in the study of young children who were being sutured for a laceration. The nurse observed the child's behaviour and assigned ratings at several predetermined intervals during the suturing procedure. The scale is presented in Table 5-1.

TABLE 5-1	Uncooperative Behaviour Scale
Score	**Behaviour**
0	No crying or physical protest
1	Mild verbal protest (e.g. ouch) or quiet crying
2	More prominent verbal protest/crying with movement of body parts; still complies with physician request
3	Protest and movement makes the procedure difficult
4	Protest stops the procedure and behaviour is addressed before procedure can be reinitiated
5	General prolonged protest verbal and body movement with no compliance

Adapted from Venham L et al (1980). Interval rating scales for children's dental anxiety and uncooperative behaviour. *Pediatric Dentistry* 2(3):195.

Psychological measurements are used to collect data about knowledge, feelings and attitudes. Because these variables cannot be directly observed, an instrument is used that asks the subject to self-report on these variables. Such instruments include questionnaires and interviews. Questionnaires pose a series of questions for the subject to answer. In a quantitative study, the questions are usually closed-ended. This means that the subject is asked to select from a range of choices. Box 5-7 contains several closed-ended questions that might appear on a questionnaire. Questionnaires are easy to administer; relatively inexpensive; can be mailed to a large, widely dispersed sample; and offer anonymity to the respondent.

> **BOX 5-7** Sample Questions on a Questionnaire
>
> Please circle the answer that best describes you.
> 1. Are you
>   a. Male
>   b. Female
> 2. Are you currently
>   a. Single (never married)
>   b. Married
>   c. Separated
>   d. Divorced
>   e. Widowed
> 3. What is your birth order?
>   a. Only child
>   b. Oldest child
>   c. Middle child
>   d. Youngest child

Questionnaires used in research generally contain some type of scale designed to measure a certain psychological variable. Scales are instruments that assign numerical values to a set of responses on a series of questions or statements. These numbers are then added together for a score. This score is used as a measurement of the variable. The most common scale type is the Likert scale. Subjects are given a series of statements and several ranges of agreement or disagreement to choose from. Box 5-8 gives an example of a few items from a Likert scale measuring the variable commitment to nursing. The response to each item is assigned a number and the numbers from all the items are added to reflect the overall degree of agreement with the concept being measured.

> **BOX 5-8** Sample Likert Scale
>
> **SA** Strongly Agree
> **A** Agree
> **U** Uncertain
> **D** Disagree
> **SD** Strongly Disagree
>
> Please circle your degree of agreement or disagreement with the following statements:
>
> 1. My most common reaction to nursing is enthusiasm.   SA   A   U   D   SD
> 2. I am disenchanted with nursing.   SA   A   U   D   SD
> 3. I consider nursing a rewarding profession.   SA   A   U   D   SD
> 4. I cannot imagine being in any other profession.   SA   A   U   D   SD
> 5. Nursing plays a major role in my life.   SA   A   U   D   SD
>
> Adapted from Langford R (1979). The relationship between student sense of commitment to the profession of nursing and their perceptions of powerlessness in the academic setting. Doctoral dissertation. University of Houston, Texas.

Interviews used to collect data in a quantitative study usually consist of a series of highly structured questions later assigned numbers for statistical analysis. A structured interview is much like an oral questionnaire. However, it offers the advantage of allowing the interviewer to clarify responses and to ensure that all questions are answered. The chief disadvantage is the added time and expense involved in the interview process.

Appropriate instruments must be selected to measure each variable being studied. This includes desired descriptive variables (e.g. gender, education level, marital status), independent and dependent variables, and pertinent extraneous variables (e.g. variables that must be controlled using statistics). Choices are made based on criteria such as the category of data (e.g. physiological, behavioural, psychological) and the cost, availability and skill required to administer the instrument. It is important that the instrument chosen is appropriate for the data category and the best the researcher has access to.

Evaluate instrument quality

Instrument quality plays a big role in the selection of an appropriate instrument. The researcher is looking for 'good' instruments to measure the variables in the study. What is a 'good' instrument? A good instrument is one that is valid and reliable. A **valid** instrument measures what it is supposed to measure. A **reliable** instrument measures the variable consistently, dependably and accurately. If an instrument is not reliable it cannot be considered valid.

Box 5-9 lists types of validity and reliability. Familiarise yourself with these terms.

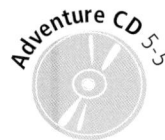

BOX 5-9 Types of Validity and Reliability

Validity

Validity is the extent to which an instrument measures what it says it measures.

Content validity is assessed by a logical evaluation and judgment of whether the instrument adequately reflects the content of the concept. A blueprint may be used to construct the instrument, or a panel of judges may be asked to evaluate the instrument. This is a weak form of validity.

Criterion validity is assessed using statistical measures. Instrument scores are correlated to scores on measures of selected external criteria. Also called *concurrent* or *predictive validity*, this is a stronger form of validity.

Construct validity is assessed using a combination of logic and statistical measures. It looks for the underlying meaning of the construct being measured. This is the strongest form of validity.

Reliability

Reliability is the degree of consistency or dependability of an instrument.

Internal consistency uses correlation statistics (e.g. Spearman's, Cronbach's alpha or Kuder-Richardson) to measure whether the subparts of an instrument all measure the same thing. Reliability values range from 0 to 1. The closer the value gets to 1, the more reliable the instrument.

Equivalence correlates two different forms of the same instrument (also called parallel forms) or the scores of two or more raters (also called interrater reliability). Reliability is reported as an 'r' value, with values ranging from 0 to 1. The closer the value gets to 1, the more reliable the instrument.

Stability correlates the scores obtained when an instrument is administered twice to the same group of subjects over a period of time. Reliability or 'r' values range from 0 to 1. The closer the value gets to 1, the more reliable the instrument.

Instruments used in research studies should be evaluated for reliability and validity before use in the study. Reliability and validity issues should be addressed in the written report of the study. Biophysical measurements are generally accepted as valid measures of the variable. However, reliability is an issue. Reliability can be addressed by ensuring that these instruments are calibrated and that the operators have sufficient expertise. Questionnaires, scales, interviews and observations all need to be assessed for some form of reliability and validity to ensure the quality and credibility of the data collected. If the data are suspect, then the study results are suspect.

Now we have covered what is involved in phase 2 of a research study, take some time to complete the following Student Challenge.

> **Student Challenge**
>
> Scrutinising Phase 2
>
> Look again at the quantitative nursing research studies you examined for phase 1. Scan these studies and see if you can identify each of the elements we have discussed in phase 2.
>
> 1. Can you identify the research design as experimental or nonexperimental? Remember that experimental studies use terms such as experimental, quasi-experimental, treatment group, control group, treatment, intervention or random assignment. Nonexperimental studies use terms or phrases such as retrospective, ex post facto, correlational, 'purpose is to describe …' or 'purpose is to explore …'.
> 2. Can you identify the sample? Can you determine what the population was? (This is harder, because it is often inferred rather than directly stated.)
> 3. Can you determine whether a probability or nonprobability sampling technique was used? Look for cue words such as 'random' for probability samples and words such as 'convenience' or 'accidental' for nonprobability samples. If the technique is not specified, chances are great that it is a nonprobability sample. What was the size of the sample in the studies you chose?
> 4. Was the setting described?
> 5. What instruments were used to measure the variables? Could you tell if the instruments were reliable and valid?

Phase 3: Conduct the study

Once the study has been conceived and designed, the planning phases are over and the researcher is ready to conduct the study. This means the researcher will now implement the study design and collect the data using the designated instruments and procedures. This is often an exciting time in the research process. The researcher begins to sense that the project is going to make it.

Get approval to use human subjects

When researchers use humans as subjects for study, they must protect them from harm. There have been a number of historical abuses of research subjects. The most famous might be the atrocities committed on prisoners of war by Nazi and Japanese physicians during World War II. More recently, several famous experiments symbolise mistreatment of research subjects. In New Zealand, 'experiments' at the

Auckland National Women's hospital in the 1950s involving women's unwitting participation in cervical cancer research led to a large cohort of women suffering and in some cases dying as a result of being in the 'limited or no treatment group' (Johnstone 1999, p 23).

Unfortunately, abuses of this type were not isolated incidents. In the 1980s in New Zealand, fetal cervixes were collected from stillborn female babies for histological studies; pancreases removed from aborted fetuses and large numbers of newborn baby girls subjected to vaginal swabs (in vain, as it turned out), all without parental consent (Johnstone 1999). In Australia, quite recently there have been reports in the media on the medical practice of removing human parts from cadavers (dead bodies) without consent. Accounts of unethical research have surfaced internationally. In the US, for example, mentally handicapped children were injected with a hepatitis virus at Willowbrook Institution in Staten Island, New York in the 1950s and 1960s. Live cancer cells were injected into elderly patients at Jewish Chronic Disease Hospital in Brooklyn, New York in 1963. US Government involvement in experiments using prisoners, soldiers and civilians to test the effects of radiation, chemical, viral and neurological agents as potential weapons have also been revealed.

Because of persistent reports of abuse in research, in the US the National Commission for the Protection of Human Subjects of Biomedical and Behavioral Research was formed in the 1970s. This group issued the Belmont Report (1979), which articulated three ethical standards that must be observed in the conduct of research. These principles form the basis for most statements on ethical conduct. In 1964 the Declaration of Helsinki published by the World Medical Association laid the foundation for many international documents related to ethics since that time (NH&MRC 1999). In Australia, research is guided by the National Health and Medical Research Council (NH&MRC) National Statement on Ethical Conduct in Research Involving Humans (1999). Research involving Aboriginal and Torres Strait Islander peoples is considered to require particular attention to ethical issues and is governed by separate guidelines (refer NH&MRC Guidelines on Ethical Matters in Aboriginal and Torres Strait Islander Health Research 1991).

In New Zealand there is considerable emphasis on ensuring that all research meets ethical standards, and particular effort is made to ensure that the interests of vulnerable groups are not compromised. As part of the Treaty of Waitangi, Maori cultural and ethical values are protected. The Health Research Council of New Zealand provides guidelines on ethics in health research at http://www.hrc.govt.nz/download/pdf/ethgdlns.pdf.

The three ethical standards articulated by the Belmont Report (1979) are:

1 *Beneficence*: Individuals who might become subjects in a research study have the right to freedom from harm. The researcher is obligated to protect subjects from potential injury, disability or death because of involvement in a study (NH&MRC Statement 1999).

2 *Justice:* Researchers need to consider the potential for injustice where because of convenience or other such factors some groups are frequently selected as research subjects and are therefore more likely to benefit from the use of public funding for research (NH&MRC Statement 1999).
3 *Respect for persons:* Individuals have the right to know and choose. Researchers must fully disclose the potential risks and benefits associated with the study and allow the individual free choice in deciding whether to participate. Individuals have the right to privacy and fair treatment. Researchers must guarantee that all identifying factors collected during the study will remain confidential. Researchers must also strive to ensure that all study participants are treated fairly, courteously and sensitively (NH&MRC Statement 1999).

The NH&MRC requires that all institutions involved in the conduct of research on humans or animals convene a relevant institutional ethics committee (IEC). The NH&MRC sets certain guidelines for membership of IECs and may audit all documentation that comes through an IEC. Institutional **ethics committees** are review groups that have been established by various research funding bodies and institutions involved in research to ensure that individual researchers adhere to these ethical standards. The first step in this phase is to obtain approval from an IEC for the use of human subjects. The researcher submits a written proposal of the research study to the committee, whose members review the proposal and grant or deny authorisation for the conduct of the study. When authorisation is granted, the researcher can then start the process of recruiting subjects for data collection. However, the researcher remains answerable to the IEC, who retain the authority to stop a project at any time if they have concerns about the conduct of a study.

Recruit subjects

If the sample units are inanimate objects, such as bacterial cultures or similar, then this step is omitted or is greatly simplified. However, since most clinical nursing studies involve human subjects, the researcher must find individuals who are willing to participate in the study. As subjects are recruited, it is the researcher's job to inform each of them about the study, the demands it will make, and the potential risks and benefits of participation. This allows individuals adequate information to make an informed choice about whether to participate in the research study. Those who opt to become subjects sign a statement that indicates they have been briefed on the study, they understand the risks and benefits, and they are willing to participate. This process is known as **informed consent**. It is very similar to the process that patients go through when agreeing to medical or surgical treatment. Box 5-10 describes the elements contained in a typical consent form. Some studies do not require written informed consent. Frequently, when written questionnaires are used, return of the questionnaire is used to imply consent. Institutional ethics committees may allow researchers to conduct observational studies without the consent of the subjects as long as the researcher shows strong evidence that identifying information about participants will be kept confidential.

> **BOX 5-10 Elements of Informed Consent**
>
> General statement of study purpose
> Description of study procedures
> List of potential risks and benefits
> Assurance of anonymity or confidentiality
> Statement that participation is voluntary
> Assurance that subject may withdraw without penalty
> Contact information of researcher with offer to answer any questions about the study

Collect data

Once permission has been obtained from the appropriate ethics committee and subjects have been recruited, **data collection** may proceed. At this point, the researcher puts the design into action and carries out the prescribed procedures for the study in the appropriate research setting. Treatments are conducted, instruments are administered, and data are generated and recorded. After the data are collected, the researcher organises it into an appropriate form for analysis, and phase 3 is brought to a close.

> **Student Challenge**
>
> Conduct the Study
>
> Look again at the quantitative research studies you examined for phases 1 and 2. Look for evidence of the steps in phase 3. (Direct evidence of this phase is hard to see in published research articles. It is easier to see in theses and dissertations.)
>
> 1 Were the rights of human subjects protected in these studies? What evidence did you find to support this?
> 2 Is there evidence of ethics committee approval?
> 3 Was informed consent obtained?
> 4 Was any information provided about what occurred during collection of the data?

Phase 4: Analyse the study

Data cannot be reported to research consumers in raw form. The results would be too cumbersome and would not provide a very good picture of the sample or a clear answer to the research questions or hypotheses proposed. Thus we come to the phase that strikes fear and trepidation into the hearts of many research students—statistical analysis and interpretation of the data. Before we discuss the steps involved in this phase, a little background information is needed. To statistically analyse variables, they must be measurable. This means the variables must be represented in number form.

Measurement is a set of rules used to assign numbers to variables. The level of measurement guides the kinds of statistical analyses that can be performed on a variable. There are four levels of measurement: nominal, ordinal, interval and ratio. Box 5-11 presents these four levels. For statistical purposes, interval and ratio data are treated the same.

BOX 5-11 Levels of Measurement

Nominal variables are broken into two or more categories and assigned arbitrary numbers. These numbers have no rank order (i.e. no sense of one category being ranked at a higher level than another).

Example:
Gender: male = 1, female = 2
Marital status: single = 1, married = 2, separated = 3, divorced = 4, widowed = 5

Ordinal measurement reflects a rank order among the categories, but we do not know how much greater than or less than.

Example:
Pain: ranked on a scale of 1 to 10 with 10 being the worst pain and 1 being no pain
Anxiety: ranked on a 5-point scale from low to high

Interval categories are made up of 'real' numbers that allow us to order the numbers and to know the distance between those numbers. The intervals between the categories are equal.

Example:
Temperature: the interval between the numerical values of 76 and 77 degrees is the same as the interval between the values of 44 and 45 degrees. A degree is a precise interval.
Time: hours, minutes and seconds are precise intervals.

Ratios have the same properties as interval data, except that the measurement scale for the variable possesses a meaningful zero. This means that when zero is reached on the scale, the variable is absent.

Example:
Weight, height: zero means no weight or no height.

Describe the sample

When analysing the data, the researcher wants to derive a picture or description of the sample. This description is obtained through statistical analysis and the use of descriptive statistical tests. **Descriptive statistics** group the data in ways to make it easier to understand. There are four common ways to describe data using statistics: (1) frequencies, (2) measures of central tendency, (3) measures of spread (dispersion), and (4) measures of shape.

One thing we can do is count the times that scores or categories of a variable occur. Frequency counts can then be turned into percentages (number in a category divided by the number for the variable). Table 5-2 presents sample frequencies and percentages taken from a sample of 90 nursing students.

TABLE 5-2 Frequencies and Percentages

Variable	Frequency	Percentage
Gender		
Female	82	91%
Male	8	9%
Current marital status		
Single	46	51%
Married	34	38%
Separated	2	2%
Divorced	8	9%
Satisfaction with school		
Very dissatisfied	2	2%
Dissatisfied	9	10%
Uncertain	18	20%
Satisfied	45	50%
Very satisfied	16	18%
Age		
19–21	16	18%
22–24	27	30%
25–27	36	40%
28–30	11	12%

$n = 90$

In the examples in Table 5-2, we can see that the majority of students in this sample were single females 22 to 30 years of age who were satisfied with school. Frequencies are most useful with nominal and ordinal data. Interval or ratio data make reporting frequencies for each score a little cumbersome. So, we can group several scores together and report the frequency and percentage of the groups as we did with the variable 'age' in Table 5-2. Frequencies for interval and ratio data can also be plotted on a graph to form a frequency distribution (Fig 5-4).

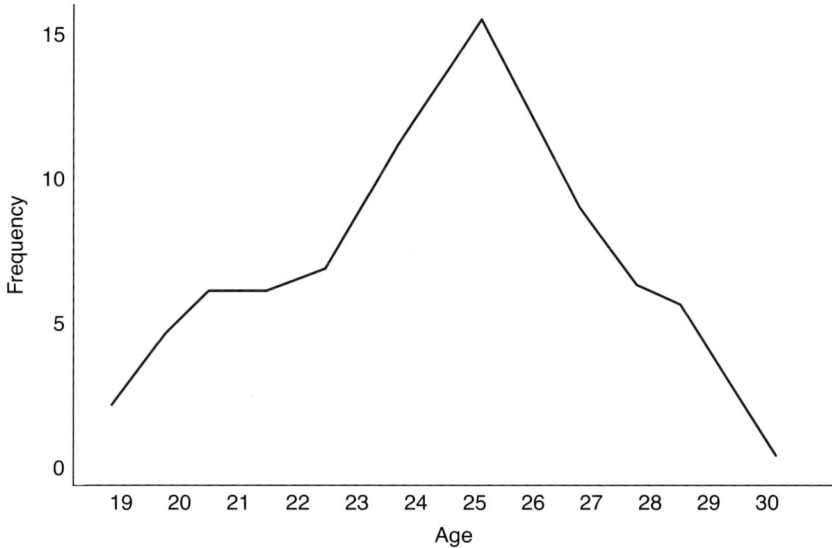

Figure 5-4 *Example of a frequency distribution*

We can also use statistics to describe how data are distributed along the number continuum of a frequency distribution. We can describe how data clump or cluster together, how they spread apart, and what shape the frequency distribution forms. These statistics are defined in Box 5-12. All these statistics let us reduce large amounts of data about a variable down to a very manageable description whose meaning is commonly understood. Imagine if you tried to make sense out of the reported ages for 5000 subjects if you had no precise way to count them, group them, or talk about how much the subjects were alike or different in age.

BOX 5-12 Descriptive Statistical Measures

Measures of central tendency are statistical tests that describe how data for a variable tend to cluster together in a distribution.
1. Mode (Mo) is the numerical value that occurs most often for a particular variable.
2. Median (Md) is the middle value in a frequency distribution of numbers.
3. Mean (M, X) is the average of all the scores.

Measures of dispersion are statistical tests that describe how data for a variable tend to spread out in a distribution.
1. Range is the distance between the highest and lowest scores for a variable.

> **2** Variance (V, s²) is the average area of spread under a frequency distribution curve.
> **3** Standard deviation (SD, s) is the average distance of spread in a frequency distribution. It tells us how much, on the average, the scores are spread out from the mean.
>
> **Measures of shape** are statistical tests that describe the shape of the distribution for a variable.
> **1** Skewness reflects the degree of symmetry or asymmetry of the distribution curve (e.g. Is the distribution symmetrical or asymmetrical?).
> **2** Kurtosis is the height of the distribution (e.g. How tall or flat is the distribution curve?).

Answer the research questions

Once the researcher has described the sample, the next step is to analyse the data to answer the research questions or to see whether the hypothesis was true. This is the step when the researcher discovers the answer the study was designed to uncover. If the study was a descriptive one, the researcher uses the same kinds of statistics used to describe the sample. Now, however, the variables of interest are those from the research questions. Remember the research questions from Example 1 in Box 5-4 about elderly individuals in the ED? These questions were answered using descriptive statistics. The question 'What percentage of total ED visits are by elderly individuals?' was answered using frequencies and percentages. The question 'What are the presenting chief complaints of the elderly?' was answered by categorising all the reported chief complaints and then reporting frequencies and percentages of each category.

If the study asked questions or stated hypotheses that looked at the relationships or differences between variables, then statistics that analyse those relationships or differences are used. A wide variety of statistics are available for such analysis. The easy access to personal computers with sophisticated statistical software has increased the complexity of statistical tests used. Many studies now identify and examine greater numbers of variables because analysis of multiple variables is now readily available. This means that reports of statistical analysis and study are increasingly complicated, making reading and understanding the results section of most studies difficult. For most studies you will read, there is little chance that you will recognise or understand why particular statistics were selected. Moreover, you will probably have little understanding of the precise meaning of the numbers generated by those statistics.

> **HINT** Most hospitals and universities have statisticians who can help you to understand statistical issues.

This does not mean that you should give up without a fight. You *can* decipher study results, with patience and armed with a few strategic pieces of information.

1 **Different statistics have different requirements for use**. Selection of the appropriate statistic is based on several factors, including the number of variables to be analysed, the level of measurement of the variables, the nature of the question asked (e.g. testing relationships or differences), and the sampling procedure used.
2 **Research hypotheses may be translated into statistical hypotheses**. This is merely a restatement of the research hypothesis in symbol form and is used as a decision-making tool.
3 **The result of a statistical test is reported as a number**. (e.g. $t = 4.26$, $F = 3.98$, $r = .68$). The letter gives a clue about the statistical test used (e.g. t is a t test, F is an ANOVA test, r indicates a correlation). Many multivariate statistics generate a series of numbers that tell the researcher about several variables and how they vary as part of a multiple variable set.
4 **These numbers are either significant or not significant**. Significance is reported using a p value (e.g. $p = .17$, $p = .03$, $p = .01$). A p value of less than .05 is generally considered significant. Some researchers use a p value of less than .01 to decide if a value is significant. Sometimes, nonsignificance is reported by using the letters NS.
5 **A significant p value (.05) means the relationship or difference found between the variables was probably not caused by chance**. In other words, there really is a high degree of certainty that the difference or a correlation exists between the variables tested.
6 **Statistical results are often displayed in table form**.

When you read the results section, do not panic over the numbers and the discussion of those numbers. The researcher will translate the statistical results into text at some point in the presentation of results. This is what you are looking for as you read. Search to see how the research questions or hypotheses were answered. Were the variables related or not? Was group A different from group B?

In Example 2 in Box 5-4, the research question is: 'Will there be a difference between the anxiety levels and disruptive behaviours of young children whose parents are present during laceration repair versus those with no parental presence?' A Hotelling T square test was used and no significant difference was found in behaviour or anxiety between the group of children with parents present and the group without parents present.

Remember we said that the effects of extraneous variables were sometimes controlled using statistics? Well, in this study, age was identified as an extraneous variable that might influence whether parental presence made a difference. So another statistical test (ANCOVA) was used to look at differences while controlling for the extraneous variable age. This analysis found that both behaviour and anxiety in younger children were significantly different between those with parents present and those without. Younger children were less anxious and more cooperative with a parent present. As children became older, parental presence did not affect anxiety or behaviour.

In Example 3 in Box 5-4, the research hypothesis is 'Premature infants who receive extratactile stimulation will have higher Po_2 levels than those who do not.' A *t* test was used to examine the differences in Po_2 between the group of infants who got stimulation and the group who did not. The resulting *t* value was significant. This indicated that there was a difference between the Po_2 levels of the two groups. A look at mean Po_2 levels showed that infants who received tactile stimulation had higher Po_2 levels.

Interpret the results

Once the statistical analysis has been performed and the results have been examined, the researcher must interpret the results. This means making sense of the findings and how they fit into the existing research literature. Findings from descriptive studies are used to secure a tentative picture. There is very little to interpret because no relations were tested among the described variables. Findings from exploratory studies that ask questions about relationships or differences among variables provide a starting point for the researcher to explain why relationships or differences were or were not present.

Findings from studies in which relationships or differences were predicted in the form of hypotheses need the most interpretation. An explanation of the findings is straightforward if the hypothesis was supported. The researcher used theoretical evidence to make a guess about variable relations, and the guess was supported. All came out as anticipated. The study lends more proof to the underlying theoretical foundations. However, if the hypotheses were not supported, the researcher must try to explain what happened. Was there a problem with the theoretical structure for the study, or was there a problem with the research design? Answers to these questions are usually presented in a discussion section and lead to the final phase of the process.

Student Challenge

Seeking Statistics

Examine your chosen research studies for the analyses used and the results of the analyses.

1. Can you locate a description of the sample? (Hint: Some studies include the description when discussing the sample and sampling techniques in the methods or research design section of the study.)

> **2** Can you find the answers to the research questions or hypotheses that were posed?
>
> **3** Can you locate how the findings were tied to the literature?

Phase 5: Use the study

You might think that once a researcher discovers the answers to the questions posed in a study the work would be finished. However, one important phase remains. This phase completes the research process, emphasises its circular nature, and ensures results are shared with the research consumer.

Recommend further research

Once the findings are stated and discussed, the researcher must decide what those findings mean for future research. When the researcher examines what the next research study might be, **recommendations** for further research are made, to ensure the circular nature of the process. That researcher or another researcher can accelerate the advancement of nursing knowledge by beginning another research study building on the one just completed.

The researcher also examines and discusses any problems encountered while doing the study. These are known as limitations. Examples include uncontrolled extraneous variables that interfered with study results, difficulties in data collection, not enough subjects, and so forth. Identifying limitations allows future researchers to correct them when repeating or doing a similar study.

State implications for practice

The researcher must also decide what, if any, **implications** the study results have for nursing practice. This assists the research consumer (that is, all of us) in making use of the study results.

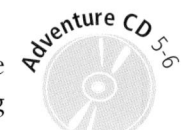

Disseminate results

The final obligation on the part of the researcher is to disseminate the results of the study. This means the researcher must communicate what was found to the research consumer. The most common forms of communication are through articles in nursing research or specialty journals or through a presentation at a conference. An article has the most widespread effect.

Once the results have been communicated, the researcher's job is finished, and the research consumer's job begins. Nurses have an obligation to keep their practices current and grounded in a solid scientific knowledge base. This means regular reading and use of the knowledge being generated through research.

> ### Student Challenge
>
> Entertaining the End
>
> 1 Examine your chosen research studies for future research recommendations and implications for nursing practice.
> 2 Rejoice in the fact that you have now scanned entire research studies.
> 3 In an upcoming chapter, we walk through more studies step-by-step, so don't worry if you still feel uncomfortable with what you're reading.

> ### Resource Kit
>
> Ethics and Research
>
> Want to view a copy of the NH&MRC National Statement on Ethical Conduct in Research Involving Humans? Want to see the official guidelines for informed consent? Want to see what Institutional Ethics Committees are responsible for? Log on to the book's Evolve website and check out the listed government websites.
>
> Research Is My Thing
>
> If you have formed an abiding interest in the research process, you can get a more in-depth view of the process by exploring the phrase 'research process' using a search mechanism on the internet. There are even complete research courses taught online.
>
> 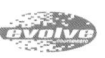 Visit the book's Evolve website at http://evolve.elsevier.com/AU/Borbasi/maze for further information.
>
> Check out the puzzles, mazes and games on your CD-ROM.
>
> Recommended Reading
>
> Johnstone MJ (1999). *Bioethics: a nursing perspective*, 3rd edn. Harcourt Saunders, Sydney.
>
> Tolich M (ed) (2001). *Research ethics in Aotearoa New Zealand*. Longman, Auckland.

References

Belmont Report: ethical principles and guidelines for the protection of human subjects of research 1978, National Commission for the Protection of Human Subjects of Biomedical and Behavioral Research, Department of Health, Education and Welfare Publication No (OS) 78-0012. US Government Printing Office, Washington, DC.

Connelly CD (1998). Hopefulness, self-esteem, and perceived social support among pregnant and nonpregnant adolescents. *Western Journal of Nursing Research* 20(2):195–209.

Erikson E (1950). *Childhood and society*. WW Norton, New York.

Gallinagh R, Nevin R, McIlroy D et al (2002). The use of physical restraints as a safety measure in the care of older people in four rehabilitation wards: findings from an exploratory study. *International Journal of Nursing Studies* 39:147–156.

Gawlinski A, Dracup K (1998). Effect of positioning on Svo_2 in the critically ill patient with a low ejection fraction. *Nursing Research* 47(5):293–9.

Jennings-Dozier K (1999). Predicting intentions to obtain a Pap smear among African American and Latina women: testing the theory of planned behavior. *Nursing Research* 48(4):198–205.

Johnstone MJ (1999). *Bioethics: a nursing perspective*, 3rd edn. Harcourt Saunders, Sydney.

King IM (1971). *Toward a theory for nursing: general concepts of human behavior*. John Wiley, New York.

Langford R (1979). The relationship between student sense of commitment to the profession of nursing and their perceptions of powerlessness in the academic setting. Doctoral Dissertation, University of Houston, Texas.

Lengacher CA, Bennett MP, Kip KE et al (2002). Frequency of use of complementary and alternative medicine in women with breast cancer. *Oncology Nursing Forum* 29(10):1445–1452.

Maslow A (1943). A theory of human motivation. *Psychology Review* 50:370–96.

Mimnaugh L, Winegar M, Mabrey Y et al (1999). Sensations experienced during removal of tubes in acute postoperative patients. *Applied Nursing Research* 12(2):78–85.

National Health and Medical Research Council (NH&MRC) (1999). National statement on ethical conduct in research involving humans. Commonwealth of Australia, Canberra. Online. Available: http://www.health.gov.au/nhmrc/publications/synopses/e35syn.htm 12 Mar 2003.

National Health and Medical Research Council (1991). *Guidelines on ethical matters in Aboriginal and Torres Strait Islander Health Research*. Commonwealth of Australia, Canberra.

Orem DE (1971). *Nursing concepts of practice*. McGraw-Hill, New York.

Pryor SK, Caruth AK, McCoy CA (2002). Children's injuries in agriculture related events: the effect of supervision on the injury experience. *Issues in Comprehensive Pediatric Nursing* 25(3):189–205.

Rogers ME (1970). *An introduction to the theoretical basis of nursing*. FA Davis, Philadelphia.

Selye H (1956). *The stress of life*. McGraw-Hill, New York.

Seyfer J (1999). Scientist faked data. Feds find no links between power lines, cancer. *Houston Chronicle* 24 July, 3 Star, A20.

Venham LL, Gaulin-Kremer E, Munster E et al (1980). Interval rating scales for children's dental anxiety and uncooperative behavior. *Pediatric Dentistry* 2(3):195–202.

http://evolve.elsevier.com/AU/Borbasi/maze

Learning Objectives

After reading this chapter and following critical reflection the student will be able to:

1. Define qualitative research.
2. Describe qualitative research classifications.
3. Discuss conceptualisation for various research designs.
4. Describe structural elements for various research designs.
5. Describe processes involved in conducting a study.
6. Identify methods used in analysing various types of studies.
7. Describe the reporting of study results and conclusions.
8. Discuss the relationships among phases of the research process.
9. Cite examples of phases of the research process.
10. Compare and contrast qualitative and quantitative research.

Chapter Outline

What Is Qualitative Research?
How Is Qualitative Research Classified?
Theoretical perspective
Research design
   Phenomenology
   Ethnography
   Grounded theory
   Historical method
   Case study
What Is the Qualitative Research Process?
Phase 1: Conceive the study
Phase 2: Design the study
   Setting
   Samples and sampling
   Data collection methods
Phase 3: Conduct the study
Phase 4: Analyse the study
   Methods
   Findings
Phase 5: Use the study
Using Qualitative and Quantitative Research Approaches Together

Chapter 6

Qualitative Research: the Whole Picture

Uh, could you tell me your life story? And make it snappy. I still have a lot of people to interview this afternoon.

Student Quote

'When I read the qualitative study we were assigned about nurses' work in the ICU, I felt like I was right there living the experience. I could really identify with what was happening.'

Abstract

Qualitative research is used to examine subjective human experiences by using nonstatistical methods of analysis. It can be classified by theoretical perspective (i.e. constructivist, interpretive, critical) or by research design. Research design classifications include phenomenology, ethnography, grounded theory, historical method and case study. Qualitative research processes vary across research methodologies. The research aim provides a broad boundary that guides the conduct of the study. Data collection occurs predominately through observation and in-depth interview, though other methods are also used. Analysis takes place using various methodologies to manage, interpret and synthesise data. With some qualitative approaches, analysis even dictates the direction and course of further data collection. Qualitative researchers search for patterns of meaning in the collected narrative, observational or other data. Findings are presented in a descriptive narrative format with excerpts from the data to illustrate key patterns and themes.

Key Terms

Qualitative Concerns

basic social process Social or psychological process identified as enduring over time regardless of environmental conditions (e.g. stages of death and dying).

bracketing Process used in some forms of phenomenology to identify and set aside personal beliefs about the phenomenon under study.

case study In-depth research study of an individual unit (e.g. a person, family, group or other identified social unit). A case study generally uses both qualitative and quantitative data.

coding One of the processes by which data may be categorised and conceptualised. It is most often seen in studies using a grounded theory approach.

collective case study Series of case studies that examine similar patterns about identified phenomena.

constant comparative method Method of analysis used in grounded theory in which categories of meaning are derived by comparing collected data incidents to one another until concepts emerge.

credibility Steps taken to make certain of accuracy, authenticity and validity of data.

critical approaches Endeavours to produce research findings to generate change of some sort. When referring to this concept of change, authors often state that their research has transformative or emancipatory potential (that is, the potential to be a catalyst for change).

data immersion Repeated engagement with primary data to become familiar with its content, feeling and tone. This can mean listening and relistening to audiotaped data, and reading and rereading text.

ethnography Qualitative research design that focuses on the world view of an identified cultural group.

field Natural setting in which investigation and data collection take place in a qualitative study.

field notes Written accounts of what a researcher sees, hears, experiences and thinks during the course of data collection in a qualitative study.

grounded theory Qualitative research that develops theoretical propositions about identified social–psychological processes from collected data.

historical method Qualitative analysis of historical events to draw additional insights or inferences about how past events affect the present.

holism Belief that for any aspect of life to be fully understood, the associated factors and context must also be recognised and understood.

phenomenology The study of lived experience. Its purpose is to understand and attribute meaning to the phenomenon of interest.

researcher journal Journal kept by a researcher in which thoughts, ideas,

> feelings and reflections are recorded. Field notes or observations may also be recorded.
>
> **saturation** Point at which sampling and data collection are stopped in a grounded theory study because the information being collected is redundant and repetitive. Is similar to the concept of theoretical redundancy.
>
> **theoretical sampling** Procedure used in grounded theory to gather additional data about emerging concepts.
>
> **triangulation** The use of both quantitative and qualitative research methodologies in a study or series of studies.

In order to engage with the nursing literature and effectively explore questions in nursing, an understanding of qualitative approaches as well as quantitative approaches is necessary. This chapter defines qualitative research, compares qualitative and quantitative approaches, explores various ways in which qualitative research can be classified and identified, and discusses phases of qualitative research processes.

What Is Qualitative Research?

Nursing and nurses have an interest in questions and issues that involve human subjectivity and in developing holistic understandings of people and their experiences. These interests mean that nurses have embraced qualitative methods because they provide researchers with methodical and rigorous pathways to exploring and making meaning from life experiences. They rely heavily on inductive reasoning processes and seek to examine and understand the whole of a phenomenon. The focus of the research is on the process by which concepts are attributed with meaning in a given context rather than on cause and effect, or measurement of the concepts and their relationships. Qualitative researchers view reality as a subjective, multifaceted experience rather than as a single, fixed, objective actuality. Complex phenomena closely tied to the human experience or subjects about which little is known are readily understood using a qualitative approach.

Qualitative research uses multiple data collection procedures that rely heavily on researcher involvement. It produces findings that are arrived at using analytical procedures that are nonstatistical in nature. Qualitative researchers may seek to examine individual lives and their stories and behaviour; organisations and their functioning; role relationships and intercommunications; or cultures and their conduct, interactions and social movement. Qualitative research is generally characterised by small sample sizes and rich descriptive data.

> No singularly defined scientific approach governs qualitative research.

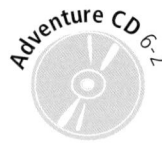

No singularly defined scientific approach governs qualitative research. It is driven by multiple methods across various disciplines. Therefore, many aspects of qualitative research are not as clear-cut as those for quantitative research. While traditional quantitative research has concentrated on trying to establish relationships and differences within a narrow, controlled frame of reference, qualitative research permits multiple ways to explore the depth, richness and complexity inherent in most phenomena. Table 6-1 presents some of the differences between the two approaches.

TABLE 6-1 Differences Between Qualitative and Quantitative Research

Quantitative	Qualitative
Focuses on small number of specific concepts and their relationships and differences.	Attempts to understand the entirety or whole of some phenomenon within a prescribed context.
Set on a predefined theoretical foundation. 'Educated guesses' made about relationship of concepts and study outcomes.	No preconceived theoretical boundaries or preconceived notions about study outcomes.
Researcher controls and interprets data.	Focuses on people's interpretations of events and circumstances rather than researcher's.
Tends to use larger samples.	Uses smaller samples.
Describes people in the study as 'subjects'.	Describes people in the study as 'participants', 'informants' or sometimes 'co-investigators'.
Uses language in a way that implies neutrality, such as writing in the third person.	Can be written up using the first person.
Uses structured procedures and formal instruments to collect information.	Collects information without formal structured instruments.
Collects information under conditions of control and manipulation.	Doesn't attempt to control the context of research, but attempts to capture it in its entirety.
Emphasises objectivity in collection and analysis of information.	Attempts to capitalise on the subjective as a means of understanding and interpreting human experiences.

Qualitative researchers do not claim that their findings are generalisable. Because the study methodology embraces the examination of subjective phenomena, findings are considered to be idiosyncratic to a particular situation. That means they are considered to be representative of a particular person (or people), in a particular context or setting, and not necessarily reflective of experiences of other people in other contexts or settings. Many people assume that qualitative research is easily performed and fail to receive adequate education in qualitative methodologies before embarking on qualitative studies. Conducting qualitative research studies requires every bit as much expertise as conducting quantitative research studies and may take longer because of the nature of recruitment and data collection.

The research problem statement and the nature of the inquiry should guide selection of the research approach. Other issues to consider are access to a sample, and the expertise and philosophical grounding of the researcher. This is crucial because of the advanced knowledge required to successfully conduct a qualitative study.

How Is Qualitative Research Classified?

Several terms are used to describe or classify qualitative research. We explore some of the more common classifications and terms so they will be familiar to you when you encounter them in the literature. Qualitative research may be classified by theoretical perspective or by research design (Box 6-1).

BOX 6-1 Classification Systems for Qualitative Research

Theoretical perspective:
1. Postpositivist
2. Constructivist–interpretive
3. Critical
4. Poststructural

Research design:
1. Phenomenology, ethnomethodology
2. Ethnography, participant observation
3. Grounded theory
4. Historical method
5. Case study

Adapted from Denzin NS, Lincoln YS (1994). *Handbook of qualitative research*. Sage Publications, Thousand Oaks, Calif.

Theoretical perspective

When theoretical perspectives are used to classify qualitative research they indicate the underlying belief systems that informed the research. Postpositivist research is informed by the quantitative tradition and often uses language and approaches closely aligned with the quantitative research process. On the other hand, the interpretive tradition seeks understanding of the world through the perspective of people who have lived a particular experience (e.g. women who have had a mastectomy), or who have a particular way of being in the world (such as those from a particular cultural or social background). Critical theorists are agents of change. They are interested in the social construction of experience and the material resources, power dynamics and ideologies of societies, and use research to develop transformative knowledge (knowledge to effect positive and empowering change). Poststructural and postmodern studies may also be concerned with concepts such as culture, gender, power and oppression, and how these are represented in everyday life through language and structures such as large institutions and other constructs of social governance. They may be concerned with ingrained social stereotypes and prejudices.

Research design

Classification by research design provides us with a little more direction as to what a qualitative study might be all about. These are the classifications you are most likely to see in the nursing literature.

Phenomenology

Phenomenology is the study of **lived experiences**. The researcher examines human experiences through interviews and descriptions that come from the people who have lived the experience. This type of research seeks to describe the entirety of an experience as it is lived and to understand the subjective meaning of the experience. It is based on the premise that the way individuals 'know' is through their perceptions. Therefore reality is perceived as subjective and unique to individuals based on their experience.

Types of questions that might be asked in a phenomenological study are 'What is it like to experience …?' or 'Tell me about your experiences of …'. For example, 'What is it like being the mother of a child in the neonatal intensive care unit?' Interviews and observations are most frequently used to collect data. Analysis occurs by searching the data for themes and patterns. Reflections are drawn on the meaning of the whole of the experience.

Recent examples of published Australian phenomenological studies can be found in articles by Lillibridge, Cox & Cross (2002), who adopted a phenomenological approach to gain insights into the experiences of nurses who misuse substances, and Eckert & Jones (2002), who used phenomenology to explore the lived experience of patients with implantable cardioverter defibrillators and their families. In keeping with a phenomenological approach, both studies involved unstructured in-depth interviews, and used thematic analysis to analyse narrative data. Study findings are presented as a series of themes in both cases.

Ethnography

Ethnography is the systematic study of cultures or subcultures. It has its roots in anthropology. 'Culture' is a broad term whose meaning could range from study of a community in Western Samoa, to examination of a neighbourhood in Melbourne or Auckland, or investigation of the culture of a hospital, or of a group of people such as those who are homeless. Ethnography focuses on the study of the symbols, rituals and customs of an identified cultural group. It provides a picture of that identified group through observation and documentation of interactions in their daily lives.

Research questions in ethnography focus on issues such as the following:
- What procedures does a person follow that makes them part of a group?
- What practices do group members engage in that result in an end product?
- What kinds of work do members engage in to accomplish the goals of the group?

Ethnography focuses on group interactions and activities rather than on individual behaviours. Researchers immerse themselves in the culture or group to be studied. Data are gathered through observation and interview, and are analysed for cultural patterns in an attempt to grasp the lifeways of a particular group in a particular environment.

Leininger is a prominent nurse ethnographer who has conducted a lifetime of ethnographic studies that examine the phenomenon of 'caring' from various cultural perspectives. She views caring as the central and unifying theme for the practice of nursing (Leininger 1981). Recent examples of ethnographical studies in nursing can be found in a study by Carr & Fogarty (1999) entitled 'Families at the bedside: an ethnographic study of vigilance'. This study examines the day-to-day experiences of families who remain at the bedside of hospitalised relatives. Another study, entitled 'The experience of nursing home life' (Fiveash 1998), uses an ethnographic approach to paint a picture of life in a nursing home.

Grounded theory

In **grounded theory** research, data are collected, analysed and used to develop a theoretical explanation and generate hypotheses for further research. Thus, the theory is generated from and 'grounded' in the data. Grounded theory is used to examine basic social processes that occur in a given phenomenon. Pertinent factors, elements and bits of data are collected. Core concepts and dominant processes occurring in interactions are identified. Then the researcher attempts to discover explanations for these concepts and processes.

Research questions revolve around the chief concern or problem of individuals in a defined area. Examples of research questions that might be asked in a grounded theory study are 'How do people prepare themselves emotionally for surgery?' or 'How do cancer patients achieve hopefulness?'. Data are collected using observational and interview techniques. **Coding** helps the researcher conceptualise the underlying patterns of the pieces of data collected. Categories of data are then developed. Analysis uses a process known as *constant comparison* whereby each piece of data is compared to data already collected. Concepts are developed as data are blended into larger and larger categories. Relationships between concepts are examined and then linked into a conceptual framework. The literature is then consulted to determine whether any similar associations have already been uncovered.

Recent Australian examples of grounded theory studies can be seen in a number of areas. A grounded theory design was used to develop a new way of approaching and shaping clinical consultations in the area of sexually transmitted infections (Browne, Minichiello & Plummer 2002). Fenwick, Barclay & Schmied (2001) used a grounded theory approach to look at ways in which nurses support women to take up mothering in a neonatal nursery.

Historical method

Historical method research examines social phenomena by studying their historical context or their past. A historical study analyses a defined event, identifies key concepts and relationships, and draws inferences in an attempt to understand the impact of that event on the present. Historical research involves revisiting a historical event, viewing it from a fresh perspective, and searching for new meaning. Historical research is used to investigate past similar events or phenomena and derive common theoretical explanations of those events. For example, a historical study might try to explain a nursing shortage by examining past cycles of nursing shortages.

Historical researchers look at what has been, what is, and what should be. The researcher begins with an acknowledged philosophical or interpretive point of view. This is important because this point of view influences how information is gathered, read and interpreted. Thus different researchers with varying points of view could revisit the same set of historical events and interpret them differently.

Historical research is somewhat different from the other forms of qualitative research discussed thus far. Rather than observing or interviewing people in the present, the historical researcher relies on historical documents and past written records. These might include diaries, letters, newspapers, articles, books, audio or videotapes, government or professional records, and archives. People might be interviewed, but it would be to elicit their recollections of a past event. This type of interview is generally known as an *oral history*.

Historical research is not nearly as prevalent in the qualitative nursing research literature as some of the other classifications we have discussed. However, an excellent example can be found in an article by Biedermann et al (2001) in a paper about the experiences of Australian nurses in the Vietnam war. The researchers used oral history inquiry as a framework for gathering first-hand narrative data from nurses who had served during the conflict, and data from various archival collections held in Australia were also gathered.

Case study

A **case study** is an in-depth examination of certain phenomena in an individual or in small numbers of individuals. It has also been used to examine the workings of a group, organisation or institution. It is a study of the particular. Nursing and medicine have long used this approach to detail what happens when a person has a certain disease. Medicine focuses on the disease and its processes, while nursing focuses on how the individual responds to the disease, the treatment and the environment. Much of the early research reported in the nursing literature used a case study approach.

Many researchers would argue that a case study is not a qualitative research design at all, but a sampling choice (Denzin & Lincoln 1994). Most often the case study method uses both qualitative and quantitative elements of research (Denzin & Lincoln 1994). For example, if you study an ill individual, some characteristics can be quantified or measured (e.g. vital signs, frequency of signs and symptoms). Other characteristics are better qualified or described in narrative fashion (e.g. the feelings associated with illness).

Remember: a case can be any social unit … an individual, a couple, a family, a street, a school, a town, a hospital ward, a clinic, a hospital and so on.

The case study is used to examine one entity in depth and to study and analyse patterns occurring in that one case. When researchers study more than one unit (e.g. individual, group or institution) they are really doing what is termed a **collective case study** or a series of case studies. This is done to see if patterns carry over from one case to the next. Case studies provide a way to study and analyse phenomena that are relatively rare. Case studies are not seen as frequently in the nursing literature as they once were, but examples can still be spotted. Irving (2002) used an in-depth case study approach to interpret how the use of restraints is legitimised despite the ethical and practical concerns surrounding their use. The 'case' she studied was an acute teaching hospital. Blue & Fitzgerald (2002) conducted a collective case study of four rural health services (they carried out a case study at each site) to explore the interpersonal working relationships between nurses and doctors.

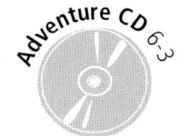

> **Student Challenge**
>
> Scrutinising Study Classifications
>
> 1. Go to the library and look up the research studies cited as examples in the previous paragraphs. Can you tell why they are classified as they are?
> 2. Now choose several other current qualitative nursing research articles. See if you can locate one study in each of the five qualitative research design categories. (Hint: Use the design category as your search term and limit the results to one or two years.)
> 3. Observe the general look and feel of the articles you've located. Note how they differ from quantitative reports. Note how they differ from one another.

What Is the Qualitative Research Process?

As you have already observed, qualitative and quantitative research look different in final written report format. The conduct is also different, with the processes of qualitative research being less segmented and therefore providing more scope for creative, expressive and innovative dimensions. Several phases of a given process frequently occur simultaneously or are revisited numerous times during the course of a study. Many of the decisions about various aspects of the process are made or altered as data are collected and certain trends or patterns are noted. There is an artistry and responsiveness to qualitative research, with a much greater focus on writing and rewriting in order to create a text representative of the phenomenon under examination.

In quantitative research, the conception and design of the study form a detailed blueprint for conducting, analysing and interpreting the study. In qualitative research, conceptualisation and design form only a broad umbrella-like structure for the study. Data collection and analysis dictate detailed study decisions. We will use the broad research phases identified in Chapter 5 as we discuss the qualitative research process. However, keep in mind that the phases are more fluid and less distinct for qualitative research and that the process varies for the different research classifications we have identified. You will see that there are common issues to be addressed for all classifications of qualitative research. This section discusses those common features using the phases of the research process identified in Chapter 5.

> Qualitative research focuses on writing and rewriting in order to create a text that is representative of the phenomenon under examination.

Phase 1: Conceive the study

As with quantitative research, the first task a qualitative researcher faces is to make a decision about what to study. The activities in this phase focus on identifying the phenomenon to be studied. This means an identification of some 'whole' or 'whole process' the researcher is interested in studying. This differs from quantitative studies in which specific measurable concepts are identified. Table 6-2 presents specific examples by research design.

TABLE 6-2 Identification of Phenomenon

Research Design	Identification of Phenomenon
Phenomenology	Lived experience
Ethnography	Issue(s) of interest within a defined culture
Grounded theory	Basic social process
Historical method	Past event
Case study	Broad area for case(s) selection

The initial identification of the phenomenon to be studied is done in the broadest sense. Phenomenological studies identify a phenomenon to be explored and seek individuals with experience of the phenomenon to be interviewed. Examples are parents of children in an intensive care unit or people who have undergone heart transplant surgery. The ethnographer may choose a group of people or a field setting with a broad statement of what is to be investigated. For example, the health beliefs and practices of Vietnamese immigrants or older residents of a nursing home might be selected. Grounded theorists begin with a broad area of social interest with no specific problem in mind. For example, the area of interest might be hopefulness and cancer. Historical research begins with a broadly defined historical event such as the influence of Nightingale's system of nurse education in Australia and New Zealand.

Although all researchers bring their own frame of reference and belief systems to their work, qualitative researchers acknowledge and accept the role of subjectivity and intersubjectivity. This means that qualitative researchers may state their preconceived notions or ideas about the study at the outset, while others will 'bracket' them or set them aside during the actual investigation. A hypotheses-driven design is not a feature of qualitative research. However, historical research is a possible exception and may propose broadly stated hypotheses about expected relationships among historical phenomena.

Most qualitative designs do a literature review at this point. The review serves various purposes depending on the study classification. For example, Phenomenological researchers may do a literature review to ascertain whether the area of interest (i.e. the lived experience) has been previously researched and there is a demonstrated need for such a study. They may also do a literature review to see how other researchers have used phenomenological ideas in the design and conduct of research. Ethnographers may do a literature review to help identify a culture or to identify a particular aspect of a culture that has not been previously researched. When a culture has been selected, they may do an extensive literature review for any available information about that defined culture.

Literature review is an integral part of historical research and the selection of the event to be studied. Historical researchers often conduct extensive literature reviews to place limits on the final topic to be studied. In fact, the initial literature review and narrowing of the event and the historical time span considered often requires a large investment of time. Some case studies do an extensive literature review for all information available on the identified area of interest (e.g. a disease process). Others may review the literature as data are collected. Grounded theory researchers make a point not to look at the literature before beginning the study. Literature review occurs after data collection and analysis has begun and theory has emerged from the data. Then the literature is reviewed and related to the developing theory. This is done to avoid contamination of the data with preconceived concepts and notions about what might be relevant.

Once the phenomenon of interest is selected, a research aim is formulated. This might be expressed in the form of a research question, purpose or objective. The aim is generally broad and serves as a general focus or guide for the study. More defined focal areas of the research often emerge as data are collected and analysed. Table 6-3 presents sample research aims for each design using the previously cited articles in the discussion on design classification.

TABLE 6-3 Sample Research Aims

Research Design	Sample Purpose
Phenomenology	To describe the experience of being a nurse with a substance abuse problem.
	To explore the effect of implantable cardioverter defibrillators on the lives of patients and their families.
Ethnography	To examine the meaning of vigilance in families who remain at the bedside of a hospitalised family member.
	To explore the experience of nursing home living.

Grounded theory	To investigate the processes used when STI health workers interact with patients. To develop a theory for supporting mothers to practise mothering skills in a neonatal nursery.
Historical method	To illuminate and record the experiences of Australian nurses in the Vietnam war.
Case study	To examine the use of restraint in an acute teaching hospital. To examine the interpersonal working relationships between nurses and doctors in rural health services.

Do the following Student Challenge and see if you can identify the researcher's intent in some sample studies.

> **Student Challenge**
>
> Reading Research Aims
>
> Use the studies you found in the previous Student Challenge.
>
> 1 For the studies that were identified in this book, see if you can locate where we came up with the research aims listed in Table 6-3. Notice that some of the studies specifically state the aim or purpose, while others imply it.
> 2 Now look at the other studies you located. Can you determine the research aim for each of them?
> 3 Examine the literature review. Can you tell when it was done? Is the review more comprehensive in some studies than in others?

Phase 2: Design the study

Once the phenomenon has been identified and the general aim of the study is determined, the next phase is to design the study. The chosen design dictates the general structure of the study and includes initial decisions about setting, sample selection and data collection methods. Remember, the qualitative process is fluid, and sampling and data collection methods may evolve during the course of data collection.

Setting

The setting in qualitative research is often referred to as the 'field' because the study is set 'in the field' (i.e. the natural setting where the phenomenon under investigation occurs). Settings vary by type of research design. The selected setting assumes more importance in some research designs than in others. The data collection method may also influence the selected setting. Phenomenological research settings are usually chosen based on convenience for the people who are being studied. Since most of the data are collected through a series of interviews with individual participants, setting is secondary.

Ethnographical studies take place in a setting where the researcher can readily observe and interact with a grouping of people of a particular culture. If the culture of interest is institutionalised people, a prison or nursing home might be an appropriate setting. If the culture of interest is the critically ill, the setting might be an intensive care unit. It is important that the setting in ethnographical research allows the researcher to see and interact with the people collectively.

Grounded theory research takes place in a setting that allows the researcher to observe the selected social processes in action. This means an ability to observe both the environment and the selected participants in the study. Case study settings allow the researcher to view and interact extensively with the chosen case. Historical studies have no real setting. Data are collected from records, relics and artefacts located, for example, in libraries, museums, personal collections or boxes in storage. Table 6-4 lists the settings for the studies we've been following.

TABLE 6-4 Examples of Research Settings

Research Design	Sample Settings
Phenomenology	Acute care setting for cardiac patients
Ethnography	Hospital Two 80-bed nursing homes
Grounded theory	STI outpatient clinic Neonatal nursery
Historical method	Community
Case study	Acute teaching hospital Four rural health settings

Samples and sampling

Samples in qualitative research tend to be small and selected using purposive or convenience sampling techniques (see Box 5-6 in Chapter 5). The researcher is concerned that the selected sample be what is termed 'information rich'. This means the selected sample provides a powerful picture of the phenomena under study. Several other sampling techniques can be used to help provide an 'information rich' sample. These include snowball, extreme, intensity, maximum variety and critical case (Denzin & Lincoln 1994). Box 6-2 discusses these techniques.

> **BOX 6-2** Qualitative Sampling Techniques
>
> **Samples of convenience and purposive sampling** As described in the previous chapter, these are also commonly seen in qualitative designs.
> In addition, the following may be seen:
> **Snowball sampling** This method involves getting recruited participants to help identify and recruit additional participants.
> **Extreme (deviant) sampling** Selection of subjects who exemplify the phenomena to be studied (e.g. in a study about the 'experience of pain', extreme sampling would choose those in extreme pain).
> **Intensity sampling** Selection of subjects who are experiential experts or authorities about the selected phenomena (e.g. in the pain study, intensity sampling might choose those who have chronic pain).
> **Maximum variety sampling** The deliberate selection of subjects who are different, who come from different backgrounds, for the purpose of observing commonalties of experience. (This is particularly helpful when exploring abstract phenomena such as love, joy or hope.)
> **Critical case sampling** Selection of subjects identified as demonstrating what has been identified as a 'critical incident' while collecting and analysing data. (Once critical cases have been identified, additional purposive sampling is conducted to find cases that confirm or disconfirm the critical case.)

Grounded theory studies use a sampling technique called **theoretical sampling**. In theoretical sampling, the researcher begins by collecting and analysing data on an initial sample. This sample is called an open sample because the sampling process is not guided by data analysis. As data are collected and analysed (coded), concepts begin to emerge that will help form an evolving theory. These concepts are called categories and are identified by their repeated presence or absence in the data. The researcher then samples again, looking for additional data to support identified categories. The researcher continues sampling, data collection and analysis until all identified categories are fully explored or **saturated**.

Sample selection in historical research is unique because the sample comprises data sources rather than people. The sampling process occurs simultaneously with data collection and analysis and is ongoing as the researcher refines the study topic. As the topic becomes more clearly defined, the pertinent data sources become more readily identified. This sampling process can cover an extended period of time. Initially the needed data are known only generally. The researcher spends time collecting and reading data sources, which allows the researcher to add greater clarity and definition to the chosen historical topic, which in turn allows the researcher to more clearly identify needed data sources. Sampling and data collection cease when no new information is uncovered from several successive sources.

Data collection methods

Data for qualitative studies are gathered chiefly by use of observation and interview. When a researcher desires to study behaviour, activity and sequences of interaction, or the context or environment in which these behaviours and actions take place, observation is used. Observations may be classified by several features such as structure, participation of the researcher, and visibility of the researcher. Box 6-3 presents a fuller description of these classifications. Ethnographic studies use an unstructured participant approach. Grounded theory uses a combination of observational approaches.

BOX 6-3 Classification of Observation Features

Structure
1. *Structured:* Specified behaviours are predetermined and listed on a checklist to be counted or checked off during an observation period.
2. *Unstructured:* Behaviours are described and recorded as or after they occur using a journal, diary or field notes. A detailed descriptive picture is recorded.

Participation of the researcher
1. *Participant:* The researcher is an active part of the activities or behaviours engaged in by the participants being observed.
2. *Nonparticipant:* The researcher is a bystander or passive participant in the activities being observed.

Visibility of the researcher
1. *Concealed:* The nonparticipant observer is hidden from those being observed. The activities might be recorded on videotape for later viewing and analysis, or activities might be viewed from a concealed space such as behind a two-way mirror.
2. *Nonconcealed:* The observer is in full view of the participants. Participants are aware of being observed.

Interviews allow the researcher to tap into the opinions, attitudes and belief systems of participants. Interviews can be on a continuum from structured to unstructured. Highly structured and focused interviews are used primarily in quantitative research and were discussed in Chapter 5. In-depth semistructured or unstructured interviews are generally used in qualitative research. Unstructured interviews are guided by the general aim of the research and are conducted in a conversational, storytelling style. The researcher might begin with a very broad, open-ended request such as 'tell me about …'. As the person being interviewed tells his or her story, the interviewer may ask additional questions to encourage elaboration on a certain part of the story.

The real instrument in a qualitative study is the researcher. This is because the amount, type and quality of data retrieved are due in large part to the skills and abilities of the researcher, who must be able to enter the field and gain the trust of the people in that environment. Qualitative interviewing requires considerable skill and particularly so because it is often about sensitive or potentially distressing topics. Participants are therefore vulnerable. Narrative is often the primary source of data, and poor interviewing skills will compromise the quality of data and therefore the study itself. The researcher must have well-honed interviewing skills, with a good feel for the ebb and flow of conversation, and be able to keep the interview flowing with well-placed responses and cues. Interviewing requires active listening and the ability to pick up and follow up on subtle leads or clues dropped in the course of the interview. The researcher must be able to put the participant at ease and know how to elicit information that the participants may find hard to express. The researcher must have an eye for detail and be attuned to variations and changes when observing. The researcher needs to be able to capture in depth what has been seen and heard. Finally, the researcher must have a good grasp of self. This means being aware of and able to recognise and reflect on feelings and beliefs that may influence the data collection and analysis. In short, quality data collection in a qualitative study demands a very skilled researcher.

> Quality data collection demands specialised skills on the part of the researcher.

Researchers use several tools to record their observations or interview results. These include audio and video recordings and field notes. Audio and video recordings are later transcribed for closer analysis. **Field notes** are a written account of what the researcher sees, hears, experiences and thinks during the course of data collection. Field notes can be classified into four basic types. The first is a brief description of what has occurred. Notes of this type contain key phrases and major events and are often jotted down in the field. The second type of notes is an expansion of the first type. These are recorded immediately after a data collection session and expand on the brief notes, adding detail. A reflective journal is also kept by many researchers, and contains descriptions of personal thoughts and feelings that occur during the process of data collection. Finally, any insights, analysis of observations, judgments and interpretations made in the field are recorded and kept.

Qualitative researchers are concerned with the accuracy and comprehensiveness of the data they collect. Data are considered **reliable** when what is recorded matches what actually occurred. The use of audio and video recordings and multiple samplings helps ensure data are reliable. **Validity** is used in qualitative research to examine whether or not the explanation or interpretation of data matches what has been described or recorded. Validity then is a question of **credibility**.

Validity may be examined and cross-checked through the use of two techniques: member checks and audit trails (Denzin & Lincoln 1994). Though controversial (St Pierre 1999), member checks are made by having study participants review the material once it has been analysed and interpreted. Audit trails (decision trails) ensure that adequate documentation is available about the data collection and analysis processes. Enough detail should be provided to enable another researcher to repeat the study. This is known as auditability.

> **Student Challenge**
>
> Scrutinising Phase 2
>
> Look again at the qualitative nursing research studies you examined for phase 1. Scan these studies and see if you can identify each of the elements we have discussed in phase 2.
>
> 1. Identify the settings.
> 2. Identify the sample and sample size.
> 3. Did any of the studies use snowball, extreme, intensity, maximum variety, critical sampling or theoretical sampling techniques?
> 4. What data collection methods were used?
> 5. Did any of the studies address the issues of reliability and validity? (Hint: Look for key words such as accuracy, credibility, member checks or audit trails.)

Phase 3: Conduct the study

This phase receives a lot of time and attention in qualitative research. The conceptualisation and planning stages are usually preliminary and broadly defined, in order to lay a broad set of boundaries for data collection. As data collection begins, data analysis may also occur. Data collection and analysis can lead to ongoing conceptualisation and planning about further collection and analysis. So we again see the fluid and repetitive nature of the qualitative research process.

The issues of human subjects' approval and informed consent as they apply to qualitative research differ from those of quantitative research. Most of the guidelines and procedures used by institutional ethics committees were designed for quantitative research methods. Although qualitative studies do not involve invasive, potentially 'risky' procedures such as trialling drugs or treatments, there are still ethical considerations. Like other researchers, investigators using qualitative approaches have to be able to demonstrate that procedures of informed consent are addressed, and also that participation is voluntary, and that participants are able to withdraw from the study at any time. Frequently, too, the focus of qualitative research is on things that are very personal and even traumatic in nature, so participation in qualitative studies can involve participants being asked to recall (and therefore in a way relive) very traumatic life events. This means there is the potential for emotional distress. Institutional ethics committees will expect to see some strategies for dealing with the possibility of emotional distress in participants.

Consent forms often do not contain a detailed description of the study or the risks and benefits because they are not known at the time of data collection. Permission is obtained for interviews and for the use of audio and video recording equipment. Confidentiality is assured. Consent may need to be renegotiated with participants as data collection progresses and information emerges that sends the collection process in a new direction.

Subjects of qualitative research studies are often called participants or informants rather than subjects. Many qualitative researchers see the term 'subject' as too closely associated with the concept of experimentation and the connotation that people are being experimented on like laboratory specimens. The term 'participant' or 'informant' is used to convey the sense of mutual participation and trust-building that occurs between the researcher and the people being researched.

Data collection is a lengthy process in most qualitative studies. Data collection in typical quantitative studies might take from several minutes to several weeks, whereas data collection in qualitative studies may last for months or even years. The process of data collection is often described in more detail in qualitative studies because the collection process is often used to make decisions about the credibility of the data. Take the following challenge.

Student Challenge

Study Conduct

Look again at the qualitative research studies you examined for phases 1 and 2. Look for evidence of the steps in phase 3.

1. Were the rights of human subjects protected in these studies? What evidence did you find to support this?
2. Is there evidence of approval by an institutional ethics committee?
3. Was informed consent obtained?
4. What information was provided about what occurred during data collection?

Phase 4: Analyse the study

Analysis of data in qualitative studies is an inductive process and involves examining words, descriptions and processes. Analytical procedures vary according to the design, but all require the researcher to read and reread field notes and transcripts, to ensure familiarity with the data. This is often called **data immersion** or dwelling with the data. It lets the researcher get in touch with not only the content but also the feeling, tone and emphasis being communicated.

Initial analysis efforts are directed at setting up a system to make large volumes of data more manageable. A system is needed that allows the researcher to file, code and easily retrieve needed data. Computer programs can assist in this management and analysis process. The researcher searches for themes, patterns and meaning in the data and arranges the data in some way that classifies or categorises it.

Methods

Several specific formats and methods have been developed to analyse the data collected for various types of qualitative research. Common techniques used in phenomenological research include methods by Giorgi (1970); Spiegelberg (1976); Colaizzi (1978); van Kaam (1984); Parse, Coyne & Smith (1985); and van Manen (1990). All these methods are similar, requiring qualitative researchers to immerse themselves in the data and use inductive reasoning to sort and make sense of, and to extract and synthesise meaning from, the data. Once it is more manageable, the researcher begins to refine categories and to assign meaning to the data. Data are compared and contrasted, similarities and differences noted, and processes and relationships defined. Finally, descriptions are constructed that represent the synthesis of material. These descriptions may take the form of a metaphor or an analogy or may be presented as a common theme.

Grounded theory has a very well-defined method of data collection and analysis described by Strauss (1987) and Strauss & Corbin (1990). The key is the use of techniques known as theoretical sampling and the **constant comparative method**. Theoretical sampling was discussed earlier in the sampling section. In the constant comparative method of analysis, the researcher categorises units of meaning through a process that compares recorded incident to recorded incident until concepts and categories of concepts begin to emerge. As this occurs, theoretical constructs and relationships are developed and a theory emerges.

Ethnography uses several analytic methods such as ethnoscience, life history, network and event analysis, and the natural history method to examine conceptual and structural patterns in an identified culture. Ethnoscience techniques are designed to explore the 'mental maps' that people use to navigate everyday life (Dobbert 1984). Examination takes place at four levels. Data are described, classified, compared and explained. Description occurs using a technique known as domain analysis; classifications are made through taxonomic analysis; and comparisons are made through componential analysis. Explanation occurs by using the information from the first three analytic steps to make sense of the cultural patterns that emerge. (Spradley (1979, 1980) provides a good basic discussion of the four levels used in the ethnoscience approach.) A life history gathers in-depth information about an informant's life and examines how similar or different individual patterns are from surrounding cultural patterns. Network and event analysis techniques are used to examine social structures.

Historical studies use analytic techniques that examine the documents gathered to determine their importance and their reliability and validity. Initial importance may be judged in various ways including a gross classification into three categories such as: 'clearly valuable', 'mildly interesting' and 'not valuable'. Valuable documents are included in the write-up. Interesting documents are re-reviewed and nonvaluable documents are deleted from the study.

Case studies use a content analysis methodology that allows the researcher to search for patterns or themes in the data using a specific set of rules governing coding and the formation of categories and category relationships.

Findings

The findings in most qualitative studies are presented in a way more immediately understandable to the novice reader (you) than the results in most quantitative studies. This is because the language used is commonly in a descriptive narrative form. However, you will notice that many qualitative researchers have a very sophisticated use of language and you will see words used that you may not be familiar with. You will also notice that many of these papers present very complex ideas and may require reading, reflection and rereading in order to fully grasp their meaning. Frequently findings are illustrated with the use of excerpts of participants' narratives. A good qualitative presentation of findings leaves the reader with a clear, cohesive picture of the phenomena under study.

Student Challenge

Analysis and Results

Examine your chosen research studies for the analyses used and the results of the analyses.

1. Can you identify the specific analytic methods employed?
2. Were the results understandable? Did you get a sense of what had been uncovered in the study?
3. Did you find the results easier to decipher than those in the quantitative studies you examined in Chapter 5?

Phase 5: Use the study

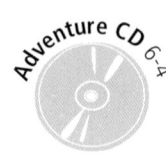

In qualitative studies researchers also reach conclusions about their research findings. However, the inferences drawn from the conclusions may not be as easily applied to clinical practice. The reader is often left with the task of applying the results. Because qualitative researchers are often studying poorly understood aspects of human existence they usually have recommendations for further work. Recommendations for further research may include ideas for both quantitative and qualitative studies. Consumers of research (such as you, the reader) need to be able to satisfy themselves that the findings are credible and trustworthy. Ensuring the trustworthiness of the study and its findings is crucial if qualitative research is to be accepted by the scholarly community. Although the notion of rigor is contentious, qualitative researchers have developed concepts such as adequacy and credibility to ensure that qualitative studies meet the criterion of scientific rigor.

The qualitative researcher is under the same obligation as the quantitative researcher to disseminate the results of the research study. The avenues for this dissemination are much the same and include journal articles and conference presentations. However, many qualitative studies may be found in monograph or book form because of the length of presentation. These formats allow fuller description and use of a greater number and variety of example illustrations obtained from data collection.

Student Challenge

Entertaining the End

Examine your chosen research studies.

1. What did you glean from the studies' conclusions that might be helpful in the practice of nursing?
2. How would you compare your overall experience of reading qualitative research studies with reading quantitative research studies? Did you find one type easier to read and comprehend than the other?

Using Qualitative and Quantitative Research Approaches Together

One question students frequently raise is whether quantitative and qualitative methods can be used together. Some researchers do combine the two methodologies to study certain phenomena. This approach is known as **triangulation**. Both methods may be used at the same time in one study (simultaneous triangulation), or one method at a time may be used in a series of studies (sequential triangulation).

When simultaneous triangulation is used, the researcher must use either a qualitative or a quantitative approach as a foundation. The other approach then provides additional or complementary data. For example, in a quantitative study unstructured interviews or observations might initially be used to help develop more structured and hence measurable questions or behaviours. Qualitative researchers might use statistics to describe a sample of informants or to count frequencies of certain categorised events. A qualitative researcher might also use a quantitative scaled instrument to add an additional dimension to data on a particular concept.

> ### Resource Kit
>
> Want to Know More About Qualitative Research?
>
> Try entering 'qualitative research' as a search phrase using a search engine on the internet. A variety of interesting websites are devoted to qualitative research.
>
> 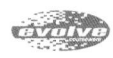 Visit the book's Evolve website at http://evolve.elsevier.com/AU/Borbasi/maze for further information.
>
> Check out the puzzles, mazes and games on your CD-ROM.

References

Biedermann N, Usher K, Williams A et al (2001). The wartime experience of Australian Army nurses in Vietnam, 1967–1971. *Journal of Advanced Nursing* 35(4):543–549.

Blue I, Fitzgerald M (2002). Interprofessional relations: case studies of working relationships between registered nurses and general practitioners in rural Australia. *Journal of Clinical Nursing* 11(3):314–321.

Browne J, Minichiello V, Plummer D (2002). Guided reflection: transcending a routine approach in the management of sexually transmissible infections. *International Journal of STD & AIDS* 13(9):624–632.

Carr JM, Fogarty JP (1999). Families at the bedside: an ethnographic study of vigilance. *Journal of Family Practice* 48(6):433.

Colaizzi P (1978). Psychological research as a phenomenologist views it. In: Vaille RS, King M, eds, *Existential phenomenological alternatives for psychology*. Oxford University Press, New York; 48–71.

Denzin NS, Lincoln YS (1994). *Handbook of qualitative research*. Sage Publications, Thousand Oaks, Calif.

Dobbert ML (1984). *Ethnographic research: theory and application for modern schools and societies*. Praeger, New York.

Eckert M, Jones T (2002). How does an implantable cardioverter defibrillator (ICD) affect the lives of patients and their families? *International Journal of Nursing Practice* 8(3):152–157.

Fenwick J, Barclay L, Schmied V (2001). Chatting: an important clinical tool in facilitating mothering in neonatal nurseries. *Journal of Advanced Nursing* 33(5):583–593.

Fiveash B (1998). The experience of nursing home life. *International Journal of Nursing Practice* 4(3):166.

Giorgi A (1970). *Psychology as a human science: a phenomenologically based approach*. Harper & Row, New York.

Irving K (2002). Governing the conduct of conduct: are restraints inevitable? *Journal of Advanced Nursing* 40(4):405–412.

Leininger MM (1981). *Caring: an essential human need*. Charles B Slack, Thorofare, New Jersey.

Lillibridge J, Cox M, Cross W (2002). Uncovering the secret: giving voice to the experiences of nurses who misuse substances. *Journal of Advanced Nursing* 39(3):219–229.

Parse RR, Coyne AB, Smith MJ (1985). *Nursing research qualitative methods*. Brady Communications Bowie, Md.

Spiegelberg H (1976). *The phenomenological movement*. Martinus Nijhoff, The Hague.

Spradley JP (1979). *The ethnography interview*. Holt, Rinehart & Winston, New York.

Spradley JP (1980). *Participant observation*. Holt, Rinehart & Winston, New York.

St Pierre (1999). The work of response in ethnography. *Journal of Contemporary Ethnography* 28(3):266–287.

Strauss AL (1987). *Qualitative analysis for social scientists*. Cambridge University Press, New York.

Strauss AL, Corbin J (1990). *Basics of qualitative research: grounded theory procedures and techniques*. Sage Publications, London.

van Kaam A (1984). *Existential foundation of psychology*. Doubleday, New York.

van Manen M (1990). *Researching lived experience: human science for an action sensitive pedagogy*. State University of New York Press, New York.

http://evolve.elsevier.com/AU/Borbasi/maze

Learning Objectives

After reading this chapter and following critical reflection the student will be able to:

1. Identify reputable research and clinical nursing journals with a research focus.
2. Describe the elements found in a standard research article format.
3. Discuss the relationship between a standard article format and the quantitative and qualitative research processes.
4. Describe a strategy that can be employed to more effectively read and comprehend research articles.
5. Apply the specified reading strategy to survey, examine, critically read and evaluate a sample quantitative article and visualise practice applications.
6. Apply the specified reading strategy to survey, examine, critically read and evaluate a sample qualitative article and visualise practice applications.

Chapter Outline

Reporting Research
Research and clinical journals
Journal presentation format
   Title, abstract and key words
   Introduction/background
   Methodology or methods
   Results/findings
   Discussion/conclusions
   References
How to Read a Research Article
Research reading strategy
Using the reading strategy with sample research studies
   Quantitative research example
   Qualitative research example

Chapter 7

Reading Research: Critical Approaches to Effective Understanding

Well the directions did say 'select a conducive environment!'

Student Quote

'I thought reading the article three times was going to be a colossal waste of time; but when I followed the strategy I really did come away with a better understanding of what the researcher was doing.'

Abstract

Research results are disseminated primarily through journal articles and are generally (but not always) presented in a standard format that includes a title, abstract and key words, introduction, methodology or methods, results, discussion and references. These sections encompass the steps of the research process. A reading strategy can improve comprehension and use of research results. The described reading strategy consists of five phases. The article is read three times: once to survey the study, once to examine it for key ideas, and once to identify key elements of the research process. The study is then evaluated, and practice applications are visualised. Sample quantitative and qualitative articles are used to illustrate the use of the research reading strategy.

> **Key Terms**
>
> **Reading Strategy Rhetoric**
>
> **abstract** Summary of the essential characteristics of something more extensive (e.g. a summary of a research article).
>
> **critically read** Step 3 of the research reading strategy; designed to focus on key steps in the research process.
>
> **evaluate** Step 4 of the research reading strategy; designed to judge the quality of the article.
>
> **examine** Step 2 of the research reading strategy; designed to identify key ideas and sort out the meaning of the article.
>
> **research critique** Detailed critical examination and evaluation of the theoretical and methodological merits of a given research study.
>
> **research reading strategy** Five-step process designed to increase comprehension and application of research studies. The steps are survey, examine, critically read, evaluate and visualise.
>
> **survey** Step 1 of the research reading strategy; designed to provide a general overview and feel for the article.
>
> **visualise** Step 5 of the research reading strategy; designed to apply research results to practice.

Now that we have honed your library, internet and reading skills and introduced you to the world of research, you can begin to integrate this knowledge. This chapter helps you examine and critically read research articles. We look at the typical presentation format of research articles and introduce a set of criteria and a strategy to use when reading. We then dissect some sample articles using the reading strategy and evaluation criteria.

Reporting Research

Research and clinical journals

The most common way to disseminate research findings is by publishing a research article. We have already identified several nursing research journals. In addition, several clinical specialty journals devote at least half of their journal space to presentation of nursing research articles. There are also journals that review and critique the current state of nursing research. Box 7-1 lists some of the more common journals where research studies or discussions of studies are located. As discussed in Chapter 6, some qualitative studies are presented in monograph or book form because the presentation is lengthy and not suited to an article format. Our focus is on research reports presented in article format.

BOX 7-1 Journals with a Research Focus

Nursing Research Journals
Journal of Advanced Nursing
Australian Journal of Advanced Nursing
Nursing Research
Research in Nursing and Health
Nursing Science Quarterly
*International Journal of Nursing Practice**
Journal of Nursing Scholarship
Scholarly Inquiry for Nursing Practice
International Journal of Nursing Studies

Clinical Nursing Journals
Australian Critical Care
AORN Journal
Australian Journal of Holistic Nursing
Nursing Praxis in New Zealand
*International Journal of Nursing Practice**
Heart and Lung: Journal of Acute and Critical Care
International Journal of Mental Health Nursing
Oncology Nursing Forum
Rehabilitation Nursing

Research Review Nursing Journals
Annual Review of Nursing Research
Online Journal of Knowledge Synthesis for Nursing
Research for Nursing Practice

*International Journal of Nursing Practice fits the profile for both a research and a clinical nursing journal.

Student Challenge

Journal Set-ups

1 Peruse several of the research and clinical journals listed in Box 7-1. What do you see? What kinds of articles are present in addition to research articles?

2 Locate research articles in several different research and clinical journals. Compare the formats for presentation. Do you see similarities? Do the journals differ in emphasis? What about the formats within a specified journal? Are they similar or different?

As you have probably discovered, even research journals contain more material than just research studies. They may discuss ethical, statistical or methodological concerns, report on the development and testing of new research instruments, or discuss reliability or validity concerns of established instruments. They may even report on the reanalysis of old studies using a statistical technique known as meta-analysis. They may also contain major literature reviews about particular topics. Clinical journals often contain anecdotal, clinical experience and theoretical articles in addition to research articles.

Journal presentation format

You have probably also discovered that the format of a research article differs somewhat from the steps of the research process we discussed in Chapters 5 and 6. However, the format is very similar among the various journals. This format comes out of a quantitative research tradition and has six major sections: (1) title, abstract and key words, (2) introduction or background, (3) methodology or methods, (4) results or findings, (5) discussion, and (6) references. Slight variations in this format may be seen, but the sections are usually recognisable. Table 7-1 identifies the steps of the research process usually delineated under these section headings.

TABLE 7-1 Relationship Between the Research Process and the Format of Research Articles

Article Section	Quantitative Process
Introduction/background	Problem statement/purpose Literature review Theoretical framework Hypotheses/research questions/objectives
Methodology or methods	Research design Sample and setting Data collection method Instrument quality Data analysis procedures Description of sample
Results/findings	Presentation of results
Discussion/conclusions	Interpretation of results Recommendations for research Implications for nursing
References	

Qualitative articles are often adapted to this format to provide consistency in journal presentation. However, as qualitative research finds broader acceptance in nursing, we are beginning to see presentations much truer to the nature of qualitative processes. Thus, increasing numbers of qualitative articles are presented in a narrative format appropriate to the nature of the study. The following discussion presents the typical quantitative presentation format and provides comments about qualitative studies when applicable.

Title, abstract and key words

The title of the study is the first thing you are likely to notice in any research article. It should capture the essence of the study. It typically states the variables or phenomena and population studied. The title section often lists the names and credentials of the researchers. Credentials may also be found at the end of an article.

Just below the title is the abstract for the study. The **abstract** is a clear, concise summary of the study. In about 100 to 300 words, the abstract describes the study purpose, research design, methodology, findings and implications. It serves as an overview and should give you a brief outline of what to expect in the article.

In many journals a list of key words immediately follows the abstract. The key words are a list of five to ten words that most closely capture the content of the paper. These words are useful in that they provide a very quick and clear idea of the content of the paper and can also be very useful as triggers to conduct database searches for additional related articles.

Introduction/background

The introduction is the first section in the body of the article. It may or may not be labelled as such. The introductory section serves to acquaint you, the reader, with the research problem and its context. In a quantitative study, the following basic elements are included in the introduction:
- Research problem
- Research questions or hypotheses
- The need for the study
- Review of literature
- Theoretical framework.

Remember, the problem statement may be in either interrogative or declarative form and may be couched as a statement of purpose. It is typically located at the beginning or the end of the introductory section. The problem may then be broken down into smaller research questions or hypotheses. In some studies you may see these stated in the results section rather than the introductory section. The introduction often begins with a statement of need followed by a brief presentation of the current literature and identification of the theoretical framework. Sometimes the literature review and/or framework are set out under separate headings. Many studies do not articulate a theoretical framework. The reported review of literature may not be complete because of space constraints. Therefore, only the most critical and current studies are cited.

Qualitative studies use the introductory section to present a broad overview and context of the phenomena under study. Study objectives may be identified and pertinent literature cited. When you finish reading the introduction of a study, you should have a good feel for what is being studied and why such a study is important.

Methodology or methods

Methodology and methods are two terms seen in research papers. 'Methodology' identifies and (briefly) describes the approach the researcher(s) used, while 'methods' describes the actual conduct of the study. All this information is usually subsumed under a heading of methodology or methods. In a quantitative study, this section usually identifies the research design; describes the subjects, sampling techniques, inclusion criteria and setting; and discusses instrumentation. This section may also contain a rationale for what was done, thus informing the reader of why the selected approaches were used for the study. Research journals generally place a greater emphasis on this section than clinical journals do. Qualitative studies also identify the research design at this point, as well as providing some statement as to why a particular methodology was selected. This section should also clearly describe the nature of the interview or observation techniques, how the samples were selected, and the setting. A detailed description of the analysis process will also be provided. At the end of this section it is usual to see a description of the nature of the sample. This can be as brief as the provision of basic demographic information, or as detailed as providing pseudonyms and rich descriptive information about each participant.

Results/findings

The results section presents the key research findings. In quantitative studies, the results section is fairly short. The data are presented in succinct form with little discussion. Studies often begin by describing sample characteristics here. In other studies, this description is included in the methods section. The focus is centred on answering the research questions or hypotheses. The statistical test(s) used is identified, and the value of the calculated statistic and the r value are reported. A brief narrative translation of these statistical results is included. Much of the statistical information may be displayed in table or graph form.

The results section in qualitative studies is generally longer because the results are presented in narrative form. In addition, the researcher often uses this section to describe the themes, processes or structures that emerged from the analysis and to integrate them into the researcher's theoretical perspective. A pertinent literature review is often seen in this section. Grounded theory studies use this section to present the theory that has emerged from the data analysis.

Discussion/conclusions

The discussion section focuses on interpreting the results and is sometimes labelled 'conclusions'. The researcher explains what the results mean and how they fit into the existing body of literature. This means that study findings are discussed in relation to the existing literature. Points of agreement and divergence from the literature are identified and discussed. If the research results are unexpected (for example, the hypotheses are not supported in a quantitative study), the researcher may try to explain why things turned out the way they did.

Recommendations are also given in this section and these are most often presented as implications for clinical practice and/or education, and recommendations for further research. Limitations of the study are also identified in this section.

References

Journal articles conclude with a list of references. This includes journal articles, books and other sources cited in the text of the article. The reference section can be a very valuable tool for a reader who is interested in further information on a given area of study. It provides a starting point for a preliminary review of the literature on that topic. When reading the reference list, note some of the characteristics of the literature the researcher has drawn on. For example, does the author cite original sources? Were the majority of citations less than five years old at the time the article was published? Does the researcher mainly draw on research articles, opinion pieces or non-refereed sources?

> **Student Challenge**
>
> ### Qualitative and Quantitative Comparisons
>
> Choose a quantitative article and a qualitative article that use the general format described earlier. Select an additional qualitative article that does not follow the prescribed format.
>
> 1. View each of the first two articles. Identify each of the major sections. Note how the information is presented under each section. Were the sections readily identifiable?
> 2. Did you notice differences between the qualitative and quantitative approaches?
> 3. Now look at the two qualitative articles. Which approach seemed more readable to you? Which approach did you like better?

How to Read a Research Article

The primary reason we read research articles is to determine whether the findings will be helpful to our own professional practice. As we discuss effective ways to read research articles, you might want to quickly review Chapter 3. We introduce a reading strategy and a set of criteria to help you read research articles effectively and critically. The reading strategy as applied to research articles is outlined in Box 7-2. Criteria for increasing your comprehension of quantitative and qualitative studies are outlined in Boxes 7-3 and 7-4.

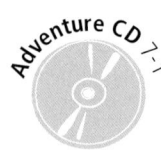

BOX 7-2 Research Reading Strategy

Get prepared. Select a conducive reading environment and a time when you are mentally alert. Have a glossary of research terms available for reference. Follow the steps listed below.

1. **Survey** the article to get a general feel for what is being studied and the overall outcomes.
   a. *Examine the title* to give you a good idea of the study area and to identify the major concepts or phenomena under investigation. Identify authors and author qualifications.
   b. *Pay careful attention to the abstract* to help you determine the type of study you're reading and whether this particular study is pertinent to you and your nursing practice. The abstract also provides a quick sketch of the research results.
   c. *Skim the major sections of the article* to pick up the general flow and article highlights. Try not to get bogged down by unfamiliar terms or statistical treatments.
   d. *Look at the reference list.* Do the articles cited seem comprehensive, relevant to the topic, and current?
2. **Examine** the article. Go back and read the article more carefully. Proceed one section at a time. Draw out the key idea in each paragraph. Write down questions about terminology, concepts or ideas that are puzzling. Consult needed resources to answer the questions you've raised.
3. **Critically read** the article. Using the criteria listed in Box 7-3 or 7-4 as a guide, read the article once more and locate the key elements of the study. Write them down as you find them.
4. **Evaluate** the article. Was the study a good one? Can the results be applied to practice?
5. **Visualise** practice applications. Think about the results and how you might use them in your own nursing practice. Make written notes of your ideas.

BOX 7-3 Guidelines to Aid in the Comprehension of Quantitative Research Studies

Introduction

Determine what is being studied:
- Locate a problem statement and/or statement of purpose.
- Locate the hypotheses and/or research questions.
- Identify the research variables and the population.

Determine why the study is important:
- Locate the rationale for the study.

Examine how the study contributes to existing knowledge:
- Look at the literature review and the theoretical/conceptual framework.

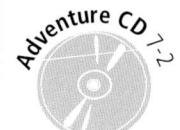

Methods

Determine how the study was conducted:
- Identify the research design (e.g. experimental or nonexperimental? descriptive, exploratory, explanatory or predictive?)
- Identify sampling issues (e.g. probability or nonprobability? number of subjects used?)

Identify the study setting (i.e. where did data collection occur?):
- Locate instruments used and reported reliability and validity measures.

Determine how the study was analysed:
- What statistical measures were used?

Results

Examine a description of the subjects. (Remember, this may be in the Methods section.)

Determine the answers found by the study:
- Were the statistical results significant or not? What does that mean?

Discussion

Determine the implications for nursing practice:
- How were the results related to practice?
- What limitations were placed on the study results?
- How were the results tied back to existing knowledge?

> **BOX 7-4** Guidelines to Aid in the Comprehension of Qualitative Research Studies
>
> **Introduction**
> Determine what phenomena are being studied:
> - Look for a statement of purpose.
> - Locate study questions or objectives.
>
> Determine the context of the study:
> - Read the literature review.
> - Look for why the study was deemed important.
>
> **Methods**
> Determine how the study was conducted:
> - Identify the research design (e.g. phenomenological, ethnographical, historical, grounded theory or case study).
> - Identify the study setting, sampling techniques, data collection techniques, and reliability (accuracy) and validity (credibility) issues.
>
> Determine how the study was analysed:
> - Look for descriptions of the analysis process (e.g. how were data processed to establish themes, structures or processes?).
>
> **Results**
> Examine a description of the subjects. (Remember, this may be the one place you see numbers used in a qualitative study.)
>
> Determine the answers found by the study:
> - What themes, metaphors, processes or structures were identified to describe the data collected?
>
> **Discussion**
> Determine the implications for nursing practice:
> - How were the results related to practice?
> - Were the results tied back to existing knowledge?

Research reading strategy

As you can see by reviewing Box 7-2, which details the **research reading strategy**, you are going to read the article a minimum of three times. The first time you are skimming to detect the general purpose and direction of the study. The second time you are reading for understanding and to detect areas that may be confusing or present roadblocks to understanding. The third reading focuses on specific components of the research process that need your attention. As you become more proficient at reading research articles, the middle reading step is often no longer necessary. This process will seem cumbersome and tedious at first. Stick with it, and ultimately you will be able to read research articles with greater ease and understanding.

Once you have surveyed, examined and critically read the research article, the next step is to evaluate the study. This involves making judgments about the value of the study and deciding whether the study is a good one. You do not yet possess the knowledge or skills necessary to offer a critical evaluation of a reported research study. This process is commonly known as a **research critique**. It judges the theoretical and methodological merits of the study and addresses issues such as whether a study is theoretically sound, whether it was appropriately designed, and whether the methods or statistical analysis were correctly applied. These judgments require considerable knowledge of research and statistical methodologies. Your best bet is to stick to research reported in established professional journals and to rely on the editors and reviewers of the journal to make those evaluations.

However, you can ask yourself questions that have a bearing on the quality of the study. These include such queries as the following:
1. Were the key elements of the study clearly identified?
2. Could you readily follow the steps of the research process?
3. Were ideas presented concisely and comprehensively?
4. Were the study findings clearly tied to existing knowledge?
5. Do the ideas make logical or intuitive sense?

In qualitative studies, you want to ask the following questions:
1. Were the phenomena fully described?
2. Did the narrative paint a clear picture of the phenomena?
3. Were themes, structures or processes clearly presented?
4. Did these themes, structures or processes make sense?
5. Did they flow logically from the data?

When evaluating a study you are also concerned with whether the results can be applied to a particular practice setting. In a quantitative study, the question is: Are the results generalisable to subjects other than those in the study? If you remember from Chapter 5, results are generalisable to the population when the sample is a probability sample. If the sample is not a probability sample, then you must determine whether other studies have generated similar results. If more than one study is showing similar results, confidence in the results is increased. Use of a theoretical framework can also broaden the application of results to other groups of subjects. You want to ask questions such as: What sampling technique was used? Is there a theoretical framework? Were results of similar studies reviewed in the article? How similar is my practice setting to the study setting?

The applicability of qualitative results is not concerned with generalisability. The questions here are whether the results have any relevance to your particular practice. That is, does the interpretation of the data and the resulting themes, patterns, structures or processes make sense to you in your practice? Do the findings give you greater insight into an aspect of human experience that can enhance your interactions with patients or colleagues? Do the ideas make sense? Are they useful?

The final step in the reading of a research article is to visualise how the study results might be helpful in your nursing practice. The study itself will suggest some ideas for application of the research results. You need to personalise the results; that is, think about them for your own practice. If you can visualise using the results, then you are more likely to incorporate them into your ongoing practice.

Using the reading strategy with sample research studies

In this section, we use the research reading strategy and the comprehension guidelines to walk through two actual research articles step-by-step. The first article (Korniewicz et al 1989) is a quantitative study and the second (Beck 1992) is a qualitative study.

Quantitative research example

If you are ready to get started, begin with the following Student Challenge.

> **Student Challenge**
>
> Quantitative Surveying
>
> 1 Go to the CD-ROM and locate the Article Access exercise in Chapter 7. Print out the reading strategy, the guidelines for comprehending quantitative studies, and the quantitative research article entitled 'Integrity of vinyl and latex procedure gloves'.
>
>   This article is not current. It was selected because it is short, appears in a standard format, involves few variables, and covers a basic topic that would be of interest to a wide variety of nurses.
>
> 2 Take your textbook; article, strategy and guideline printouts; and notepad and pen, and find a conducive reading and study environment.
>
> 3 Note that each part of the article has been labelled with a letter and a number. The letter corresponds with the six sections of a standard research article. The numbers identify subsections of the specific section.
>
> 4 Now survey the article using Step 1 of the research reading strategy listed in Box 7-2. Print it out. Make notes of what you gleaned from your survey. After you have finished, read 'Survey the quantitative article' and compare your notes with ours.

Survey the quantitative article

The first stop on the survey is the title (labelled A1). This particular title informs us that the study examines the quality of two kinds of gloves used in procedures. This sounds like a study that could provide useful information about a product used daily in the clinical area. (Note: At the time this study was published, the use of universal precautions was just beginning to become a widespread and common practice. These are now referred to in some areas as standard precautions.)

Sections A2 and A5 (end of third page) identify four authors. All hold doctorates; three are nurses, two are postdoctoral students and two are faculty members at a university. Infectious disease and infection prevention are identified specialty areas. This information gives us confidence that these researchers have enough expertise to conduct the study. Section A4 gives us additional information about the study. It was published seven to eight months after acceptance by the journal. This means the material should still be relevant and timely at the time of publication. It was supported by an outside grant-funding source, and the results have been presented at an international conference, which lends further credence to the quality of the study.

The abstract (A3) informs us that both types of gloves were tested using three different methods. From the description it sounds as if the gloves were tested for leaks of water, bacteria and dye under simulated in-use conditions. It appears that the latex gloves performed better than the vinyl gloves across all tests. Twenty per cent of the latex gloves and 34 per cent of the vinyl gloves allowed penetration of bacteria; this raises some alarm. We need to read further to find out details about each of the testing methods and for a description of full results. After reading this far, we know this study has information that affects us personally in the clinical area.

As you skim the article, several things will be readily apparent: several pertinent articles are cited in the introduction, a purpose statement is clearly identified, the tests used seem well-described, the results are straightforward and the discussion has implications for practice. Articles included in the reference list are clearly related to the topic under study, include international sources and sources from various disciplines, and most were published in the 1980s.

Student Challenge

Quantitative Examining

1. Now that you have surveyed the article and have a general idea of what it's about, go back and read the article paragraph by paragraph.
2. Jot down the key idea in each paragraph.
3. Make a note of anything you don't understand.
4. When you have finished, consult references to clarify those things that are unclear.
5. Now read 'Examine the quantitative article' for examples of abstractions of key ideas.

Section 2: Talking the Talk

Examine the quantitative article

The key ideas for each paragraph in the article are presented below and identified by their assigned code. See how they compare to your notes. Things that might raise questions about the research process are highlighted in bold.

B1 Fear of HIV exposure led to reevaluation of glove standards and practices that were designed to prevent the spread of hepatitis B virus (HBV).

B2 Several condom studies recommend latex condoms for protection against HBV and HIV, but we don't know if these results are applicable to gloves.

B3 Most of the studies on gloves have been done to test sterility during surgery.

B4 Data about the protective abilities of latex and vinyl gloves are scarce. The purpose of the study is to examine the integrity of vinyl and latex gloves under in-use conditions.

C1 Twenty-eight subjects.

C2 Watertight method used to check for visible leaks in gloves. **Sensitivity of the watertight test was checked. Sensitivity is the ability of a test to adequately detect what it was designed to detect (i.e. how well the watertight test picked up leaks).**

C3 Three levels of hand manipulations (described in Table 1) were used to simulate hand activities during patient care.

C4 Each subject wore a vinyl glove on one hand and a latex glove on the other hand (left hand versus right hand was randomly assigned). **Random assignment means that the hand wearing a certain glove type was chosen by chance.** Rubber bands were worn at wrists to prevent splashing and contamination. **This is a way to control extraneous variables.** Ninety manipulation tests were done for each glove type (30 each with no, partial or full manipulation). Gloves were then tested for leaks using dye solution. Dye stains on hands were recorded by a person who was blind to (had no knowledge of) glove type. **This is a way to control bias in data recording.**

C5 *S. marcescens* cultures were used because it is not normally found on the skin. **This is another control over possible extraneous variables (e.g. contamination by bacteria already on a subject's skin).**

C6 Hands were washed and a baseline culture was done before testing.

C7 Subjects donned a vinyl and a latex glove, performed hand manipulations (no, partial, full), and then put hands into *S. marcescens* broth.

C8 Cultures were taken from each glove. Cross-contamination was controlled by frequent investigator glove changes. **This is another control over the extraneous variable of cross-contamination.**

C9 Sensitivity of the bacterial test was examined. **(See sensitivity comment above.)**

D1 Visible defects were evident in 2.7% of latex and 4.1% of vinyl gloves ($\chi^2 = .58$, $p = .44$). χ^2 **stands for chi square, the statistical test used to determine whether**

any differences in defects were visible between latex and vinyl gloves. The *p* value of .44 tells us that differences in visible defects were not significant (see Chapter 5, p 123).

D2 The watertight test was not sensitive in the deliberately punctured latex gloves but was sensitive to vinyl.

D3 Fifty-three per cent of vinyl and 3.3% of latex gloves leaked dye after full manipulation (*p* = .0004). The difference in performance between the two glove types after full manipulation was significant. Latex performed better. No difference between glove types was found for no or partial manipulation. Dye leaks occurred mainly on thumb and forefinger.

D4 All baseline cultures were negative. **This served as a pretest showing no *S. marcescens* on hands before the bacterial penetration test.** All deliberately punctured gloves were sensitive to bacterial test. Thirty-four per cent of the vinyl and 20% of the latex gloves allowed bacterial penetration ($\chi^2 = 1.83, p = .18$). **The difference between the two glove types was not significant.** The brand of latex or vinyl gloves made no difference to the permeability.

E1 Concern over infection transmission and increased acceptance of universal precautions (standard precautions) has increased glove use by healthcare workers.

E2 This study supports other evidence showing that gloves are vulnerable to bacterial penetration.

E3 Glove testing protocols are under review by the US Food and Drug Administration (FDA).

E4 Test sensitivity could be improved by use of a dye test that shows immediate results and the point of leakage with no risk of bacterial contamination to testers.

E5 Bacterial penetration tests are very sensitive but require too much time and delay test results. Contamination is a risk to testers.

E6 Both glove types provide some protection, which decreases with use. Hands should be washed after patient care even if gloves are worn and gloves should not be reused or washed between patients.

> **Student Challenge**
>
> Quantitative Critical Reading
>
> 1 Now that you have examined the article and summarised key ideas, go back and read the article a third time using the criteria outlined in the quantitative research guidelines.
> 2 Locate and record each key element of the research process.
> 3 Now read 'Critically read the quantitative article' for confirmation of what you found.

Critically read the quantitative article

This section identifies the key elements of the research process used in our sample article. It follows the quantitative guidelines. The location of the identified elements in the article is indicated by the appropriate paragraph code.

Introduction

Determine what is being studied:
- The purpose is located in B4 'The primary purpose of this study was …'.
- No hypotheses or research questions are stated.
- Variables were not labelled, but can be identified.
- Independent variables: (1) type of glove (latex or vinyl), (2) in-use condition (none, partial, full)
- Dependent variable: glove integrity
- Extraneous variables identified and controlled for:
  - Hand the glove was worn on (left or right) C4, C7
  - Dye splashing and contamination C4, C7
  - Inspection bias C4
  - Bacteria already on skin C5, C6
  - Cross-contamination C8
- Population: procedure gloves

Determine why the study is important:
- The rationale is built into paragraphs B1 to B4. Perceived risk of exposure is increasing and there are insufficient data about barrier effectiveness of gloves.

Examine how the study contributes to nursing:
- No theoretical framework is identified.
- Brief literature review in B1 to B4 supports the need for additional testing.
- Nurses use gloves for barrier protection in the clinical area.

Methods

Determine how the study was conducted:
- Research design is experimental because the independent variable (in-use condition) was manipulated.
- The way the gloves were chosen (sampled) is not described beyond what appears in D1.
- We must assume the sampling was convenience.
- Data collection sounds as if it were done in a lab, but this is not directly stated. One mention is made of a laminar flow cabinet in C7. Three biophysical tests were designed to measure glove integrity (watertight, dye and bacterial penetration).
- Reliability and validity issues of tests were not discussed. This is not uncommon with biophysical measures.

Determine how the study was analysed:
- Frequencies and percentages reported numbers of failed gloves. Differences between the vinyl and latex gloves were measured using chi square and Fisher's

exact tests. (These tests are designed to be used with nominal level data.) See D1 to D4.

Results

Examine description of subjects:

- This is confusing. A description of the people wearing the gloves is seen in C1. However, in this study, the gloves are the subjects. The only description of them is found in D1.

Determine the answers found in the study:

- The difference between the number of visible defects seen in latex gloves and those in vinyl gloves was not significant. Overall the number of leaks seen was low (2.7 to 4.1%)—see D1. Latex gloves were significantly better than vinyl gloves at protecting against dye leaks after being fully manipulated (3.3 to 53%)—see D3. Differences between latex and vinyl gloves in the number of dye leaks under no or partial manipulation were not significant—see D3. One-fifth of latex and one-third of vinyl gloves were penetrated by bacteria. This difference was not significant—see D4. The difference in protection against bacterial penetration between the brands of latex gloves or between the brands of the vinyl gloves was not significant—see D4. The bottom line is that latex is generally better than vinyl in offering protection, particularly during use. However, neither performed well at preventing bacteria from penetrating.

Discussion

Determine implications for practice:

- Practice implications are seen in E6, where it stated that hands should be washed after patient care even if gloves are worn. Limits were discussed in E5 where it was stated that bacterial test results occurred only under simulated conditions and risk of transmission was not studied. Study results were tied to the literature in E2 and E3. The bottom line is that gloves offer some barrier protection, and latex is generally better than vinyl. However, gloves should not be relied on for complete protection and should not replace handwashing.

Student Challenge

Evaluation and Visualisation

Now that you have read the article three times, it's time to do a general evaluation of the article and visualise practice applications.

1. Use the questions given in the research reading strategy earlier in this chapter to decide whether the study was a good one.
2. Think about how these results might be applied to your own practice.
3. Now read 'Evaluate and visualise the quantitative article' for a sample evaluation of the article and sample practice applications.

Evaluate and visualise the quantitative article

This section evaluates the quality of the sample article and then discusses how the results might be used in clinical practice. Your evaluation may differ from ours, just as our levels of comprehension and understanding differ. Thus what seems clear-cut to us may not seem so clear to you. Your ideas for application to your clinical practice may also differ. The applications stated here are general. Hopefully, yours is individualised to your personal situation.

This article is good. The key elements of the study are easy to identify, and the steps of the process generally are easy to follow. The ideas are presented clearly. The introductory argument clearly leads to the primary purpose of the article. Methods are described clearly. There is some confusion over the sample and sampling technique, but the procedure is discernible. Reliability and validity issues could have been directly addressed. The results are succinctly presented and logical. The study findings are easy to understand and are clearly tied to existing knowledge. Convenience sampling means the results must be confined to the gloves tested. However, because these results are consistent with other study results, the findings can be applied to clinical situations with some degree of confidence.

As nurses, we should use gloves to provide some measure of barrier protection against disease. Latex is a better choice than vinyl. However, we should not rely on gloves to provide complete protection against bacteria. Thorough and frequent handwashing is still essential before and after patient contact, whether or not gloves are worn.

Qualitative research example

You have made it through the research reading strategy process using a quantitative article as an example. Now we are going to repeat the process using a qualitative article. So, if you are ready to move ahead, try the following Student Challenge.

> **Student Challenge**
>
> Qualitative Survey and Examination
> 1. From the CD-ROM, print the qualitative research comprehension guidelines and the qualitative research article entitled 'The lived experience of postpartum depression: a phenomenological study'. This article was selected because it is relatively short, appears in the same format as the previous article, and is written for an audience not familiar with the phenomenological method.
> 2. Each part of the article has been labelled with a letter and a number (e.g. A1). The letter corresponds to the six sections of a standard research article. The numbers identify subsections of the specific section.

> 3 Now survey the article using Step 1 of your research reading strategy. Make notes of what you gleaned from your survey.
>
> 4 Now reread the article and jot down the key idea in each paragraph, making note of anything confusing. After you have finished, read 'Survey and examine the qualitative article'.

Survey and examine the qualitative article

The title (A1) tells us this study is a qualitative phenomenological study and the phenomenon under investigation is postpartum depression. The author (A2, A5) holds a doctorate, is a certified nurse midwife and a faculty member at a college of nursing. The article was published five months after acceptance. The abstract (A3) succinctly identifies the study design, purpose, sample size, method of analysis and results. An immediate picture is painted of postpartum depression as a distressing experience. After we finished with the abstract, we were hooked and wanted to know the details of life for these women.

A quick survey of the article reveals a well-organised approach to presentation of the study. Elements of the research process are clearly labelled and well-defined. Each theme is identified, discussed and illustrated with a concrete example from actual data. References cover the 1960s to the mid-1980s, are clearly related to the topic under study and include international sources and sources from various disciplines, as well as several references about the phenomenological research process.

At this point you should be getting pretty good at pulling key ideas from a paragraph, so the following are selected examples from identified paragraphs.

C1 Purposive sample of seven women from a postpartum support group for whom the researcher was a facilitator. Sample description: 22 to 38 years old, high school/college educated, primiparas/multiparas, vaginal/C-section, all but one under psychiatric care.

C7 Data analysis—interview transcripts analysed using Colaizzi's six-step method **(specific method used in phenomenological analysis)**: (1) read, (2) extract phrases directly related to postpartum depression, (3) formulate meaning, (4) organise into themes, (5) integrate data analysis, (6) return to participants to validate.

C8, C9 Credibility, auditability and fittingness were addressed using member checks and audit trails. **(These are specific terms used by phenomenologists to look at the confirmability of results. *Confirmability* is a concept parallel to the concepts of credibility [validity] and accuracy [reliability], which were discussed in Chapter 6. *Fittingness* is a somewhat vague concept that refers to whether the study results fit the data and are understood by the reader.)**

D2 Theme 1: Loneliness

D3 Loneliness because women felt no one understood, pleas for understanding ignored, so began to isolate selves.

D4 Theme 2: Death seen as hope.

D5 Death seen as a way out of living hell.

D6 Theme 3: Consumed by obsessive thoughts of experience and being a bad mother.

D7 Obsessive thinking left them mentally and physically exhausted, but sleep was not possible because of racing thoughts.

Student Challenge

Qualitative Critical Reading

1. Now that you have examined the article and summarised the key ideas, go back and read the article a third time using the qualitative research comprehension guidelines.
2. Locate and record each key element of the research process.
3. Now read 'Critically read the qualitative article' for confirmation of what you found.

Critically read the qualitative article

This section identifies the key elements of the research process used in our sample article. It follows the qualitative guidelines. The location of the identified elements in the article is indicated by the appropriate paragraph code.

Introduction

Determine what phenomena are being studied:
- The purpose of the study is stated in the abstract (A3) and in the introduction at the end of the paragraph B3. A research question is also present in B3 and stated as 'What is the essential structure of the lived experience of postpartum depression?' The phenomenon is postpartum depression.

Determine the context of the study:
- Literature review is used to establish a need and clarify terms (B1 to B4). Study importance is developed in paragraphs B1, B3 and B4. Depression occurs in 10 to 26 per cent of mothers (B1). No qualitative research is available on the experience (B3). Results could be used to enhance content validity of quantitative instruments (B4).

Methods

Determine how the study was conducted:
- Phenomenological research design was used (A1, A3, C2). A description of phenomenology as a philosophy is described in C2, and phenomenology as a research design is described in C3.
- Sampling is purposive (C1); sample was taken from a postpartum support group (C1, C4).

- Data were collected using interviews (C4) and bracketing (C5).
- Interviews were taped and transcribed (C6).
- Collection continued until repetition occurred with no new themes (C6). Setting was a private home or private interview in a psychiatric clinic (C6).
- Reliability and validity issues are covered in C8.
- Credibility was examined using a member check and auditability (audit trail).
- Accuracy was examined by using tape recordings, verbatim transcriptions and an independent judge experienced in phenomenological analysis to check each stage of analysis.

Determine how study was analysed:
- Analysis used Colaizzi's method (C7). Significant statements are presented in Table 1 and decision trail examples in Table 2.

Results

Examine a description of the subjects:
- Description is found in C1. Mothers who were in a support group, 22 to 38 years of age, high school or college educated, both primiparas and multiparas, both vaginal and caesarian section (C-section) deliveries. Six were under psychiatric care.

Determine the answers found by the study:
- Results were discussed as identified themes. Themes can be found in D2 to D26. Eleven themes are identified and discussed. Specific examples are quoted. The eleven themes are loneliness, suicidal thoughts, obsessive thoughts, grieving over loss of normalcy, emptiness of life, guilt and fear, inability to concentrate, going through the motions, uncontrollable anxiety, loss of emotional control, and need to be mothered.

Discussion

Determine the implications for nursing practice:
- A direct relationship to practice is not discussed. The focus is on using results to improve quantitative instruments (E1 to E3). Results are related to existing tools.

Student Challenge

Evaluation and Visualisation

Now that you have read the article three times, it is time to do a general evaluation of the article and visualise practice applications.

1. Use the questions given in the research reading strategy earlier in this chapter to decide whether the study was a good one.
2. Think about how these results might be applied to your clinical practice.
3. Now review 'Evaluate and visualise the qualitative article' for a sample evaluation of the article and sample practice applications.

Evaluate and visualise the qualitative article

This study is easy to follow. The steps of the process are identified easily and described clearly. After reading the results, a picture emerges as to what it might be like to suffer from postpartum depression. Included data support the identified themes. It would have been helpful if the discussion had included uses of the results in clinical practice.

The themes are relevant to clinical practice. The picture painted of postpartum depression enhances the nurse's ability to identify and more adequately assess signs and symptoms of potential postpartum depression. It allows for greater identification, understanding and empathy with a client who has postpartum depression. The themes can lend direction to interventions, including such actions as referral for support or counselling and suicide precautions. For a psychiatric or maternal–child nurse who participated in individual or group support sessions, this information might help facilitate such sessions.

Resource Kit

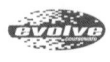

Visit the book's Evolve website at http://evolve.elsevier.com/AU/Borbasi/maze for further information.

Check out the puzzles, mazes and games on your CD-ROM.

References

Beck CT (1992). The lived experiences of postpartum depression: a phenomenological study. *Nursing Research* 41(3):166.

Korniewicz DM, Laughon B, Butz A et al (1989). Integrity of vinyl and latex procedure gloves. *Nursing Research* 38(3):144.

Section 3

Walking the Walk

Applying Research Results in a Variety of Clinical Practice Situations … Practise, Practise, Practise

The ability to consistently read and apply nursing research requires that you become comfortable with your new strategic skills. This means practising these skills with research articles from various sources across a wide range of clinical practice situations. This will allow you to become more proficient at using the strategic reading technique, and to discover a wide range of uses for research results. This section is designed to let you practise and develop your skills as a research consumer, by examining and applying example research results across the lifespan. Finally, the concept of research utilisation is explored, and you are provided with approaches, criteria and strategies to enhance your research utilisation capabilities.

http://evolve.elsevier.com/AU/Borbasi/maze

Learning Objectives

After reading this chapter and following critical reflection the student will be able to:

1. Identify maternal–infant clinical nursing journals that publish research articles.
2. Discuss clinical and research priorities in the practice of maternal–infant nursing.
3. Use research literature to clarify identified maternal–infant practice problems.
4. Explore examples of research studies conducted in various areas of maternal–infant clinical practice.
5. Discuss the application of sample research results in clinical practice.
6. Apply the reading strategy to survey, examine, critically read and evaluate sample research articles on maternal–infant care.

Chapter Outline

What Research Resources Are Available on Mothers and Infants?
What Approaches Can Be Used for Review of the Research Literature?
Addressing clinical and research priorities
Using issues that arise from clinical practice
Scanning available resources
What Current Research Is Available?
Nursing research journals
Clinical nursing journals
Other journals
Summarising and using scanning results
How to Read and Evaluate a Research Article on Maternal–Infant Care

Chapter 8
Reading and Using Research in Maternal–Infant Care

I know the study said we needed to improve patient–staff ratios, but we seem to be taking it just a bit too far.

Student Quote
'In clinical conference, we discussed a research article that I had found on how to improve feeding patterns in a premie. I really felt like I was contributing to better care.'

Abstract
Several research sources publish articles pertinent to maternal–infant care. These sources can be used to view the latest research on maternal–infant care and research priorities, address identified problems and questions uncovered in clinical practice, or provide a broad view of currently available maternal–infant research. Abundant current research studies are available for use in the clinical practice of maternal–infant care. Samples of current studies are reported, and clinical applications are discussed. The use of the research reading strategy is illustrated with one maternal–infant research article.

You now have a reading strategy, and we have tentatively tested that strategy on two sample articles. The next four chapters are designed to allow you the opportunity to develop and hone your abilities to find, read, interpret and apply research findings in specified clinical situations and settings. This and the next three chapters are divided using a lifespan schema. Chapter 8 covers maternal–infant care, Chapter 9 looks at children and adolescents, Chapter 10 discusses adults, and Chapter 11 addresses older adults.

In this chapter we identify additional publications that contain nursing research on maternal–infant care, explore strategies to simplify the search process and target relevant research articles, and preview sample selections of currently published research. Finally, we dissect a sample article using the reading strategy and evaluation criteria presented in Chapter 7.

What Research Resources Are Available on Mothers and Infants?

To effectively view the current research in maternal–infant care, it is helpful to be able to identify resources that are likely to contain research articles on the maternal–infant experience. All the research journals we have discussed in previous chapters contain articles on maternal–infant care. Several clinical specialty journals also regularly publish research articles on maternal–infant care. Clinical journals in other specialty areas such as paediatrics, community health or mental health nursing also occasionally contain research articles relevant to maternal–infant care. The journals listed in Box 8-1 are most likely to contain research relevant to the practice of maternal–infant care.

BOX 8-1 Journals Containing Maternal–Infant Nursing Research

Nursing Research Journals
Nursing Research
Australian Journal of Advanced Nursing
International Journal of Nursing Practice
Journal of Advanced Nursing
Research in Nursing and Health
Applied Nursing Research
Nursing Science Quarterly
Journal of Nursing Scholarship

Clinical Journals that Regularly Contain Research Articles About Maternal–Infant Care
Neonatal, Paediatric and Child Health Nursing

MCN: The American Journal of Maternal Child Nursing
Journal of Obstetric, Gynecologic, and Neonatal Nursing
Neonatal Network. Journal of Neonatal Nursing
Pediatric Nursing

Student Challenge

Perusing Specialty Journals

1. If some of the journals listed in Box 8-1 are unfamiliar to you, take time to locate those available in your library. Scan two or three issues of each journal.
2. Note how they are organised. What types of articles are prevalent? Can you readily distinguish research articles from other featured articles? Do you notice a difference in the focus of the various journals?
3. Where might you locate a description of the journal's focus or purpose? (Locate one electronic and one print source.)
4. Do you see any differences between articles in research journals and research articles in clinical journals? Can you detect differences in presentation and article selection among the various research journals? What about differences in the content and style of research articles in the various clinical journals? Are some journals more readable than others? More helpful?

As you become more familiar with the various clinical and research journals you should begin to note which provide the most useful information for improving maternal–infant care. You should also discover that journals have varying foci and purposes, as well as differing formats and reading levels. Discover which journals are most helpful to you.

What Approaches Can Be Used for Review of the Research Literature?

There are three major ways we might approach the current research literature to help guide and enhance our clinical practice for mothers and infants.
- One is dictated by the clinical and research priorities that have been identified in the area of maternal–infant health care.
- A second is dictated by problems you routinely encounter in your day-to-day clinical practice with mothers and their infants.
- A third approach is to regularly scan the readily available published resources.

Addressing clinical and research priorities

Keeping informed of the current clinical and research priorities in a given area can help direct and guide your practice with whatever target population you choose to work on. Let's use mothers and infants as an example. The overall goal in maternal–infant care is focused on improving outcomes for mothers and infants. Priority issues in maternal–infant care and research can be drawn from several sources. These sources include Australian-specific sources such as the National Health and Medical Research Council (NH&MRC) Strategic and Priority Driven Research (SPDR) objectives, and the Commonwealth Department of Health and Ageing, as well as international and global sources such as the (US) National Institute of Nursing Research (NINR), and the World Health Organization global nursing research priorities.

Research priorities assist you in identifying areas of concern in your own practice as well as letting you know what areas of care receive funding priority for research. The NH&MRC identify research that focuses on pregnancy and maternal–infant care for Australia's Indigenous people as a priority area and this is a response to poorer maternal–infant outcomes in Indigenous communities than are seen in other Australian communities. Internationally, the American Association of Women's Health, Obstetrical, and Neonatal Nurses (AWHONN) has generated a list of clinically relevant areas that are viewed as research priorities. These can be viewed by visiting their website (http://www.awhonn.org) and include research on preventing unintended pregnancy, cardiovascular health, weight management, cancer screening, women's health and stress management. Although many professional and consumer organisations don't have published research priorities, they all have some sort of clinical, educational or outcomes-based aims and these also can give you an insight into the types of research areas they would support.

> **BOX 8-2** Some Organisations Concerned with Maternal–Infant Care
>
> Australian College of Midwives
> Perinatal Research Centre (Royal Women's Hospital Foundation and University of Queensland)
> New Zealand College of Midwives Inc
> Karitane
> Australian Neonatal Nurses Association
> Women's and Children's Hospitals
> Australian Breastfeeding Association
> La Leche League
> Pregnancy and Newborn Services Network (NSW)

> **Student Challenge**
>
> Checking Maternal–Infant Priorities
>
> 1 Go to the SIDS Australia website (http://www.sidsaustralia.org.au/). Have a look at the areas that have been researched to try to find the causes and the ways of preventing SIDS. Can you identify any current priorities?
>
> 2 Look at the list of organisations in Box 8-2. Visit some of the websites and look for research priorities related to maternal–infant care.
>
> 3 Can you locate any other sources or organisations that list or discuss priorities in maternal–infant care or research?
>
> 4 Choose one of the priority areas that you have discovered. Run a literature search for the years 2000 to the present and see what, if any, nursing research has been conducted in your selected area. Did you find anything that might be applicable to the clinical area of maternal–infant care?

Using issues that arise from clinical practice

When you practise in a particular clinical setting and interact on a regular basis with mothers and their infants, certain questions and problems routinely arise in the course of providing care. Answers to some of these problems may be found in the research literature. When a problem surfaces you may wish to define that problem by certain parameters before going to the literature. If you have a clear frame of reference from which to think about nursing care, it makes the search and use of research materials much easier. You need to ask yourself questions such as who is the target of care—the mother, the infant, the mother–infant dyad or the family unit? You might clarify what phase of care is involved (e.g. antepartum, intrapartum or postpartum for the mother; fetus, newborn or neonate for the infant). What level of care is involved? Is the problem one of prevention, acute care or chronic care? The aspect of care is also important. Are you concerned with physical, psychological, sociocultural or spiritual needs? Finally, what care setting did the problem arise in—a clinic, physician's office, home or the hospital?

For example, we may be working in a hospital postnatal ward. We notice that many of our patients have trouble establishing breast feeding and develop cracked nipples. We wonder if there is anything we can do to assist these women in establishing breast feeding and maintaining nipple integrity. The target of concern is mothers. The care setting is a hospital postnatal ward. A search using Journals@Ovid with the key words 'maternal', 'breast feeding' and 'cracked nipples' for the years 1999–2001 produces six articles. Five are about HIV transmission and breast feeding, and the other is about hepatitis C transmission. We find no research articles to help guide our practice. If we include 1998 in the search, additional articles are retrieved. Of these, two are about HIV transmission (Tess et al 1998a, 1998b), one reports a trial of wound dressings versus conventional care for women with sore nipples (Brent et al 1998), one is about supplements to breast feeding (Campbell 1998) and the other is about promoting breast feeding (Rossiter 1998). None of these shed much light on our problem. We can see that this is an area where research is needed.

We might work in a neonatal intensive care unit and be concerned about the fact that many of the premature infants seem to have patches of skin loss as a result of various treatments and procedures. This is raised at a clinical care review meeting in the unit and we wonder if there are things we can do to decrease this problem. Currently there is no skin protocol in the unit. A MEDLINE search for three years using the key words 'premature', 'infant' and 'skin' yields a total of five articles. Two are research articles (Maguire 1999, Munson et al 1999). One discusses skin care protocols or management in infants (Lund 1999), another reviews the existing literature on neonatal skin care from 1993 to 1999 (Lund et al 1999) and the final one discusses the thermoregulation and fluid maintenance problems associated with the congenital absence of skin in some preterm infants. This last article is deemed irrelevant. The third and fourth articles serve to provide baseline data from which to better read the two research articles.

The first research article (Maguire 1999) is a quantitative descriptive survey of registered nurses from 215 different neonatal intensive care units (NICUs) in the United States. The nurses were asked questions to describe and measure the incidence of skin breakdown in low-birthweight infants in their units and to describe interventions to treat or prevent breakdown. Findings determined that about 20 per cent of low-birthweight infants suffered from skin breakdown across the 215 units. Those nurses reporting the least breakdown followed skin care protocols that limited use of tape and made liberal use of Aquaphor as a skin barrier. Recommendations included further study of the effectiveness of various products used to treat breakdown. This study might lead the way for us to propose to the clinical care committee that the unit adopt a standard skin care protocol and perhaps try Aquaphor as a skin breakdown prevention measure.

The second research article (Munson et al 1999) is a descriptive survey of 104 hospitals that deliver at least 2500 babies a year and have a level III NICU with at least 20 beds. The purpose of the survey was to ascertain current skin care practices and protocols. This study reinforced the fact that 25 per cent of the surveyed hospitals had no standard protocols, and the others surveyed showed a wide variation in their approach to skin care.

The identification of a specific clinical problem often sheds more light on the research that still needs to be conducted than on the research that is available. Literature searches targeted at specifically identified clinical problems can still prove worthwhile and may provide much needed help for a vexing clinical situation.

> **Student Challenge**
>
> Chasing Maternal–Infant Challenges
>
> 1. Review your experiences in maternal–infant nursing and think about a situation you wish to explore in the current research literature.
> 2. Identify appropriate search parameters for the subject material and conduct a library search for the year 2000 to the present.
> 3. What did you find? (Hint: If your search yielded too many entries, try one of the following ideas. If you conducted an electronic MEDLINE search, try creating a specialised journal list. List only those journals found in Box 8-1. Then perform your search. The search mechanism will be confined to those journals. If you are conducting an electronic CINAHL search, try limiting results to research by checking that option on the search page. If you had too few entries, broaden your search parameters or check the related reference option available on MEDLINE.)
> 4. If your search was fruitful, retrieve one or two promising articles. (Remember, abstracts and key words are very helpful in deciding if an article is worth retrieving.)
> 5. Review the article. How might the results of the study be helpful to you in your clinical practice or your clinical learning?

Scanning available resources

As you have just seen, your clinical practice and the concerns that arise from day-to-day experience often lead to a search for research literature that may prove helpful and be of interest. However, many students say such things as, 'I don't know enough yet to identify areas of concern in practice' or 'I can identify things that need attention, but I'm not sure what the standard of care is, let alone the new or changing care'. One way to get connected to the research literature in a particular area such as maternal–infant nursing is to regularly scan the tables of contents and the abstracts of the research and clinical specialty journals listed in Box 8-1. Look at what is available. Ask yourself if any of the articles seem relevant to what you are currently learning or practising in the clinical area. If so, check out the full article. Use the research results you have found in your nursing care plans and in clinical conferences. Bring relevant articles into your workplace and let others see them. Some wards and units have journal clubs and journal discussion groups to encourage nurses to engage with the literature and keep up with new research findings.

Your Student Challenge asks you to look at two journals for a period of one year. However, an effective scan must take into account several journals that are likely to contain maternal–infant research. You can conduct a fairly rapid scan of several journals through the use of the internet and your electronic library resources. Several publishing websites on the internet allow you to peruse the tables of contents and abstracts for various journals. Your library may also permit you to access the current abstracts of several journals. Some of these journals even have the entire article available online for reading and/or downloading. The publishing company websites usually charge a fee for these services, but they are often free through your library if you are a cardholder. In addition we know of at least one full-text collection that can be programmed to run an automatic search for a selected topic(s) and post any new citations to your email address (ask your librarian about this service). Check out the Resource Kit at the end of this chapter for a list of helpful publishing company journal sites, and then use the book's Evolve website to get a link to one of these journals.

Activity 13

Armed with these tools plus MEDLINE and CINAHL search capabilities, it is possible to do a periodic journal scan from the comfort of your own home. You need only go to the library once you have pinpointed articles (not available online) that seem relevant to your practice. Some libraries will even allow you to pay a fee for delivery of articles to your doorstep. We suggest conducting a scan about once every six months. When you get proficient, you can conduct a scan of all of the journals listed in Box 8-1 in about two hours.

> **Student Challenge**
>
> Scanning Maternal–Infant Journals
>
> 1. Select one research journal and one clinical journal from those listed in Box 8-1 that are available in your library.
> 2. Scan the year 2000 table of contents for each of these journals and note those articles that seem relevant to maternal–infant care.
> 3. Read the abstracts for the selected articles. Weed out any articles that are not clinically relevant. How long did this take you? Did you use electronic resources or the actual journal?
> 4. Save these articles. We will use them again in the next exercise.

What Current Research Is Available?

The following are specific examples of pertinent maternal–infant research articles that we found by simply scanning the 2001 issues of the research and clinical journals listed in Box 8-1. Selected articles are briefly summarised and clinical implications are discussed. The articles are arranged by journal. This allows you to see which of the journals might provide you with the most insight about various maternal–infant clinical topics.

Nursing research journals

The articles found by scanning the tables of contents of the various research journals yielded the list of possibly relevant maternal–infant articles shown in Box 8-3.

> **BOX 8-3** Relevant Maternal–Infant Article Titles in Research Journals
>
> **Nursing Research**
> Goodwin LK, Iannacchione M, Hammond W et al (2001). Data mining methods find demographic predictors of preterm birth. *Nursing Research* 50(6):340–345.
> Holditch-Davis D, Miles MS, Burchinal M et al (2001). Parental caregiving and developmental outcomes of infants of mothers with HIV. *Nursing Research* 50(1):5–14.
> Nantais-Smith LM, Covington CY, Nordstrom-Klee BA et al (2001). Differences in plasma and nipple aspirate carotenoid by lactation status. *Nursing Research* 50(3):172–176.
> Zhou Q, O'Brien B, Soeken K (2001). Rhodes Index of nausea and vomiting-form 2 in pregnant women: A confirmatory factor analysis. *Nursing Research* 50(4):251–257.
>
> **Australian Journal of Advanced Nursing**
> Harvey J, Moyle W, Creedy D (2001). Women's experience of early miscarriage: a phenomenological study. *Australian Journal of Advanced Nursing* 19(1):8–14.
> Scott D, Brady S, Glynn P (2001). A new mothers group as a social network intervention: consumer and maternal and child health nurse perspectives. *Australian Journal of Advanced Nursing* 18(4):23–29.
>
> **International Journal of Nursing Practice**
> No relevant articles
>
> **Journal of Advanced Nursing**
> Baggens C (2001). What they talk about: conversations between child health centre nurses and parents. *Journal of Advanced Nursing* 36(5):659–667.
> Bailey J, Rose P (2001). Axillary and tympanic membrane temperature recording in the preterm neonate: a comparative study. *Journal of Advanced Nursing* 34(4):465–474.
> Baker A, Ferguson SA, Roach GD et al (2001). Perceptions of labour pain by mothers and their attending midwives. *Journal of Advanced Nursing* 35(2):171–179.

Burrows J (2001). The parturient woman: can there be room for more than 'one person with full and equal rights inside a single human skin'? *Journal of Advanced Nursing* 33(5):689–695.

Cahill HA (2001). Male appropriation and medicalization of childbirth: an historical analysis. *Journal of Advanced Nursing* 33(3):334–342.

Davies MM, Bath PA (2001). The maternity information concerns of Somali women in the United Kingdom. *Journal of Advanced Nursing* 36(2):237–245.

Fenwick J, Barclay L, Schmied V (2001). 'Chatting': an important clinical tool in facilitating mothering in neonatal nurseries. *Journal of Advanced Nursing* 33(5):583–593.

Hanna B (2001). Negotiating motherhood: the struggles of teenage mothers. *Journal of Advanced Nursing* 34(4):456–464.

Huang Y-C, Mathers N (2001). Postnatal depression—biological or cultural? A comparative study of postnatal women in the UK and Taiwan. *Journal of Advanced Nursing* 33(3):279–287.

Hung C-H, Chung H-H (2001). The effects of postpartum stress and social support on postpartum women's health status. *Journal of Advanced Nursing* 36(5):676–684.

Kearney PM, Griffin T (2001). Between joy and sorrow: being a parent of a child with developmental disability. *Journal of Advanced Nursing* 34(5):582–592.

Mander R (2001). The perfect baby: parenthood in the new world of cloning and genetics. *Journal of Advanced Nursing* 36(5):711.

Pridham KF, Kosorok MR, Greer F et al (2001). Comparison of caloric intake and weight outcomes of an ad lib feeding regimen for preterm infants in two nurseries. *Journal of Advanced Nursing* 35(5):751–759.

Pridham KF, Schroeder M, Brown R et al (2001). The relationship of a mother's working model of feeding to her feeding behaviour. *Journal of Advanced Nursing* 35(5):741–750.

Robinson JJ, Wharrad H (2001). The relationship between attendance at birth and maternal mortality rates: an exploration of United Nations' data sets including the ratios of physicians and nurses to population, GNP per capita and female literacy. *Journal of Advanced Nursing* 34(4):445–455.

Symon A (2001). A social history of wet nursing in America. *Journal of Advanced Nursing* 36(3):478.

Wilson HV (2001). Power and partnership: a critical analysis of the surveillance discourses of child health nurses. *Journal of Advanced Nursing* 36(2):294–301.

Nursing Science Quarterly
No relevant articles

Journal of Nursing Scholarship
Domian EW (2001). Cultural practices and social support of pregnant women in a Northern New Mexico community. *Journal of Nursing Scholarship* 33(4):331–336.
Gaffney KF (2001). Infant exposure to environmental tobacco smoke. *Journal of Nursing Scholarship* 33(4):343–347.
Gantt CJ (2001). The theory of planned behavior and postpartum smoking relapse. *Journal of Nursing Scholarship* 33(4):337–341.
Horowitz JA, Bell M, Trybulski J et al (2001). Promoting responsiveness between mothers with depressive symptoms and their infants. *Journal of Nursing Scholarship* 33(4):323–329.

Scholarly Inquiry for Nursing Practice
No relevant articles

A scan of the 2001 issues of *Nursing Research* reveals four potentially relevant articles. An examination of the titles quickly reveals a study that focuses on parental caregiving and infant developmental outcomes where the mother has HIV (Holditch-Davis et al 2001). Nausea and vomiting in pregnancy was the focus of another of the articles (Zhou et al 2001). One study looks at demographic predictors for preterm birth (Goodwin et al 2001), while the remaining one scrutinised lactation and its effect on the transportation of the dietary antioxidant carotenoid into the micro environment of the breast (Nantais-Smith et al 2001). Further examination of article abstracts shows that all six articles might provide relevant information for varying clinical situations. Further selection would need to be based on your own clinical position, setting and interests.

Issues of the *Journal of Advanced Nursing* published in 2001 contain 17 articles of interest to maternal–infant nurses. These focused on a range of topics, including infant feeding (Pridham 2001), postpartum stress and social support (Hung & Chung 2001), women's and midwives' perceptions of labour pain (Baker et al 2001), and a comparative study of tympanic and axillary temperature recording in premature neonates (Bailey & Rose 2001). Relationships between nurses and midwives and mothers was the focus of two of the papers; one explored chatting in nurseries as a way of facilitating mothering (Fenwick et al 2001), and the other looked at the nature of the talk between nurses and mothers in child health centres (Baggens 2001). Special groups of mothers were the focus of two of the papers, with one raising issues related to teen mothers and the other to a group of Somali women in the United Kingdom (Davies & Bath 2001). One paper examines the experiences of parents who have a child with a developmental disability (Kearney & Griffin 2001). Huang & Mathers (2001) authored a paper reporting a comparative study on postnatal women in the UK and Taiwan, and raised questions about culture and its relationship to postnatal depression. Several of these articles are published reports of research conducted in Australia.

The *Australian Journal of Advanced Nursing* had two relevant articles in 2001. One was a phenomenological study of women's experiences of early miscarriage (Harvey et al 2001). The other reported the perspectives of nurses and mothers on first-time parent groups. The researchers looked in particular at how nurses facilitated these groups, the role of the groups in developing social networks, and the self-sustainability of these groups (Scott et al 2001).

The *Journal of Nursing Scholarship* contained four articles of interest. Two of these pertained to tobacco smoking: one looked at infant exposure to tobacco smoke (Gaffney 2001), while the other focused on postpartum relapse of smoking (Gantt 2001). The other two focused on particular groups of mothers. One of these considered issues related to culture and social support for pregnant women in a particular geographic location (Domian 2001), and the other looked at responsiveness interactions between infants and mothers with depressive symptoms (Horowitz et al 2001). No relevant articles were found in the *International Journal of Nursing Practice* or *Nursing Science Quarterly*.

Examining the titles of the articles across all the research journals revealed a total of 27 articles, and these included a majority on mothers, three on infants, two on maternal–infant dyads, and five about ethics and other philosophical issues of interest. The papers on mothers covered a range of issues including care in labour, postpartum depression, social support and maternal mortality. Of the three articles on infant care, two focused on the preterm infant. Published papers reported both qualitative and quantitative studies.

Clinical nursing journals

The articles found by scanning the tables of contents of the clinical journals yielded the list of possibly relevant maternal–infant research articles shown in Box 8-4.

> **BOX 8-4** Relevant Maternal–Infant Research Article Titles in Clinical Journals
>
> **MCN: The American Journal of Maternal Child Nursing**
> Armstrong D (2001). Exploring fathers' experiences of pregnancy after a prior perinatal loss. *The American Journal of Maternal Child Nursing* 26(3):147–153, 160–161.
> Barton SJ (2001). Infant feeding practices of low-income rural mothers. *The American Journal of Maternal Child Nursing* 26(2):93–97.
> Callister LC (2001). Giving birth: perceptions of Finnish childbearing women. *The American Journal of Maternal Child Nursing* 26(1):28–32.

Davis RE (2001). The postpartum experience for Southeast Asian women in the United States. *The American Journal of Maternal Child Nursing* 26(4):208–213.

DiMarco MA (2001). Evaluating a support group for perinatal loss. *The American Journal of Maternal Child Nursing* 26(3):135–140, 160–161.

Dombrowski MA (2001). Kangaroo (skin-to-skin) care with a postpartum woman who felt depressed. *The American Journal of Maternal Child Nursing* 26(4):214–216.

Evers DB (2001). Teaching mothers about childhood immunizations. *The American Journal of Maternal Child Nursing* 26(5):253–256.

Fogel CI (2001). Psychological risk factors in pregnant inmates: a challenge for nursing. *The American Journal of Maternal Child Nursing* 26(1):10–16.

Foss GF (2001). Maternal sensitivity, posttraumatic stress, and acculturation in Vietnamese and Hmong mothers. *The American Journal of Maternal Child Nursing* 26(5):257–263.

Gale J (2001). Measuring nursing support during childbirth. *The American Journal of Maternal Child Nursing* 26(5):264–271.

Steward DK (2001). Behavioral characteristics of infants with nonorganic failure to thrive during a play interaction. *The American Journal of Maternal Child Nursing* 26(2):79–85.

Wu T (2001). Growth of immigrant Chinese infants in the first year of life. *The American Journal of Maternal Child Nursing* 26(4):202–207.

Journal of Obstetric, Gynecologic, and Neonatal Nursing

Adams C (2001). Breastfeeding trends at a community breastfeeding center: an evaluative survey. *Journal of Obstetric, Gynecologic, and Neonatal Nursing* 30(4):392–400.

Callister LC (2001). Culturally competent care of women and newborns: knowledge, attitude, and skills. *Journal of Obstetric, Gynecologic, and Neonatal Nursing* 30(2):209–215.

Clemmens D (2001). The relationship between social support and adolescent mothers' interactions with their infants: a meta-analysis. *Journal of Obstetric, Gynecologic, and Neonatal Nursing* 30(4):410–420.

Coyer SM (2001). Mothers recovering from cocaine addiction: factors affecting parenting skills. *Journal of Obstetric, Gynecologic, and Neonatal Nursing* 30(1):71–79.

Gagnon AJ (2001). Indicators nurses employ in deciding to test for hyperbilirubinemia. *Journal of Obstetric, Gynecologic, and Neonatal Nursing* 30(6):626–633.

Gill SL (2001). The little things: perceptions of breastfeeding support. *Journal of Obstetric, Gynecologic, and Neonatal Nursing* 30(4):401–409.

Gupton A (2001). Complicated and uncomplicated pregnancies: women's perception of risk. *Journal of Obstetric, Gynecologic, and Neonatal Nursing* 30(2):192–201.

Hulsey TM (2001). Association between early prenatal care and mother's intention of and desire for the pregnancy. *Journal of Obstetric, Gynecologic, and Neonatal Nursing* 30(3):275–282.

Lund CH (2001). Neonatal skin care: evaluation of the AWHONN/NANN Research-Based Practice Project on knowledge and skin care practices. *Journal of Obstetric, Gynecologic, and Neonatal Nursing* 30(1):30–40.

Lund CH (2001). Neonatal skin care: clinical outcomes of the AWHONN/NANN Evidence-Based Clinical Practice Guideline. *Journal of Obstetric, Gynecologic, and Neonatal Nursing* 30(1):41–51.

McCarter-Spaulding DE (2001). Parenting self-efficacy and perception of insufficient breast milk. *Journal of Obstetric, Gynecologic, and Neonatal Nursing* 30(5):515–522.

Macke JK (2001). Analgesia for circumcision: effects on newborn behavior and mother/infant interaction. *Journal of Obstetric, Gynecologic, and Neonatal Nursing* 30(5):507–514.

Maloni JA (2001). Antepartum bed rest: effect upon the family. *Journal of Obstetric, Gynecologic, and Neonatal Nursing* 30(2):165–173.

Martell LK (2001). Heading toward the new normal: a contemporary postpartum experience. *Journal of Obstetric, Gynecologic, and Neonatal Nursing* 30(5):496–506.

Mellien AC (2001). Incubators versus mothers' arms: body temperature conservation in very-low-birth-weight premature infants. *Journal of Obstetric, Gynecologic, and Neonatal Nursing* 30(2):157–164.

Riordan J (2001). Breastfeeding care in multicultural populations. *Journal of Obstetric, Gynecologic, and Neonatal Nursing* 30(2):216–223.

Roberts L (2001). Birth center outcomes reported through automated technology. *Journal of Obstetric, Gynecologic, and Neonatal Nursing* 30(1):110–120.

Ruiz RJ (2001). Specialized care for twin gestations: improving newborn outcomes and reducing costs. *Journal of Obstetric, Gynecologic, and Neonatal Nursing* 30(1):52–60.

Spellacy CE (2001). Urinary incontinence in pregnancy and the puerperium. *Journal of Obstetric, Gynecologic, and Neonatal Nursing* 30(6):634–641.

Neonatal Network. Journal of Neonatal Nursing

Blackburn S (2001). Neonatal thermal care, part I: survey of temperature probe practices. *Neonatal Network. Journal of Neonatal Nursing* 20(3):15–18.

Blackburn S (2001). Neonatal thermal care, part II: microbial growth under temperature probe covers. *Neonatal Network. Journal of Neonatal Nursing* 20(3):19–23.

> Blackburn S (2001). Neonatal thermal care, part III: the effect of infant position and temperature probe placement. *Neonatal Network. Journal of Neonatal Nursing* 20(3):25–30.
>
> Dye E (2001). Use of translation cards to increase communication with non-English-speaking families in the NICU. *Neonatal Network. Journal of Neonatal Nursing* 20(7):25–29.
>
> Franck LS (2001). The safety and efficacy of peripheral intravenous catheters in ill neonates. *Neonatal Network. Journal of Neonatal Nursing* 20(5):33–38.
>
> Kellam B (2001). Tenderfoot Premie vs a manual lancet: a clinical evaluation. *Neonatal Network. Journal of Neonatal Nursing* 20(7):31–36.
>
> Pearson J (2001). Evaluation of a program to promote positive parenting in the neonatal intensive care unit. *Neonatal Network. Journal of Neonatal Nursing* 20(4):43–48.
>
> Pressler JL (2001). Behaviors of very preterm neonates as documented using NIDCAP observations. Newborn Individualized Developmental Care Assessment Program. *Neonatal Network. Journal of Neonatal Nursing* 20(8):15–24.

The scan netted 12 relevant research articles from *MCN: The American Journal of Maternal Child Nursing,* 19 articles from *Journal of Obstetric, Gynecologic and Neonatal Nursing,* and 8 articles from *Neonatal Network. Journal of Neonatal Nursing.* Of course, in addition to research reports, these journals contained numerous case studies, updates and other items of interest.

A survey of the research titles revealed 15 studies about infants, 20 on mothers, and 1 on fathers. The infant studies contained a number about the care of premature neonates, and focused on a range of issues including skin care, thermal regulation, the behaviour of these infants, and intravenous access. Other studies looked at full-term infants and these were about diverse issues including infant growth (Wu 2001), failure to thrive (Steward 2001), circumcision and infant feeding. The study about fathers looked at fathers' experiences of pregnancy after a perinatal loss (Armstrong 2001). Of the studies that dealt with mothers, several looked at aspects of breast feeding (see, for example: Adams 2001, Gill 2001, McCarter-Spaulding 2001), one concentrated on antepartum bedrest (Maloni 2001), while others looked at aspects of the postpartum period (see, for example: Dombrowski 2001, Spellacy 2001). It was very interesting to note that four of the papers explored maternal issues from the perspectives of various cultural groups such as Hmong (Foss 2001), Vietnamese (Foss 2001, Davis 2001) and Finnish women (Callister 2001). Other articles explored issues related to mothers with special needs and these special needs groups included adolescent mothers (Clemmens 2001) and expectant mothers in prison (Fogel 2001). Another paper reported an evaluative study of birthing centre outcomes. There was a mix of quantitative and qualitative research reported, with quite a number of studies concerned with women's experiences of pregnancy and birthing.

Other journals

Five other journal articles pertinent to maternal–infant care were also found across various other journals. The results are listed in Box 8-5. Of these five papers, three were qualitative and two quantitative, and various issues were explored. These included research reports of an action research approach to developing a clinical pathway for women requiring caesarian sections (Moody et al 2001); support for women caring for infants with sleep problems (Hanna & Rolls 2001); prevalence of exposure of Australian infants to cigarette smoke (Wiggers et al 2001); and risk factors for mastitis in breast feeding women (Kinlay et al 2001). So remember these likely ancillary sources when scanning for current maternal–infant research literature.

> **BOX 8-5** Relevant Maternal–Infant Research Article Titles from Miscellaneous Nursing Journals
>
> **Contemporary Nurse**
> Hanna B, Rolls C (2001). How do early parenting centers support women with an infant who has a sleep problem? *Contemporary Nurse* 11(2/3):153–162.
> Moody G, Choong Y, Greenwood J (2001). An action research approach to the development of a clinical pathway for women requiring caesarian sections. *Contemporary Nurse* 11(2/3):195–205.
>
> **Australian and New Zealand Journal of Public Health**
> Kinlay JR, O'Connell DL, Kinlay S (2001). Risk factors for mastitis in breastfeeding women: results of a prospective cohort study. *Australian and New Zealand Journal of Public Health* 25(2):115–120.
> Wiggers JH, Considine RJ, Daly JB (2001). Infant exposure to environmental tobacco smoke: a prevalence study in Australia. *Australian and New Zealand Journal of Public Health* 25(2):132–137.
>
> **Nursing Praxis in New Zealand**
> Smythe E (2001). The meaning of 'being responsible' for safe care in childbirth. *Nursing Praxis in New Zealand* 17(1):34–41.

Summarising and using scanning results

Two of the identified research articles have been selected to serve as examples of how research articles might be summarised and how the findings could be used to enhance knowledge that is useful in clinical practice. We have selected articles that focus on care provision in different settings. One reports a study that was undertaken in a hospital setting, and the other reports a study that took place in a residential early parenting centre.

Some of the articles looked at ways in which maternal–infant care delivery could be enhanced and made more efficient while still achieving positive and desired outcomes. Moody, Choong & Greenwood (2001) reported their use of a multi-disciplinary action–research approach to initiate and establish a clinical pathway for women admitted to Westmead Hospital (NSW) for caesarian section. Initial data were collected through review of the literature, focus groups of staff, and patient questionnaire. Reflective and planning processes were then used to develop and refine the clinical pathway prior to its implementation. Evaluative processes were thorough and revealed that use of the clinical pathway assisted with the women's need for knowledge about what would happen to them in hospital and how they could expect recovery to progress. Moody et al (2001) noted that experienced staff found no real benefit in using the clinical pathway because they were already confident and practised in the care of women undergoing caesarian section. However, the pathway was found to have a role in orientation of nurses, with student midwives and new staff finding it particularly helpful. This was because there was an improvement in the documentation and recording of day-to-day care received by the women. The researchers also reported that use of the pathway enhanced relationships among members of the multidisciplinary team, in that a greater sense of being part of a team was reported by the staff involved.

Other articles examined common maternal or infant problems. A study by Hanna & Rolls (2001) looked at infant sleep disturbance, its effects on family life, and how early parenting centres could best assist families. A qualitative focus group approach was used to collect data from parents admitted to a residential care facility to participate in a parenting program. Findings revealed that persistent infant sleep disturbances have a deleterious effect on family life, with participants reporting exhaustion, mood disturbance, friction and family disharmony. Women participants reported feeling overwhelmed by feelings of weariness and isolation, and feelings of failure as a mother. Male participants reported that arriving home from work was stressful. Participants reported trying various strategies to deal with the problem but some of these led to further family difficulties. For example, altering the family sleeping arrangements was one solution that was used, but this contributed to a loss of intimacy between the partners, and further jeopardised partner communications. Hanna & Rolls (2001) concluded that early parenting centres have a positive role in assisting parents who are experiencing difficulties with infant sleeping.

Now you have seen some examples of how studies are able to contribute to maternal–infant care across various settings. Practise with some articles of your own by completing the following Student Challenge.

> **Student Challenge**
>
> Using Data from Journal Scans
>
> Use the articles that resulted from your journal scan.
>
> 1. Read the articles to determine what and who was studied and what the study results were. Write a brief summary of each article as we have done with the articles by Moody et al (2001), and Hanna & Rolls (2001).
> 2. Read the discussion sections of the articles and make a quick determination of how the results might be used in a clinical practice setting. Write out how the findings might be used and by whom.

How to Read and Evaluate a Research Article on Maternal–Infant Care

Now that you have warmed up, we are going to examine one research article on maternal–infant care in more depth. We use the research reading strategy and the research study comprehension guidelines introduced in Chapter 7.

The CD-ROM exercises guide you through the critical reading, evaluation and visualisation of the selected research article. When you finish you will be able to print your answers and our responses to the exercises. You should be feeling more confident about reading a research article and pulling out the key ideas.

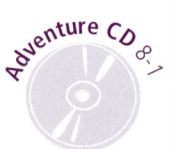
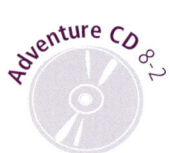
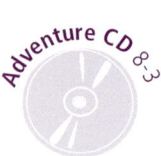

> **Student Challenge**
>
> Surveying and Examining a Maternal–Infant Research Study
>
> 1. Log on to your CD-ROM and look for the 'Survey, examine and critically read' exercise in Chapter 8. Print out the reading strategy and the research article entitled 'Testing an intervention to prevent further abuse in pregnant women'.
> 2. Take your text, the article, the strategy and a notepad and pen (or your computer), and find a conducive reading and study environment.
> 3. Survey the article using the strategy guidelines. Make notes of what you gleaned from your survey.
> 4. Now go back and read the article paragraph by paragraph and jot down the key idea in each paragraph. Be sure to note anything that you don't understand. (We know this takes time and may be tedious, but trust us, it helps in the long run.)
> 5. When you have finished, consult references to clarify those things that are unclear.
> 6. When you have completed these steps, go back to the CD-ROM and complete the 'Survey, examine and critically read' exercise, the 'Study evaluation' exercise, and the 'Application visualisation' exercise for Chapter 8.

Resource Kit

Web Sources that Include Content About Maternal–Infant Research or Researchable Areas

The American Association of Women's Health, Obstetrical, and Neonatal Nurses

The Perinatal Research Centre, Royal Women's Hospital Foundation and University of Queensland

Australian College of Midwives

New Zealand College of Midwives Inc

Karitane

Australian Institute of Family Studies

Australian Neonatal Nurses Association

Women's and children's hospitals

The Australian Breastfeeding Association

La Leche League

The Pregnancy and Newborn Services Network (NSW)

AWHONN: AWHONN's Research and Grant Priorities

Web Sources for Relevant Journal Tables of Contents and Abstracts

Nursing Research

Research in Nursing and Health

Journal of Obstetric, Gynecologic, and Neonatal Nursing (JOGNN)

MCN: The American Journal of Maternal Child Nursing

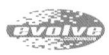 Visit the book's Evolve website at http://evolve.elsevier.com/AU/Borbasi/maze for further information.

References

Brent N, Rudy SJ, Redd B et al (1998). Sore nipples in breast-feeding women: a clinical trial of wound dressings vs conventional care. *Archives of Pediatrics and Adolescent Medicine* 152(11):1077–1082.

Campbell CMA (1998). Breast feeding does not always work: Various supplements to breast feeding are possible. *British Medical Journal* 316(7137):1093–1094.

Lund C (1999). Prevention and management of infant skin breakdown. *Nursing Clinics of North America* 34(4):907.

Lund et al (1999). Neonatal skin care: the scientific basis for practice. *Neonatal Network* 18(4):15.

Maguire DP (1999). Skin protection and breakdown in ELBW infant: a national survey. *Clinical Nursing Research* 8(3):222.

Munson KA, Bare DE, Hoath SB et al (1999). A survey of skin practices for premature low birth weight infants. *Neonatal Network* 18(3):25.

Rossiter JC (1998). Promoting breast feeding: the perceptions of Vietnamese mothers in Sydney, Australia. *Journal of Advanced Nursing* 28(3):598–605.

Tess BH, Rodrigues LC, Newell M-L et al (1998a). Breastfeeding, genetic, obstetric and other risk factors associated with mother-to-child transmission of HIV-1 in Sao Paulo State, Brazil. *AIDS* 12(5):513–520.

Tess BH, Rodrigues LC, Newell M-L et al (1998b). Infant feeding and risk of mother-to-child transmission of HIV-1 in Sao Paulo State, Brazil. *Journal of Acquired Immune Deficiency Syndromes and Human Retrovirology* 19(2):189–194.

http://evolve.elsevier.com/AU/Borbasi/maze

Learning Objectives

After reading this chapter and following critical reflection the student will be able to:

1. Identify clinical nursing journals that publish research articles relevant to children and adolescents.
2. Discuss clinical and research priorities in the care of children and adolescents.
3. Use research literature to clarify identified clinical practice problems about children and adolescents.
4. Explore examples of research studies conducted in various areas of clinical practice with children and adolescents.
5. Discuss the application of sample research results in clinical practice.
6. Apply the reading strategy to survey, examine, critically read and evaluate sample research articles on the care of children and adolescents.

Chapter Outline

What Research Resources Are Available for Children and Adolescents?
What Approaches Can Be Used for Review of the Research Literature?
Addressing clinical and research priorities
Using issues that arise from clinical practice
Scanning available resources
What Current Research Is Available?
Nursing research journals
Clinical nursing journals
Other journals
Summarising and using scanning results
Reading and Evaluating a Research Article on Children

Chapter 9
Reading and Using Research in the Care of Children and Adolescents

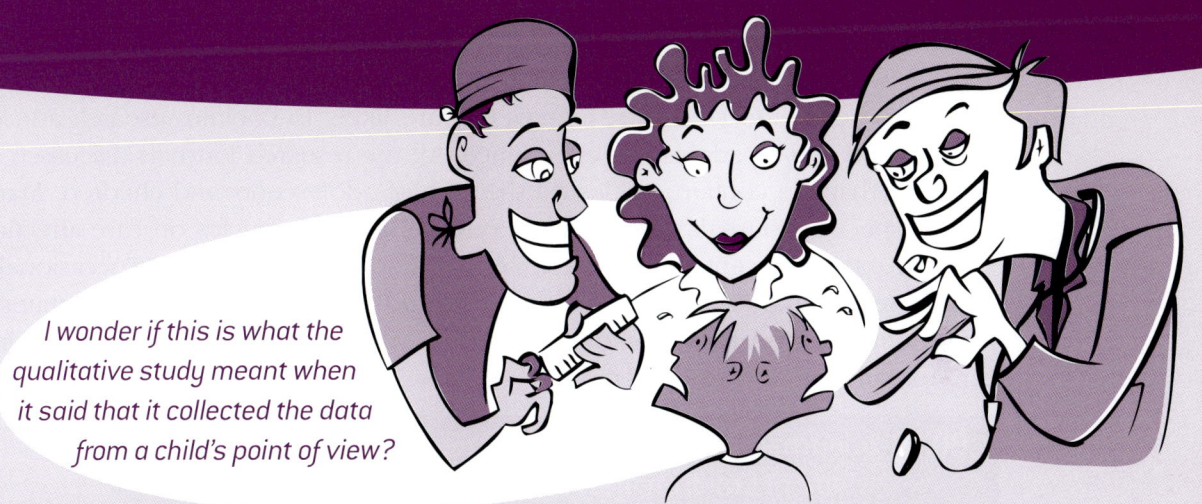

I wonder if this is what the qualitative study meant when it said that it collected the data from a child's point of view?

Student Quote

'I read a research article about letting kids blow on a pinwheel to make getting a jab less upsetting ... and I tried it and it worked!'

Abstract

Several research sources publish articles pertinent to the care of children and adolescents. These sources can be used to pinpoint priorities and current concerns in the care and research of child and adolescent problems, address identified problems and questions uncovered in clinical practice, or to provide a broad view of currently available research about children and adolescents. An abundance of current research studies is available for use in clinical practice with children and adolescents. Samples of current studies are reported, and clinical applications are discussed. The use of the research reading strategy is presented, with one research article on children.

In this chapter, we identify publications that contain nursing research on the care of children and adolescents, explore strategies to simplify the search process and target relevant research articles, and preview sample selections of currently published research. Finally we dissect a sample article using the reading strategy and evaluation guidelines.

What Research Resources Are Available for Children and Adolescents?

To effectively view the current research in care for children and adolescents, it is helpful to be able to identify resources that are likely to contain research articles on the child and/or adolescent experience. All the research journals discussed in previous chapters contain articles on the care of adolescents and children. Many clinical specialty journals also regularly publish research articles on care affecting children and adolescents. Clinical journals in other specialty areas also occasionally contain research articles relevant to children and adolescents. Box 9-1 contains a list of journals most likely to contain research relevant to the practice of nursing care for children and adolescents.

> **BOX 9-1** Journals Containing Nursing Research Relevant to the Care of Children and Adolescents
>
> **Nursing Research Journals**
> *Nursing Research*
> *Australian Journal of Advanced Nursing*
> *International Journal of Nursing Practice*
> *Journal of Advanced Nursing*
> *Research in Nursing and Health*
> *Applied Nursing Research*
> *Nursing Science Quarterly*
> *Journal of Nursing Scholarship*
>
> **Clinical Journals that Regularly Contain Research Articles About Care of Children and Adolescents**
> *Neonatal, Paediatric and Child Health Nursing*
> *Journal of Paediatrics and Child Health*
> *Australian and New Zealand Journal of Public Health*
> *Journal of Adolescent Health*
> *Issues in Comprehensive Pediatric Nursing*
> *Journal of Child and Adolescent Psychiatric Nursing*
> *Journal of Pediatric Nursing: Nursing Care of Children and Families*

Journal of Pediatric Oncology Nursing
Journal of School Nursing
Journal of the Society of Pediatric Nurses
MCN: The American Journal of Maternal-Child Nursing
Pediatric Nursing

Student Challenge

Perusing Specialty Journals

1. If any journals on the list in Box 9-1 are unfamiliar to you, take time to locate those that are available in your library. Scan two or three issues of each journal.
2. Note how they are organised. What types of articles are prevalent? Can you readily distinguish research articles from other featured articles? Do you notice a difference in the focus of the various journals?
3. Check out descriptions of the focus or purpose of any unknown journals.
4. Are some journals more readable than others? More helpful? More practical?

As you become more familiar with the various clinical and research journals, note which might provide the most useful information for improving your care to children and adolescents in various clinical settings. For example, if you are a school nurse, the *Journal of School Nursing* might be particularly helpful.

What Approaches Can Be Used for Review of the Research Literature?

In Chapter 8, we discussed three approaches to guide your use of the current research literature and help enhance your clinical practice. These three approaches also work when searching for literature about children and adolescents. We explore the clinical and research priorities that have been identified in the care of children and adolescents; identify some example problems or questions that might arise from your routine practice with children and adolescents; and finally, we scan the research literature and view what is available to enhance clinical practice.

Addressing clinical and research priorities

Keeping informed about the current clinical and research priorities in a given area can help direct and guide your practice with whatever target population you are interested in. A browse through relevant internet sites reveals several organisations and bodies in Australia and New Zealand that have research programs and health care goals and objectives for children and adolescents. These reflect priority areas for research in child and adolescent health. Some of these are given in Box 9–2. Remember, this list is not exhaustive!

> **BOX 9-2** Some Internet Sites and Web Addresses for Research Programs and/or Healthcare Goals/Objectives for Children and Adolescents
>
> - **Murdoch Children's Research Institute** aims to improve the health of infants as well as children and adolescents through its program of multidisciplinary research. The Institute has programs of laboratory and clinical research as well as a program of public health research (http://www.murdoch.rch.unimelb.edu.au/pages/about.html).
> - **The Institute for Child Health Research** has several research divisions that examine areas of concern in child health. These areas include asthma, allergies, leukaemia, child and youth mental health, infectious diseases, Aboriginal health, meningitis and meningococcal disease (http://www.ichr.uwa.edu.au/research/intro.html).
> - **The Centre for Adolescent Health** has a very comprehensive program of research that covers many areas, such as drug and alcohol use, eating disorders, research into chronic illness, youth suicide, bullying and victimisation, depression and health promotion (http://www.rch.unimelb.edu.au/cah/index.cfm?doc_id=833).
> - **The Asthma and Respiratory Foundation of New Zealand** provides an overview of research findings conducted in New Zealand into issues related to respiratory disorders in people of all ages, but there is a lot of content about research into children and young people with asthma (http://www.asthmanz.co.nz).
> - **The Paediatric Society of New Zealand** (http://www.paediatrics.org.nz/default.asp?id=1&mnu=1)

Issues viewed as high priority in the provision of care to children and adolescents include immunisation, asthma, infectious disease, nutrition, substance use, mental health (including suicide and addiction), chronic and complex illness, safety (injuries are the leading cause of disability and death for children and adolescents), child abuse and neglect, and sexuality. Ways of delivering care to make health care for children and adolescents more equitable and accessible, especially to those in remote communities or from minority groups, are also a priority. These may assist you in identifying areas of concern in your own nursing practice with children and adolescents.

> **Student Challenge**
>
> Checking Child and Adolescent Care Priorities
>
> 1. There are several government documents that outline health priorities for children and young people. Go to this activity on the Evolve website to view the National Health Plan for Young Australians. This plan terminated on 30 June 2001, so would have had a role in shaping research for the past several years. Note the seven key action areas. Do they complement the priority areas that you can see in some of the organisations listed in Box 9–2?
> 2. Go to this activity on the Evolve website and access the Murdoch Children's Research Institute web page. Look at the site and see if you can find areas of research that nurses are involved in.
> 3. Can you locate any other sources that list or discuss priorities in care of or research on children or adolescents?
> 4. Choose one of the priority areas listed or that you have discovered. Run a literature search for the years 2000 to the present and see what (if any) nursing research has been conducted in your selected area. Did you find anything that might be applicable to the care of children and adolescents?

Activity 14

Using issues that arise from clinical practice

We will look at two examples of clinical questions or problems that might arise during routine clinical practice and review the current research literature that might be helpful in addressing the identified problem. As a problem surfaces, you first need to define it by certain parameters to provide a clear frame of reference from which to think about nursing care. It can make the search and use of research materials much easier. Ask yourself the following questions: Who is the target of care—a toddler, preschooler, school-aged child or adolescent, parents, siblings or family? What level of care is involved (i.e. does the problem require health maintenance or prevention, acute care or chronic care)? The aspect of care is also important. Are you concerned with physical, psychological, sociocultural or spiritual needs? How do developmental and maturational issues come into play? Finally what care setting did the problem arise in—a clinic, doctor's office, home, school, community, institution or hospital?

For example, we may be nurses in paediatric clinics where many children with asthma are treated. We notice that many of the children and their families have trouble keeping their asthma under control. We wonder if any research is available that would shed light on how to assist children to more successfully follow their treatment protocols. Using the questions above as a guide we decide we are interested in toddlers through to adolescents. We identify this as a health maintenance/illness prevention problem. We also decide that developmental issues will have an effect on interventions.

We do a CINAHL search using the key words 'asthma' and 'children' and limit the search to research reports in the years 2000–2002. We get 29 citations. Seven are from nursing journals, and cover a range of issues such as patterns of family adaptation to childhood asthma, home management of childhood asthma, children with asthma and their parents' decision making, increasing awareness of asthma and resources for asthma in the community, the effects of nurse teaching on mothers and asthmatic children's health status, evaluation of a multimedia educational package, and the development of the Child Resilience Model. The search also reveals three papers reporting Australian studies. One is about the management of children presenting to hospital with acute asthma, but not requiring admission, one reports a study of asthma camps for young people, and the other is about the experiences of children with respiratory and allergic illnesses in day care. We can see that some of these papers will give us valuable information about health maintenance and illness prevention.

The remaining studies detail various medical treatments, and look at a whole range of issues including allergens in the home, prevalence and management of asthma, use of peak flow meters, and under-use of prescribed medications because of economic problems. Now we return to the original search and drop the research limitation. This gives us several additional studies. Three of these are pertinent to nursing and asthma management. One is an overview of asthma and current trends in management, another looks at issues around hyperactivity and the use of bronchodilators in preschoolers, while a third looks at educating children with asthma.

Now, say we are paediatric rehabilitation nurses in an acute rehabilitation centre and want to update our knowledge on nursing care for children with head trauma. We are interested in all ages of children and adolescents and are looking for research that addresses all care aspects (physical, psychological, sociocultural, developmental or spiritual). A CINAHL search using the key words 'head injury' and 'children' and limited to 2000–2002 yields a total of seven articles. One reports a research study that aimed to determine the factors associated with vomiting following minor head injury in children. There are also two case studies: one on severe head injury in children and one on vomiting and serious head injury. Other papers discuss management of raised intracranial pressure, assessment of head injury in young children, and activity restrictions for children hospitalised with traumatic head injury.

As with the maternal–infant examples, identification of clinical problems in child health often sheds more light on the research that still needs to be conducted than on the research that is available. Literature searches targeted at specifically identified clinical problems can still prove worthwhile and may provide much-needed help for a vexing clinical situation.

> **Student Challenge**
>
> ### Chasing Paediatric Challenges
>
> 1 Review your experiences in caring for children and think about a situation that you wish to explore in the current research literature.
> 2 Identify appropriate search parameters for the subject material and conduct a library search for the years 2000 to the present. What did you find?
> 3 If your search was fruitful, retrieve one or two promising articles.
> 4 Review the articles. How might the results of the studies be helpful in clinical practice?

Scanning available resources

Let's explore what is available in the paediatric research literature when we use our third strategy and scan the tables of contents and the abstracts of the research and clinical specialty journals listed in Box 9-1. Do the following Student Challenge to explore a sample of what is currently available, then continue reading to see what a scan of articles in the year 2001 reveals. Check out the Resource Kit at the end of this chapter to find websites that allow you to see the tables of contents and abstracts of relevant journals.

Activity 15

> **Student Challenge**
>
> ### Scanning Paediatric Journals
>
> Select one research journal and one clinical journal from those listed in Box 9-1 that are available in your library.
>
> 1 Scan the 2002 table of contents for each of these journals and note those articles that seem relevant to the care of children and adolescents.
> 2 Read the abstracts of the selected articles. Weed out any articles that are not clinically relevant. How long did this take you? Was the task easier this time than when you tried it for Chapter 8? Save these articles. You will use them again in the next exercise.

What Current Research Is Available?

The following are specific examples of pertinent research articles on the care of children and adolescents that we found by scanning the 2001 tables of contents of the research and clinical journals listed in Box 9-1. Selected articles are briefly summarised and clinical implications are discussed. The articles are arranged by journal. This allows you to see which of the journals might provide the most insight about various paediatric clinical topics.

Nursing research journals

The articles found by scanning the tables of contents of the various research journals yielded the paediatric article titles listed in Box 9-3.

BOX 9-3 Relevant Paediatric Article Titles in Selected Research Journals

Australian Journal of Advanced Nursing
No relevant articles

International Journal of Nursing Practice
McKinley D, Blackford J (2001). Nurses' experiences of caring for culturally and linguistically diverse families when their child dies. *International Journal of Nursing Practice* 7(4):251–256.
Puotiniemi T, Kyngas H, Nikkonen M (2001). Factors associated with the coping of parents with a child in psychiatric inpatient care. *International Journal of Nursing Practice* 7(5):298–305.

Journal of Advanced Nursing
Clendon J, White G (2001). The feasibility of a nurse practitioner-led primary health care clinic in a school setting: a community needs analysis. *Journal of Advanced Nursing* 34(2):171–178.
De Jonge A (2001). Support for teenage mothers: a qualitative study into the views of women about the support they received as teenaged mothers. *Journal of Advanced Nursing* 36(1):49–57.
Farrell M, Ryan S, Langrick B (2001). 'Breaking bad news' within a paediatric setting: an evaluation report of a collaborative education workshop to support health professionals. *Journal of Advanced Nursing* 36(6):765–775.
Fisher HR (2001). The needs of parents with chronically sick children: a literature review. *Journal of Advanced Nursing* 36(4):600–607.
Ford K, Turner D (2001). Stories seldom told: paediatric nurses' experiences of caring for hospitalised children with special needs and their families. *Journal of Advanced Nursing* 33(3):288–295.
Hanna B (2001). Negotiating motherhood: the struggles of teenage mothers. *Journal of Advanced Nursing* 34(4):464–465.
Holm K, Li S, Spector N et al (2001). Obesity in adults and children: a call for action. *Journal of Advanced Nursing* 36(2):266–269.

Jolley S (2001). Promoting teenage sexual health: an investigation into the knowledge, activities and perceptions of gynaecology nurses. *Journal of Advanced Nursing* 36(2):246–255.

Kearney PT, Griffin T (2001). Between joy and sorrow: being a parent of a child with developmental disability. *Journal of Advanced Nursing* 34(5):582–592.

Kirk S (2001). Negotiating lay and professional roles in the care of children with complex health care needs. *Journal of Advanced Nursing* 34(5):593–602.

Laakso H, Paunonen-Ilmonen M (2001). Mothers' grief following the death of a child. *Journal of Advanced Nursing* 36(1):69–77.

Lackey NR, Gates MF (2001). Adults' recollections of their experiences as young caregivers of family members with chronic illnesses. *Journal of Advanced Nursing* 34(3):320–328.

Llahana SV, Poulton BC, Coates VE (2001). The paediatric diabetes specialist nurse and diabetes education in childhood. *Journal of Advanced Nursing* 33(3):296–306.

Long A, McCarney S, Smyth G et al (2001). The effectiveness of parenting programmes facilitated by health visitors. *Journal of Advanced Nursing* 34(5):611–620.

Olsen R, Maslin-Prothero P (2001). Dilemmas in the provision of own-home respite support for the parents of young children with complex health care needs: evidence from an evaluation. *Journal of Advanced Nursing* 34(5):603–610.

Ribeiro MO, Ciamponi MH (2001). Homeless children: the lives of a group of Brazilian street children. *Journal of Advanced Nursing* 35(1):42–49.

Sapountzi-Krepia DS, Valavanis J, Panteleakis GP et al (2001). Perceptions of body image, happiness and satisfaction in adolescents wearing a Boston brace for scoliosis treatment. *Journal of Advanced Nursing* 35(5):683–690.

Simons J, Franck L, Roberson E (2001). Parent involvement in children's pain care: view of parents and nurses. *Journal of Advanced Nursing* 36(4):591–599.

Swallow VM, Jacoby A (2001). Mothers' evolving relationships with doctors and nurses during the chronic childhood illness trajectory. *Journal of Advanced Nursing* 36(6):755–764.

Wilson HV (2001). Power and partnership: a critical analysis of the surveillance discourse of child health nurses. *Journal of Advanced Nursing* 36(2):294–301.

Yeh C (2001). Development and testing of the parental coping strategy inventory (PCSI) with children with cancer in Taiwan. *Journal of Advanced Nursing* 36(1):78–88.

Journal of Nursing Scholarship

Burkhart PV, Dunbar-Jacob JM, Rohay JM (2001). Accuracy of children's self-reported adherence to treatment. *Journal of Nursing Scholarship* 33(1):27–32.

> Rew L, Taylor-Seehafer M, Thomas NY et al (2001). Correlates of resilience in homeless adolescents. *Journal of Nursing Scholarship* 33(1):33–40.
> Rew L, Thomas N, Horner SD et al (2001). Correlates of recent suicide attempts in a triethnic group of adolescents. *Journal of Nursing Scholarship* 33(4):361–367.
> Shelton D (2001). Health policy and systems. Emotional disorders in young offenders. *Journal of Nursing Scholarship* 33(3):259–263.
> Teall AM, Graham MC (2001). Youth access to tobacco in two communities. *Journal of Nursing Scholarship* 33(2):175–178.
> Tigges BB (2001). Affiliative preferences, self change, and adolescent condom use. *Journal of Nursing Scholarship* 33(3):231–237.
> Veenema TG (2001). Children's exposure to community violence. *Journal of Nursing Scholarship* 33(2):167–173.
>
> ### Applied Nursing Research
> Dormire S, Yarandi H (2001). Predictors of risk for adolescent childbearing. *Applied Nursing Research* 14(2):81–86.
> Kelly K (2001). Assessment of dietary intake of preschool children living in a homeless shelter. *Applied Nursing Research* 14(3):146–154.
> LaMontagne LL, Hepworth JT, Salisbury MH (2001). Anxiety and postoperative pain in children who undergo major orthopedic surgery. *Applied Nursing Research* 14(3):119–124.
>
> ### Nursing Science Quarterly
> Yeh C (2001). Adaptation in children with cancer: research with Roy's model. *Nursing Science Quarterly* 14(2):141–148.

A scan revealed 2 articles in *International Journal of Nursing Practice*, 21 articles in *Journal of Advanced Nursing*, 3 articles in *Applied Nursing Research*, 1 article in *Nursing Science Quarterly*, and 7 articles in *Journal of Nursing Scholarship*. No relevant articles were found in the *Australian Journal of Advanced Nursing*.

Let's look more closely at a couple of the searches from individual journals. Of the 21 relevant articles published in *Journal of Advanced Nursing* in 2001, several also came up in the searches we did for Chapter 8. For example, an Australian study of the struggles of teenage mothers (Hanna 2001) came up in both searches because the paper is concerned with both maternal issues (being a mother), and adolescent issues (the mothers who were the focus of the study were teenagers). Similarly, the studies by Wilson (2001) and Kearney & Griffin (2001) traversed both searches. In addition to those by Hanna (2001), Wilson (2001) and Kearney & Griffin (2001), two other papers reported research carried out in Australia and New Zealand. Clendon & White (2001) reported a community needs analysis to determine the feasibility of a nurse-practitioner led primary health care clinic in a school setting.

Ford & Turner (2001) reported a study that explored nurses' experiences of caring for special needs children and their families in an acute care setting.

Relevant articles in the *Journal of Nursing Scholarship* included research reports about a broad range of health concerns using a range of methodological approaches. Shelton (2001) undertook a study of young people committed or detained by the criminal justice system to estimate rates of emotional disorder among this group. A school-based survey of sexually active adolescents about condom use revealed information that could help target nursing interventions to make them more effective and appropriate (Tigges 2001). Veenema (2001) reported results from a systematic review into children's exposure to community violence and highlighted several areas where additional research is needed. Teall & Graham (2001) undertook unannounced compliance checks of tobacco outlets in two urban US communities to determine the availability of tobacco to youth in those communities. This information was used as a basis for the design of a community-based intervention. Other papers reported research that examined children's adherence to an asthma program (Burkhart et al 2001), and a study that explored issues around resilience in homeless adolescents (Rew et al 2001).

Clinical nursing journals

The articles found by scanning the tables of contents of the clinical journals yielded several possibly relevant paediatric research articles as listed in Box 9-4.

BOX 9-4 Relevant Child and Adolescent Research Articles in Selected Clinical Journals

Neonatal, Paediatric and Child Health Nursing
No relevant articles

Issues in Comprehensive Pediatric Nursing
Amen MM, Clarke VPJ (2001). The influence of mothers' health beliefs on use of preventive child health care services and mothers' perception of children's health status. *Issues in Comprehensive Pediatric Nursing* 24(3):153–163.
Hanna KM, Guthrie D (2001). Parents' and adolescents' perceptions of helpful and nonhelpful support for adolescents' assumption of diabetes management responsibility. *Issues in Comprehensive Pediatric Nursing* 24(4):209–223.
Havener L, Gentes L, Thaler B et al (2001). The effects of a companion animal on distress in children undergoing dental procedures. *Issues in Comprehensive Pediatric Nursing* 24(2):137–152.
Hulton LJ (2001). The application of the Transtheoretical Model of Change to adolescent sexual decision-making. *Issues in Comprehensive Pediatric Nursing* 24(2):95–115.

Montgomery KS (2001). Planned adolescent pregnancy: what they needed. *Issues in Comprehensive Pediatric Nursing* 24(1):19–29.

Murray JS (2001). Self-concept of siblings of children with cancer. *Issues in Comprehensive Pediatric Nursing* 24(2):85–94.

Rew L, Taylor-Seehafer M, Fitzgerald ML (2001). Sexual abuse, alcohol and other drug use, and suicidal behaviors in homeless adolescents. *Issues in Comprehensive Pediatric Nursing* 24(4):225–240.

Sloand ED, Vessey JA (2001). Self-medication with common household medicines by young adolescents. *Issues in Comprehensive Pediatric Nursing* 24(1):57–67.

Journal of Pediatric Health Care

Berti LC, Zylbert S, Rolnitzky L (2001). Comparison of health status of children using a school-based health center for comprehensive care. *Journal of Pediatric Health Care* 15(5):244–250.

Ecklund CR, Ross MC (2001). Over-the-counter medication use in preschool children. *Journal of Pediatric Health Care* 15(4):168–172.

Jackson PL, Kennedy C, Sadler LS et al (2001). Professional practice of pediatric nurse practitioners: implications for education and training of PNPs. *Journal of Pediatric Health Care* 15(6):291–298.

Joyce BA, Keck JF, Gerkensmeyer J (2001). Evaluation of pain management interventions for neonatal circumcision pain. *Journal of Pediatric Health Care* 15(3):105–114.

Mahat G, Scoloveno MA (2001). Factors influencing health practices of Nepalese adolescent girls. *Journal of Pediatric Health Care* 15(5):251–255.

Maskell G, Powell CVE, Marks MK et al (2001). Updating asthma management: the process of change. *Journal of Pediatric Health Care* 15(1):20–23.

Murphy LMB (2001). Adolescent mothers' beliefs about parenting and injury prevention: results of a focus group. *Journal of Pediatric Health Care* 15(4):194–199.

Niederhauser VP, Baruffi G, Heck R (2001). Parental decision-making for the varicella vaccine. *Journal of Pediatric Health Care* 15(5):236–243.

Sharieff GQ, Trocinski DR, Thompson K (2001). Pediatric patients with bleeding dyscrasias: what is the cause of delays in initiating replacement therapy? *Journal of Pediatric Health Care* 15(1):10–13.

Stevens-Simon C, Barrett J (2001). A comparison of the psychological resources of adolescents at low and high risk of mistreating their children. *Journal of Pediatric Health Care* 15(6):299–303.

Wilson T (2001). A bi-state, metropolitan, school-based immunization campaign: lessons from the Kansas City experience. *Journal of Pediatric Health Care* 15(4):173–178.

Journal of Pediatric Nursing: Nursing Care of Children and Families

Azar R, Solomon CR (2001). Coping strategies of parents facing child diabetes mellitus. *Journal of Pediatric Nursing: Nursing Care of Children and Families* 16(6):418–428.

Balling K, McCubbin M (2001). Hospitalized children with chronic illness: parental caregiving needs and valuing parental expertise. *Journal of Pediatric Nursing: Nursing Care of Children and Families* 16(2):110–119.

Busen NH, Modeland V, Kouzekanani K (2001). Adolescent cigarette smoking and health risk behavior. *Journal of Pediatric Nursing: Nursing Care of Children and Families* 16(3):187–193.

Cavusoglu H (2001). Depression in children with cancer. *Journal of Pediatric Nursing: Nursing Care of Children and Families* 16(5):380–385.

Corrarino JE, Walsh PJ, Nadel E (2001). Does teaching scald burn prevention to families of young children make a difference? A pilot study. *Journal of Pediatric Nursing: Nursing Care of Children and Families* 16(4):256–262.

Fisher KM, Hupcey JE, Rhodes DA (2001). Childhood farm injuries in old-order Amish families. *Journal of Pediatric Nursing: Nursing Care of Children and Families* 16(2):97–101.

Gresham LS, Zirkle DL, Tolchin S et al (2001). Partnering for injury prevention: evaluation of a curriculum-based intervention program among elementary school children. *Journal of Pediatric Nursing: Nursing Care of Children and Families* 16(2):79–87.

Higgins SS (2001). Parental role in decision making about pediatric cardiac transplantation: familial and ethical considerations. *Journal of Pediatric Nursing: Nursing Care of Children and Families* 16(5):332–337.

Huang C, Menke EM (2001). School-aged homeless sheltered children's stressors and coping behaviours. *Journal of Pediatric Nursing: Nursing Care of Children and Families* 16(2):102–109.

Hunter AJ (2001). A cross-cultural comparison of resilience in adolescents. *Journal of Pediatric Nursing: Nursing Care of Children and Families* 16(3):172–179.

Jones FC, Broome ME (2001). Focus groups with African American adolescents: enhancing recruitment and retention in intervention studies. *Journal of Pediatric Nursing: Nursing Care of Children and Families* 16(2):88–96.

Letourneau N (2001). Improving adolescent parent–infant interactions: a pilot study. *Journal of Pediatric Nursing: Nursing Care of Children and Families* 16(1):53–62.

Lundblad B, Byrne MW, Helström A (2001). Continuing nursing care needs of children at time of discharge from one regional medical center in Sweden. *Journal of Pediatric Nursing: Nursing Care of Children and Families* 16(1):73–78.

Mu P, Ma F, Ku S et al (2001). Families of Chinese children with malignancy: the factors impact on mother's anxiety. *Journal of Pediatric Nursing: Nursing Care of Children and Families* 16(4):287–295.

Neufeld SM, Query B, Drummond JE (2001). Respite care users who have children with chronic conditions: are they getting a break? *Journal of Pediatric Nursing: Nursing Care of Children and Families* 16(4):234–244.

O'Brien ME (2001). Living in a house of cards: family experiences with long-term childhood technology dependence. *Journal of Pediatric Nursing: Nursing Care of Children and Families* 16(1):13–22.

Percy MS, McIntyre L (2001). Using touchpoints to promote parental self-competence in low-income, minority, pregnant, and parenting teen mothers. *Journal of Pediatric Nursing: Nursing Care of Children and Families* 16(3):180–186.

Ritchie MA (2001). Self-esteem and hopefulness in adolescents with cancer. *Journal of Pediatric Nursing: Nursing Care of Children and Families* 16(1):35–42.

Sadler LS, Anderson SA, Sabatelli RM (2001). Parental competence among African American adolescent mothers and grandmothers. *Journal of Pediatric Nursing: Nursing Care of Children and Families* 16(4):217–233.

Santacroce SJ (2001). Measuring parental uncertainty during the diagnosis phase of serious illness in a child. *Journal of Pediatric Nursing: Nursing Care of Children and Families* 16(1):3–12.

Shields L, King SJ (2001a). Qualitative analysis of the care of children in hospital in four countries—part 2. *Journal of Pediatric Nursing: Nursing Care of Children and Families* 16(3):206–213.

Shields L, King SJ (2001b). Qualitative analysis of the care of children in hospital in four countries—part 1. *Journal of Pediatric Nursing: Nursing Care of Children and Families* 16(2):137–145.

Vacik HW, Nagy MC, Jessee PO (2001). Children's understanding of illness: students' assessments. *Journal of Pediatric Nursing: Nursing Care of Children and Families* 16(6):429–437.

Yidiz S, Savasere S, Tatlioglu GS (2001). Evaluation of internal behaviors of children with congenital heart disease. *Journal of Pediatric Nursing: Nursing Care of Children and Families* 16(6):449–452.

Journal of Child and Adolescent Psychiatric Nursing

Elder JH (2001). A follow-up study of beliefs held by parents of children with pervasive developmental delay. *Journal of Child and Adolescent Psychiatric Nursing* 14(2):55–60.

Krueger M, Kendall J (2001). Descriptions of self: an exploratory study of adolescents with ADHD. *Journal of Child and Adolescent Psychiatric Nursing* 14(2):61–72.

Lambert LT (2001). Identification and management of schizophrenia in childhood. *Journal of Child and Adolescent Psychiatric Nursing* 14(2):73–80.

> Mainous RO, Mainous AG III, Martin CA et al (2001). The importance of fulfilling unmet needs of rural and urban adolescents with substance abuse. *Journal of Child and Adolescent Psychiatric Nursing* 14(1):32–40.
> Petti TA, Mohr WK, Somers JW, Sims L (2001). Perceptions of seclusion and restraint by patients and staff in an intermediate-term care facility. *Journal of Child and Adolescent Psychiatric Nursing* 14(3):115–127.
> Waibel-Duncan MK (2001). Medical fears following alleged child abuse. *Journal of Child and Adolescent Psychiatric Nursing* 14(4):179–185.
> Yearwood EL (2001). 'Growing up' children: current child-rearing practices among immigrant Jamaican families. *Journal of Child and Adolescent Psychiatric Nursing* 14(1):7–16, 40.

There are a number of clinical journals that regularly publish research on the care of children and adolescents. Some publish a wide variety of research results across the paediatric spectrum, while others, such as the *Journal of Child and Adolescent Psychiatric Nursing,* are highly specialised. We selected several titles to search for research-based articles that appeared in 2001 for paediatric and adolescent health. Our scan netted 8 relevant research articles from *Issues in Comprehensive Pediatric Nursing,* 7 from the *Journal of Child and Adolescent Psychiatric Nursing,* 11 from the *Journal of Pediatric Health Care,* and 24 from the *Journal of Pediatric Nursing: Nursing Care of Children and Families.* There were no relevant research articles in that period appearing in *Neonatal, Paediatric and Child Health Nursing.*

A survey of the titles revealed 50 studies about children, including 12 on adolescents; 17 on children; and 14 on mothers, parents or families of children or adolescents. The studies covered a broad range of areas such as psychological and behavioural issues, physical issues and nursing interventions. Mental health, suicide, cigarette smoking, pain and distress associated with health care, cancer, asthma, diabetes, immunisation and self-care by children and adolescents were also addressed.

Other journals

Ten research studies pertinent to the care of children or adolescents were found among various other journals. The results can be viewed in Box 9-5.

> **BOX 9-5** Relevant Paediatric Research Articles from Miscellaneous Nursing Journals
>
> **Qualitative Health Research**
> Chesler MA, Parry C (2001). Gender roles and/or styles in crisis: an integrative analysis of the experiences of fathers of children with cancer. *Qualitative Health Research* 11(3):363–384.
> Martyn KK, Hutchinson SA (2001). Low-income African American adolescents who avoid pregnancy: tough girls who rewrite negative scripts. *Qualitative Health Research* 11(2):238–256.
> Moffat BM, Johnson JL (2001). Through the haze of cigarettes: teenage girls' stories about cigarette addiction. *Qualitative Health Research* 11(5):668–681.
> Stubblefield C, Murray RL (2001). Pediatric lung transplantation: families' need for understanding. *Qualitative Health Research* 11(1):58–68.
> Young RA, Lynam MJ, Valach L et al (2001). Joint actions of parents and adolescents in health conversations. *Qualitative Health Research* 11(1):40–57.
>
> **Contemporary Nurse**
> Lord A, Ridge DT, St Leger LH et al (2001). The value of asthma camps for young people in Victoria, Australia. *Contemporary Nurse* 11(2/3):133–141.
> Monterosso L (2001). Priorities for paediatric cancer nursing research in Western Australia: a Delphi study. *Contemporary Nurse* 11(2/3):142–152.
>
> **Australian and New Zealand Journal of Public Health**
> Booth ML, Wake M, Armstrong T et al (2001). The epidemiology of overweight and obesity among Australian children and adolescents, 1995–97. *Australian and New Zealand Journal of Public Health* 25(2):162–169.
> Magarey A, Daniels LA, Smith A (2001). Fruit and vegetable intakes of Australians aged 2–18 years: an evaluation of the 1995 National Nutrition Survey data. *Australian and New Zealand Journal of Public Health* 25(2):155–161.
> Wickens K, Crane J, Kemp T et al (2001). A case-control study of risk factors for asthma in New Zealand children. *Australian and New Zealand Journal of Public Health* 25(1):44–49.

Two of these studies addressed issues related to nutrition of Australian children and adolescents (Booth et al 2001; Magarey, Daniels & Smith 2001). Two focused on issues related to asthma—one of these reported a case-controlled study of risk factors in New Zealand children (Wickens et al 2001) and the other was concerned with asthma camps for young people held in Victoria, Australia (Lord et al 2001). Two of the papers related to children, adolescents and cancer. Monterosso (2001) undertook a Delphi study to ascertain priorities for nursing research for paediatric cancer, and Chesler & Parry (2001) reported a study of experiences of fathers of children with cancer. Other studies explored teenage girls' stories of addiction to cigarettes (Moffat & Johnson 2001), parents' and adolescents' health conversations (Young et al 2001), the needs of families with a child undergoing lung transplantation (Stubblefield & Murray 2001), and avoiding adolescent pregnancy (Martyn & Hutchinson 2001).

Summarising and using scanning results

Several of the identified research articles have been selected to serve as examples of how research articles might be summarised and the findings used in practice. Several articles tested nursing interventions for effectiveness and provide concrete data about the effectiveness of certain nursing interventions, and the healthcare needs and concerns of children, adolescents or their families. We look at several of these articles in more depth.

The first article evaluated the intake of fruit and vegetables by Australian children in the 2–18 year age group. Using data from a National Nutrition Survey conducted in 1995, the authors were able to assess consumption of fruit and vegetables of 3007 children and adolescents. Findings suggested that two-thirds of Australian children in the 2–18 year age group do not have an adequate intake of fruit and vegetables (Magarey, Daniels & Smith 2001). This finding is of concern and the authors had several recommendations for health workers and workers from other sectors to facilitate the consumption of more fruit and vegetables by 2–18 year olds.

Another article aimed to establish the incidence of overweight and obesity among Australian children and adolescents. The authors used body mass index measures to assess children and young people and then categorised them as either non-overweight, overweight or obese. Findings suggested that overweight or obesity affects between 19 and 23 per cent of Australian children and adolescents (Booth et al 2001). The authors noted some differences between cultural groups.

A third article (Farrell, Ryan & Langrick 2001) reported an evaluative study of a workshop that aimed to provide preparation for health professionals to give bad news in the paediatric setting. A series of workshops were provided and participants given the opportunity to discuss bad news scenarios and reflect on issues surrounding giving people bad news. Participants used scenarios and debriefing in the workshops and then completed an evaluation questionnaire that was administered immediately after the workshop. Most participants had received no prior educational preparation for breaking bad news and all found the workshop to be helpful to them in their roles as clinicians. These findings support the importance of nurses and other health workers taking part in the ongoing education and professional development opportunities offered by healthcare organisations.

Ecklund & Ross (2001) conducted a descriptive correlational study with a convenience sample of 52 carers of preschool children. The study sought to establish how perceptions of severity of and susceptibility to illness, trust in healthcare providers, barriers to accessing health care and efficacy of over-the-counter pharmaceuticals affects carers' healthcare decision-making for preschoolers. Investigators used a questionnaire design and findings revealed significant correlations between perceived illness severity, susceptibility to illness and seeking healthcare from healthcare providers. Significant correlations were also found between age and socioeconomic status of the caregiver, the perceived efficacy of over-the-counter medications and their administration. The study authors concluded that guidelines about the use of over-the-counter preparations should be provided to parents.

In order to establish whether there were differences in gender and ethnicity in self-reported suicide attempts in adolescents from three different ethnic backgrounds, Rew et al (2001) designed a study that used secondary analysis of previously collected survey data gathered from over 10,000 high school students. Statistical analysis revealed the presence of differences relating to both gender and ethnicity, and also established significant relationships between suicide attempt and a family or social association with a person who had made a suicide attempt. A history of sexual or physical abuse was also revealed as significant. All data were collected from only one location and a self-report tool was used, so the study authors recommended that the findings be viewed with caution. However, they pointed to a need for culturally appropriate interventions when dealing with adolescents who attempt suicide.

The randomised control trial or RCT is considered the 'gold standard' when it comes to evidence to support this or that intervention for any given condition or health problem. But as research designs go, it doesn't always lend itself easily to nursing situations. Also, there can be ethical issues and difficulties associated with the RCT design that make it very difficult for nurses to gain the necessary permissions to carry out an RCT. However, over the past few years more and more reports of studies that used RCT design have become evident in the literature. Burkhart, Dunbar-Jacob & Rohay (2001) used an RCT to examine the association between self-reported and electronically monitored adherence to peak flow regime in children aged 7–11 years of age. Statistical analysis revealed a modest correlation between self-reported and electronically recorded peak expiratory flow rates, and differences in electronically monitored and self-reported adherence at some points in the study. Implications for practice and patient education are drawn from this study.

Kearney & Griffin (2001) used a phenomenological approach to explore the experiences of parents of children with developmental disabilities. The researchers used conversational-style interviews to gain experiential accounts from parents, and also derived descriptions from other sources such as books, magazines and newspaper articles. Analysis of the descriptive accounts led to the development of a visual interpretive model that captured the concepts of joy and sorrow, and many other related elements. The authors proposed that participants reported feeling joy and pleasurable feelings in their relationships with their children, but experienced sorrow in many of their other relationships, because of the perception that friends, family and professional people perhaps devalued their children and saw them only in terms of their disability. The authors concluded by reinforcing the importance of hope and optimism in clinical practice.

Student Challenge

Using Data from Journal Scans

Use the articles that resulted from your journal scan.

1. Read the articles to determine what was studied, who was studied and what the study results were. Write a brief summary of each article. Use the articles cited as examples in the previous section.

2. Read the discussion sections of the articles and make a quick determination about how the results might be used in a clinical practice setting. Write out how the findings might be used and by whom.

Reading and Evaluating a Research Article on Children

In this section, we examine in more depth one quantitative research article on a paediatric intervention. We again use the research reading strategy and the research study comprehension guidelines discussed in Chapter 7.

These exercises guide you through the critical reading, evaluation and visualisation of the selected research article. When you finish, print out your answers and our responses to the exercises. You should be feeling more confident about reading a research article and pulling out the key ideas.

Student Challenge

Surveying and Examining a Paediatric Research Study

1. Log on to your CD-ROM and find the 'Survey, examine and critically read' exercise in Chapter 9. Print out the reading strategy and the research article entitled 'Children's responses to immunisation: lullabies as a distraction'.

2. Take your text, the article, the strategy and a notepad and pen and find a conducive reading and study environment.

3. Survey the article using the strategy guidelines. Make notes of what you gleaned from your survey.

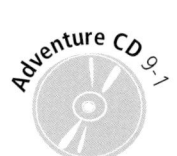
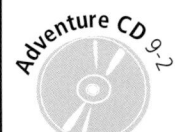

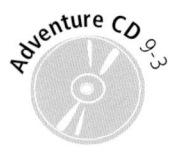

4 Now go back and read the article paragraph by paragraph and jot down the key idea in each paragraph. Note anything that you don't understand.

5 When you have finished, consult references to clarify those things that are unclear.

6 When you have completed these steps, go back to the CD-ROM and complete the rest of the 'Survey, examine and critically read' exercise, the 'Study evaluation' exercise, and the 'Application visualisation' exercise for Chapter 9.

Resource Kit

Web Sources for Child and Adolescent Research Priorities

Murdoch Children's Research Institute

Institute for Child Health Research

Centre for Adolescent Health

Asthma and Respiratory Foundation of New Zealand

Paediatric Society of New Zealand

National Institute for Nursing Research

Web Sources for Relevant Journal Tables of Contents and Abstracts

Nursing Research

Research in Nursing and Health

Child and Adolescent Mental Health

Issues in Comprehensive Pediatric Nursing

Journal of Pediatric Oncology Nursing (indexed in MEDLINE and CINAHL)

Journal of Society of Pediatric Nurses

The Journal of Child and Family Studies is an excellent source for examples of how research has been used in particular clinical settings.

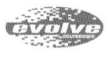
Visit the book's Evolve website at http://evolve.elsevier.com/AU/Borbasi/maze for further information.

Check out the exercises on your CD-ROM.

http://evolve.elsevier.com/AU/Borbasi/maze

Learning Objectives

After reading this chapter and following critical reflection the student will be able to:

1. Identify clinical nursing journals that publish research articles relevant to adults.
2. Discuss clinical and research priorities in the care of adults.
3. Use research literature to clarify identified clinical practice problems for adults.
4. Explore examples of research studies conducted in various areas of clinical practice with adults.
5. Discuss the application of sample research results in clinical practice.
6. Apply the reading strategy to survey, examine, critically read and evaluate a sample research article on the care of adults.

Chapter Outline

What Research Resources Are Available on the Care of Adults?
What Approaches Can Be Used for the Review of the Research Literature?
Addressing clinical and research priorities
Using issues that arise from clinical practice
Scanning available resources

What Current Research Is Available?
Nursing research journals
Clinical nursing journals
Summarising and using scan results
Reading and Evaluating a Research Article on the Care of Adults

Chapter 10

Reading and Using Research in the Care of Adults

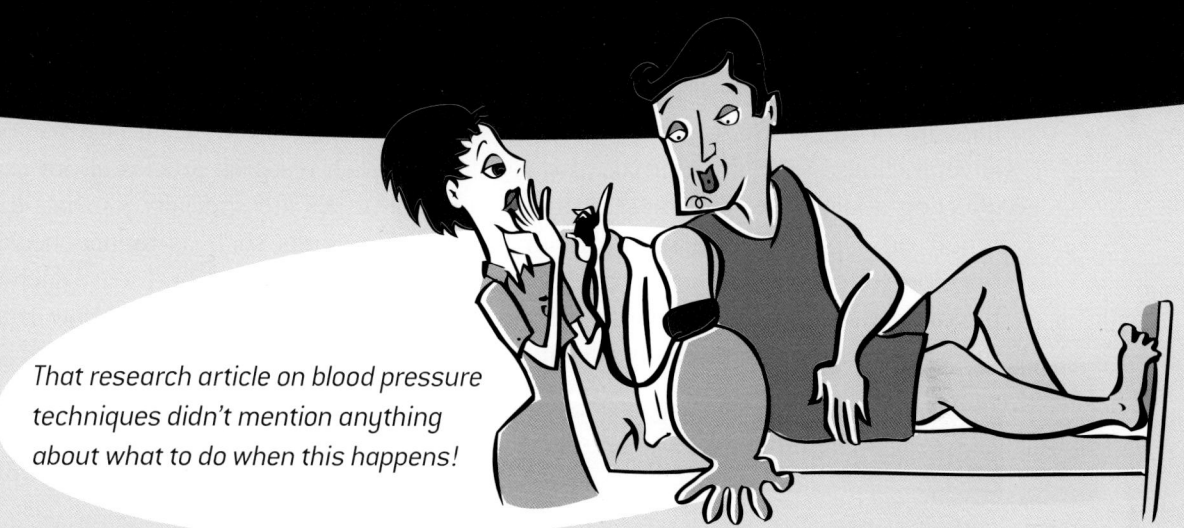

That research article on blood pressure techniques didn't mention anything about what to do when this happens!

Student Quote

'I never even thought about needing updates on basic skills procedures until we learnt about evidence-based practice in class. I've already altered the way I take blood pressures.'

Abstract

Several research sources publish articles pertinent to the care of adults. These sources tend to be identified by clinical subspecialty area and can be used to view identified priorities in the care of and research on adults, to address identified problems and questions uncovered in clinical practice, or to provide a broad view of currently available research about adults. Abundant current research studies are available for use in clinical practice with adults. Samples of current studies are reported and clinical applications are discussed. The use of the research reading strategy is illustrated with one research article on an adult population.

In this chapter we identify periodical publications that contain nursing research on the care of adults, explore strategies to simplify the search process and target relevant research articles, and preview sample selections of currently published research. Finally, we dissect a sample article using the reading strategy and evaluation criteria presented in Chapter 7.

What Research Resources Are Available on the Care of Adults?

Several resources are available that report the results of nursing research focusing on the care of adults. By now the nursing research journals should be familiar to you. Several clinical specialty journals also regularly publish research articles about care affecting adults. Note that most of these clinical journals are specialty journals that report on a particular segment of nursing care for adults such as mental health, oncology or critical care, or the care of some specific body system or disease such as the cardiovascular or pulmonary system or cancer. Box 10-1 contains a list of journals most likely to contain research relevant to the practice of nursing care for adults.

> **BOX 10-1** Journals Containing Nursing Research Relevant to the Care of Adults
>
> **Nursing Research Journals**
> *Australian Journal of Advanced Nursing*
> *Journal of Advanced Nursing*
> *Nursing Research*
> *Research in Nursing and Health*
> *Nursing Science Quarterly*
> *Journal of Nursing Scholarship*
> *International Journal of Nursing Studies*
> *Western Journal of Nursing Research*
>
> **Clinical Journals that Regularly Contain Research Articles About the Care of Adults**
> *Australian Critical Care*
> *Australian Journal of Holistic Nursing*
> *International Journal of Mental Health Nursing*
> *Heart and Lung: Journal of Acute and Critical Care*
> *Nursing Praxis in New Zealand*
> *AORN*
> *International Journal of Nursing Practice*
> *Oncology Nursing Forum*
> *Rehabilitation Nursing*

Note that there is no listing for nursing journals that occasionally contain research relevant to the adult population because research studies are scattered among many different nursing journals. Some of these studies would surface using our search strategy for a specified clinical problem. However, searching for these studies using the journal scan procedure is not a viable option. If you are interested in a listing of nursing journals with information about their function and purpose, check out the Resource Kit at the end of the chapter for a handy website address.

By now you should have begun to notice a difference between the research articles you see in clinical journals and the articles reported in research journals. Research reports in research journals tend to be geared to the knowledge and reading level of other researchers. This means they include greater detail about research methodology and statistics and use more technical language. The relevance of the studies to clinical practice may not always be immediately obvious. In short, they require more time and concentration to read and understand.

Research studies in clinical journals are targeted at clinical practitioners. The language is less technical and the methods section and statistical reporting are less detailed. The clinical relevance is usually clear-cut and easy to ascertain. In short, they are easier to read and apply, but it is more difficult to ascertain exactly how the research was conducted. However, both are equally rigorous and serve a useful purpose for you, the research consumer. So keep reading both types. Make note of the journals that provide the most useful information for improving your care to various segments of the adult population.

Student Challenge

Perusing Specialty Journals

1. If any of the journals listed in Box 10-1 are unfamiliar to you, take time to locate those available in your library. Scan two or three issues of each journal.
2. Note how they are organised. What types of articles are prevalent? Can you readily distinguish research articles from other featured articles? Do you notice a difference between the foci of the various journals?
3. Check out descriptions of the focus or purpose of any unknown journals.
4. Are some journals more readable than others? More helpful?

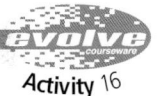
Activity 16

What Approaches Can Be Used for the Review of the Research Literature?

We again explore our three strategies for use of the research literature as it pertains to adults. We explore the relevant clinical and research priorities, identify some sample problems or questions that might arise from clinical practice with an adult population, and scan the research literature to get a feel for available research that might enhance clinical practice.

Addressing clinical and research priorities

Let's look at the care and research priorities relevant to an adult population. Health maintenance, promotion and restoration remain the key goals in the care of adults, as is combating diseases that carry high morbidity and mortality rates. There are many areas of adult health that require current and rigorous research activity. A browse of key websites such as those of the National Heart Foundation, the Cancer Council or Diabetes Australia will highlight some areas of current concern. The NH&MRC's Strategic Research Development Committee (SRDC) has formulated areas for Strategic and Priority Driven Research (SPDR). These areas are listed in Box 10-2. The Australian Department of Health and Ageing has also identified a number of research areas pertinent to promoting better health outcomes for adult Australians and the Federal Government has announced four national research priorities, including Promoting and Maintaining Good Health.

> ### BOX 10-2 NH&MRC Strategic and Priority Driven Research
>
> The research framework is arranged in three tiers:
> 1. Tier one identifies the following research priority areas:
>   - Indigenous health
>   - Ageing
>   - Mental health
>   - Oral health
>   - Systems of care for chronic diseases
> 2. Tier two relates to health services research, socioeconomic influences, rural health and palliative care.
> 3. Tier three explores avenues to develop strategic research.
>
> Source: National Health and Medical Research Council, Strategic and priority driven research. Online. Available: http://www.health.gov.au/nhmrc/research/spdres.htm. Last updated 18 Apr 2002.

> ### Student Challenge
>
> Checking Adult Care Priorities
> 1. Check out the Australian Department of Health and Ageing National Health Priority Areas. Locate the elements relevant to care for adults. Compare them to the foci in Box 10-2. Note similarities and differences.

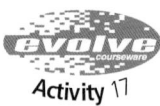
Activity 17

2 Australia's national research priorities include Promoting and Maintaining Good Health. Check out the goals associated with this research priority on the Department of Education Science and Training website. What is new or different about these objectives?

3 Locate the World Health Organization's research priorities and see how they compare with Australian government initiatives.

4 Locate the latest research priorities of at least two nursing specialty areas of interest relevant to adult care. (Hint: Use MEDLINE or CINAHL and do a search for 2000 to 2002.)

5 Choose one priority area from one of the specialty areas. Run a literature search for the year 2001 to the present and see what nursing research has been conducted in your selected area.

Using issues that arise from clinical practice

In this section, we examine another example of a clinical question that might arise during clinical practice, explore the search process, and examine the search results. We define our problem by parameters that provide guidance in viewing a nursing care problem. Ask yourself the following questions: Who is the target of care (e.g. male, female, young or middle-aged adult, family or caregiver)? What level of care is involved (e.g. does the problem require health maintenance or prevention, acute care or chronic care)? What aspect of care is involved (e.g. physical, psychological, sociocultural or spiritual)? What, if any, nursing specialty area is involved (e.g. respiratory, cardiovascular, oncology, rehabilitation or mental health)? Finally, what care setting did the problem arise in (e.g. clinic, physician's office, home, occupational setting or hospital)?

We are nurses in the outpatient clinic of a large cancer treatment centre. Regardless of cancer diagnosis or treatment, one theme—being chronically tired—is a constant for all our patients. They use phrases like 'tired to the bone', 'dead tired' and 'beyond exhaustion'. They all say they have never felt this tired or experienced this type of tiredness before. All state that they have tried getting more rest, doing less and eating better, with little effect. We check them for anaemia and make sure they see a physician if they are anaemic, but we wonder if there is any new wisdom on nursing interventions for this problem. It is obvious that the standard advice to alternate rest and activity, decrease activity, decrease stress, get enough sleep and eat a balanced diet is not helping.

We do a CINAHL search through the OVID search interface using the key words 'cancer related fatigue'. This sends us to a mapping display that gives a choice of 10 subject headings. We choose 'fatigue' and tick the Focus box. (Hint: This means the search will only consider those articles for which fatigue is a major focus.) We choose a second term in this list: 'cancer patients'. With this term we tick the Explode box. (Hint: This means that the search will look for articles with this or any related term.) Then we combine the terms by selecting the Boolean operator 'and' in the box at the top of the mapping display page. This means the search will only look for articles that deal with both 'fatigue' and 'cancer patients'. We then click Continue to run the search. Finally, we limit the search to the year 2001 and to research articles. We run the search and get 30 citations.

Twenty-two of the citations are immediately eliminated by examining the article titles. Eliminations include articles not immediately related to cancer-related fatigue, articles that focus on testing fatigue scales or other models, fatigue studies with very select contexts, and studies of children or the elderly. Reading available article abstracts and discovering that they are not applicable to our situation eliminates another five studies. Four studies confirm our patients' perceptions about fatigue and its effects, but are basically literature reviews and expert opinion. One study is a pilot project that appears to imply that fatigue is not a major concern for the participants in that particular study.

However, the final three studies offer new insights and strategies. A study by Holley & Borger (2001) evaluated the effect of a rehabilitation group intervention for people experiencing cancer-related fatigue. The treatment included weekly structured sessions over a period of eight weeks and involved instruction on topics such as exercise, energy conservation and Tai Chi as well as the sharing and support provided by the group process. Post-test results showed a significant difference in reduction of fatigue distress and quality of life scores to those of the pre-test.

Dodd et al (2001) describe a study that considered fatigue as one of a cluster of symptoms associated with cancer. Symptom clusters comprise three or more simultaneous symptoms that are related to each other. The theory is that symptom clusters may have a synergistic adverse effect on patient morbidity. In the study, pain, fatigue and sleep insufficiency were considered a cluster. Due to its potential confounding effect, the patient's age was also taken into consideration. The results showed that age, pain and fatigue were significant as predictors of change in the patient's functional status. While the study had recognised limitations, the implications are that nurses need to pay more attention to the identification of clusters of symptoms rather than isolating symptoms and treating them individually.

A study by Schwartz et al (2001) examined the relationship between an eight-week home-based exercise intervention and fatigue over the first three cycles of chemotherapy in women being treated for breast cancer. Seventy-two newly diagnosed women were instructed in a moderate-intensity aerobic exercise intervention, with 61 women completing the program. Measurements were taken at baseline and post intervention and included functional ability, energy expenditure and fatigue. The women were asked to maintain daily fatigue records.

Following statistical analysis the results showed a significant reduction in the day-to-day fatigue experienced by women who followed the low-to-moderate intensity exercise program regularly. The study was deemed limited due to its one-group design and further research was recommended. However, the researchers concluded that even minimal but regular exercise can assist in reducing fatigue in women with breast cancer who are receiving chemotherapy.

> **Student Challenge**
>
> Chasing Adult Challenges
>
> 1. Review your experiences in caring for adults and think about a situation you wish to explore in the current research literature.
> 2. Identify appropriate search parameters for the subject material and conduct a library search for the years 2001 to the present. What did you find?
> 3. If your search was fruitful, retrieve one or two promising articles.
> 4. Review the articles. How might the results of the studies be helpful in clinical practice?

Scanning available resources

Let's explore what is available in the research literature by using our third strategy and scanning the tables of contents and the abstracts of the research and clinical specialty journals listed in Box 10-1. By now you should be developing scanning skills that allow you to do journal scans more efficiently and effectively. For example, some journals and their tables of contents and abstracts of articles are available through various websites on the internet. Several of these are listed in the Resource Kit. Check the Resource Kit for a handy website that lists links to journals on the internet. These journals all have descriptive information available on the web, and many may now offer tables of contents and abstracts. These websites make scanning a particular journal as easy as sitting down with a copy of the journal itself.

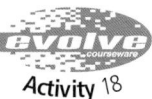

Activity 18

How do you scan journals that are not listed on the web without having actual journals in hand? Make use of CINAHL or MEDLINE electronic search features. Either search mechanism allows you to specify a specific journal or journals and put a limit on the years you are interested in. In MEDLINE, simply make a temporary personalised journal list. Search for the journals you are interested in (e.g. *Australian Journal of Advanced Nursing*) by clicking on the journal icon at the top of the screen and then entering the title in the search box. Tick the appropriate journal and run the search. The journal is now added to your search history box. To look at just the contents of a particular year you limit the search to a year range. Any search you do uses only those journal(s). Now specify the year you want (e.g. 2001). (Note: Do not enter any search parameters in the Search box.) The resulting search will retrieve all articles for the specified journals in the specified years (e.g. *Australian Journal of Advanced Nursing* for 2001). You can then do a quick title scan by clicking on Display. You can click on the Abstract link for those articles you want to see an abstract for. Pretty neat trick, huh?

CINAHL will let you do the same thing. Just specify the journal(s) and year(s) of interest in the appropriate places and run a search with no specification of subject matter. If you haven't discovered this trick yet, try it out by doing the following Student Challenge.

Student Challenge

Scanning Relevant Journals

1. Select one research journal and two clinical journals from those listed in Box 10-1 that are available in your library and that you have not previously scanned for in Chapter 8 or 9.
2. Scan the 2001 table of contents for each of these journals and note those articles that seem relevant to the clinical care of adults.
3. Read the abstracts for the selected articles. Weed out any articles that are not clinically relevant. How long did this take you? Are you getting more proficient? Save these articles. You will use them again later.

What Current Research Is Available?

The following are specific examples of pertinent research articles for the care of adults we found by scanning the 2001 tables of contents of the research and clinical journals listed in Box 10-1. Selected articles are briefly summarised and clinical implications are discussed.

Nursing research journals

The articles found by scanning the tables of contents of the various research journals yielded the articles listed in Box 10-3. By now you should be noticing features that allow you to eliminate certain articles as you perform your scan of research journals. For example, the titles should allow you to quickly eliminate articles that focus on tool development and tool reliability and validity or discuss methodological issues. Articles that focus on the education of nurses or nursing administration issues can also be eliminated. Opinion or editorial articles can also be deleted from the scan. More subtle clues also allow elimination of articles from consideration. Articles on children or adolescents are not relevant to an adult population. Though you may be tempted to discard reports from other countries, they are well worth reading. In

Australia, international research is particularly important as it can provide insights applicable to Australia's diverse society. As you refine your scanning techniques, the process becomes more efficient and more productive.

This scan produced a large array of articles, as would be expected by the breadth of the population we are using as a search parameter. Examining the titles of the articles among all the research journals reveals quite a number of articles on the adult population. When scanning for journals that publish more frequently, such as the *Journal of Advanced Nursing*, hundreds of articles/features may be displayed. Our scan of 2001, for example, revealed 391 articles for the year. In this case it was necessary to limit the search to research and the age range to adult 19–44 years and middle age 45–64 years in order to produce a more manageable list (53 articles).

This time, it is your job to examine the results of the scan. This will help you make use of the available information just by looking at the study titles. Read this list, then try the Student Challenge that follows.

BOX 10-3 Relevant Adult Titles in Research Journals

Nursing Research

Belza B, Steele BG, Hunziker J et al (2001). Correlates of physical activity in chronic obstructive pulmonary disease. *Nursing Research* 50(4):195–202.

Bliss DZ, Jung H, Savik K et al (2001). Supplementation with dietary fiber improves fecal incontinence. *Nursing Research* 50(4):203–213.

Carrieri-Kohlman V, Gormley JM, Eiser S et al (2001). Dyspnea and the affective response during exercise training in obstructive pulmonary disease. *Nursing Research* 50(3):136–146.

Cowan MJ, Pike KC, Budzynski HK (2001). Psychosocial nursing therapy following sudden cardiac arrest: impact on two-year survival. *Nursing Research* 50(2):68–76.

Dwyer KA, Coty M, Smith CA et al (2001). A comparison of two methods of assessing disease activity in the joints. *Nursing Research* 50(4):214–221.

Gulick EE (2001). Emotional distress and activities of daily living functioning in persons with multiple sclerosis. *Nursing Research* 50(3):147–154.

Johnson VY (2001). Effects of a submaximal exercise protocol to recondition the pelvic floor musculature. *Nursing Research* 50(1):33–41.

Milner KA, Funk M, Richards S et al (2001). Symptom predictors of acute coronary syndromes in younger and older patients. *Nursing Research* 50(4):233–241.

Morse GG, House JW (2001). Changes in Ménière's disease responses as a function of the menstrual cycle. *Nursing Research* 50(5):286–292.

Nyamathi A, Leake B, Longshore D et al (2001). Reliability of homeless women's reports: concordance between hearsay and self report of cocaine use. *Nursing Research* 50(3):165–171.

Tilden VP, Tolle SW, Nelson CA et al (2001). Family decision-making to withdraw life-sustaining treatments from hospitalised patients. *Nursing Research* 50(2):105–115.

Journal of Nursing Scholarship

Côté-Arsenault D, Morrison-Beedy D (2001). Women's voices reflecting changed expectations for pregnancy after perinatal loss. *Journal of Nursing Scholarship* 33(3):239–244.

Horowitz JA, Bell M, Trybulski J et al (2001). Promoting responsiveness between mothers with depressive symptoms and their infants. *Journal of Nursing Scholarship* 33(4):323–329.

Humphreys JC (2001). Turnings and adaptations in resilient daughters of battered women. *Journal of Nursing Scholarship* 33(3):245–251.

Western Journal of Nursing Research

Anderson DG, Imle MA (2001). Families of origin of homeless and never-homeless women. *Western Journal of Nursing Research* 23(4):394–413.

Beckie TM, Beckstead JW, Webb MS (2001). Modeling women's quality of life after cardiac events. *Western Journal of Nursing Research* 23(2):179–194.

Brauer DJ (2001). Common patterns of person–environment interaction in persons with rheumatoid arthritis. *Western Journal of Nursing Research* 23(4):414–430.

Ellermann CR, Reed PG (2001). Self-transcendence and depression in middle-age adults. *Western Journal of Nursing Research* 23(7):698–713.

Logsdon MC, Usui W (2001). Psychosocial predictors of postpartum depression in diverse groups of women. *Western Journal of Nursing Research* 23(6):563–574.

McCormack D, MacIntosh J (2001). Research with homeless people uncovers a model of health. *Western Journal of Nursing Research* 23(7):679–697.

Scisney-Matlock M, Watkins KW, Colling KB (2001). The interaction of age and cognitive representations in predicting blood pressure. *Western Journal of Nursing Research* 23(5):476–489.

Williamson C, Folaron G (2001). Violence, risk, and survival strategies of street prostitution. *Western Journal of Nursing Research* 23(5):463–475.

Journal of Advanced Nursing

Bergman E, Berterö C (2001). You can do it if you set your mind to it: a qualitative study of patients with coronary artery disease. *Journal of Advanced Nursing* 36(6):733–741.

Chan H (2001). Effects of injection duration on site-pain intensity and bruising associated with subcutaneous heparin. *Journal of Advanced Nursing* 35(6):882–892.

de Wit R, van Dam F (2001). From hospital to home care: a randomized controlled trial of a pain education programme for cancer patients with chronic pain. *Journal of Advanced Nursing* 36(6):742–754.

Hemsley B, Sigafoos J, Balandin S et al (2001). Nursing the patient with severe communication impairment. *Journal of Advanced Nursing* 35(6):827–835.

Koch T, Kralik D (2001). Chronic illness: reflections on a community-based action research programme. *Journal of Advanced Nursing* 36(1):23–31.

Mastaglia B, Kristjanson LJ (2001). Factors influencing women's decisions for choice of surgery for stage I and stage II breast cancer in Western Australia. *Journal of Advanced Nursing* 35(6):836–847.

Nordgren S, Fridlund B (2001). Patients' perceptions of self-determination as expressed in the context of care. *Journal of Advanced Nursing* 35(1):117–125.

Solomon MR (2001). Eating as both coping and stressor in overweight control. *Journal of Advanced Nursing* 36(4):563–572.

Thorpe K, Barsky J (2001). Healing through self-reflection. *Journal of Advanced Nursing* 35(5):760–768.

Ward T (2001). Using psychological insights to help people quit smoking. *Journal of Advanced Nursing* 34(6):754–759.

Australian Journal of Advanced Nursing

Harvey J, Moyle W, Creedy D (2001). Women's experience of early miscarriage: a phenomenological study. *Australian Journal of Advanced Nursing* 19(1):8–14.

Jannings W, Kelly M (2001). Difficulty in removing suprapubic urinary catheters in home based patients: a comparative descriptive study. *Australian Journal of Advanced Nursing* 19(2):20–25.

Kermode S, MacLean D (2001). A study of the relationship between quality of life, health and self-esteem. *Australian Journal of Advanced Nursing* 19(2):33–40.

Lo R, MacLean D (2001). The dynamics of coping and adapting to the impact when diagnosed with diabetes. *Australian Journal of Advanced Nursing* 19(2):26–32.

Scott D, Brady S, Glynn P (2001). New mother groups as a social network intervention: consumer and maternal and child health nurse perspectives. *Australian Journal of Advanced Nursing* 18(4):23–29.

van Leeuwen M, Bennett L, West S et al (2001). Patient falls from bed and the role of bedrails in the acute care setting. *Australian Journal of Advanced Nursing* 19(2):8–13.

Nursing Science Quarterly

Anderson JA (2001). Understanding homeless adults by testing the theory of self-care. *Nursing Science Quarterly* 14(1):59–67.

Jonas-Simpson CM (2001). Feeling understood: a melody of human becoming. *Nursing Science Quarterly* 14(3):222–230.

Woods SJ, Isenberg MA (2001). Adaptation as a mediator of intimate abuse and traumatic stress in battered women. *Nursing Science Quarterly* 14(3):215–221.

Research in Nursing and Health

Benfield RD, Herman J, Katz VL et al (2001). Hydrotherapy in labor. *Research in Nursing and Health* 24(1):57–67.

Blue CL, Wilbur J, Marston-Scott M (2001). Exercise among blue-collar workers: application of the theory of planned behavior. *Research in Nursing and Health* 24(6):481–493.

Kearney MH (2001). Enduring love: a grounded formal theory of women's experience of domestic violence. *Research in Nursing and Health* 24(4):270–282.

Lindgren K (2001). Relationships among maternal–fetal attachment, prenatal depression, and health practices in pregnancy. *Research in Nursing and Health* 24(3):203–217.

Mellon S, Northouse LL (2001). Family survivorship and quality of life following a cancer diagnosis. *Research in Nursing and Health* 24(6):446–459.

Moore SM, Dolansky MA (2001). Randomized trial of a home recovery intervention following coronary artery bypass surgery. *Research in Nursing and Health* 24(2):93–104.

Nyamathi A, Flaskerud JH, Leake B et al (2001). Evaluating the impact of peer, nurse case-managed, and standard HIV risk-reduction programs on psychosocial and health-promoting behavioral outcomes among homeless women. *Research in Nursing and Health* 24(5):410–422.

Pieper B, Templin T (2001). Chronic venous insufficiency in persons with a history of injection drug use. *Research in Nursing and Health* 24(5):423–432.

Stull DE, Clough LA, Van Dussen D (2001). Self-report quality of life as a predictor of hospitalization for patients with LV dysfunction: a life course approach. *Research in Nursing and Health* 24(6):460–469.

Welch JL (2001). Hemodialysis patient beliefs by stage of fluid adherence. *Research in Nursing and Health* 24(2):105–112.

Zauszniewski JA, Chung C (2001). Resourcefulness and health practices of diabetic women. *Research in Nursing and Health* 24(2):113–121.

International Journal of Nursing Studies

Galvin K, Webb C, Hillier V (2001). Assessing the impact of a nurse-led health education intervention for people with peripheral vascular disease who smoke: the use of physiological markers, nicotine dependence and withdrawal. *International Journal of Nursing Studies* 38(1):91–105.

Glacken M, Kernohan G, Coates V (2001). Diagnosed with hepatitis C: a descriptive exploratory study. *International Journal of Nursing Studies* 38(1):107–116.

Kuzu N, Ucar H (2001). The effect of cold on the occurrence of bruising, haematoma and pain at the injection site in subcutaneous low molecular weight heparin. *International Journal of Nursing Studies* 38(1):51–59.

> **Student Challenge**
>
> Sorting Out Scan Results
>
> 1. Examine the results of the scan of research journals listed in Box 10-3.
> 2. What patterns do you see in the titles of the research?
> 3. Which of these articles might be relevant to the adult research priorities we discussed in the previous section?
> 4. Can you determine which articles are qualitative and which are quantitative?
> 5. Can you distinguish the target of care, level of care, aspect of care, nursing specialty area and care setting from the titles?
> 6. Which studies seem to be research about specific nursing interventions?
> 7. Which studies do you need to see an abstract of to determine enough about the study to answer the questions raised in this challenge?

Clinical nursing journals

The articles found by scanning the tables of contents of the clinical journals yielded a number of possible relevant research articles, listed in Box 10-4. Have you been able to distinguish between research and non-research articles yet when you are scanning titles in a table of contents? Sometimes it is hard, particularly when the study uses a qualitative methodology. As you become more familiar with the different clinical journals, you will be able to zero in on the research articles more quickly. (Hint: When you are uncertain, take a quick peek at the abstract of the article. If there is no abstract, this is a clue that the article is not a research article. Remember, too, that you can always limit your search to research.) Look for other clues in CINAHL and MEDLINE citations. Article citations labelled review, editorial or opinion are not research articles.

> **BOX 10-4** Relevant Research Article Titles Using Adult Populations in Clinical Journals
>
> **Australian Critical Care (2001)**
> Boyle M, Green M (2001). Pressure sores in intensive care: defining their incidence and associated factors and assessing the utility of two pressure sore risk assessment tools. *Australian Critical Care* 14(1):24–30.
> Grech C, Pannell D, Smith-Sparrow T (2001). The delay in transfer between the emergency department and the critical care unit for patients with an acute cardiac event—in hospital factors. *Australian Critical Care* 14(4):139–145.
> Heron R, Davie A, Gillies R et al (2001). Interrater reliability of the Glasgow coma scale scoring among nurses in sub-specialties of critical care. *Australian Critical Care* 14(3):100–105.
> McKenna S, Wallis M, Brannelly A et al (2001). The nursing management of diarrhoea and constipation before and after the implementation of a bowel management protocol. *Australian Critical Care* 14(1):10–16.
>
> **Heart & Lung: Journal of Acute & Critical Care**
> Banasik, JL, Emerson RJ (2001). Effect of lateral positions on tissue oxygenation in the critically ill. *Heart & Lung: Journal of Acute & Critical Care* 30(4):269–276.
> Evangelista LS, Berg J, Dracup K (2001). Relationship between psychosocial variables and compliance in patients with heart failure. *Heart & Lung: Journal of Acute & Critical Care* 30(4):294–301.
> Mårtensson J, Dracup K, Fridlund B (2001). Decisive situations influencing spouses' support of patients with heart failure: a critical incident technique analysis. *Heart & Lung: Journal of Acute & Critical Care* 30(5):341–350.
> Matthees BJ, Anantachoti P, Kreitzer MJ et al (2001). Use of complementary therapies, adherence, and quality of life in lung transplant recipients. *Heart & Lung: Journal of Acute & Critical Care* 30(4):258–268.
> Plach SK, Heidrich SM (2001). Women's perceptions of their social roles after heart surgery and coronary angioplasty. *Heart & Lung: Journal of Acute & Critical Care* 30(2):117–127.
> Rankin JA, Fofonoff DA (2001). Atypical presentation of acute myocardial infarction in 3 age groups. *Heart & Lung: Journal of Acute & Critical Care* 30(4):285–293.
> Salyer J, Sneed G, Corley MC (2001). Lifestyle and health status in long-term cardiac transplant recipients. *Heart & Lung: Journal of Acute & Critical Care* 30(6):445–457.
> Scherer YK, Bruce S (2001). Knowledge, attitudes, and self-efficacy and compliance with medical regimen, number of emergency department visits, and hospitalizations in adults with asthma. *Heart & Lung: Journal of Acute & Critical Care* 30(4):250–257.

Song R, Lee H (2001). Effects of a 12-week cardiac rehabilitation exercise program on motivation and health-promoting lifestyle. *Heart & Lung: Journal of Acute & Critical Care* 30(3):200–209.

Walthall H, Robson D, Ray S (2001). Do any preoperative variables affect extubation time after coronary artery bypass graft surgery? *Heart & Lung: Journal of Acute & Critical Care* 30(3):216–224.

Wong HLC, Lopez-Nahas V, Molassiotis A (2001). Effects of music therapy on anxiety in ventilator-dependent patients. *Heart & Lung: Journal of Acute & Critical Care* 30(5):376–387.

Australian Journal of Holistic Nursing

Henderson J (2001). Migraine in women twenty-six to forty-five years of age. *Australasian Journal of Neuroscience* 14(2):10–17. (Originally published *Australian Journal of Holistic Nursing* (1999) 6(2):10–19.)

Nursing Praxis in New Zealand

Stephens C, Carryer J, Budge RC (2001). Decisions about starting and ceasing HRT use: information needs of women. *Nursing Praxis in New Zealand* 17(2):33–43.

International Journal of Nursing Practice

Åstedt-Kurki P, Isola A, Tammentie T, Kervinen U (2001). Importance of humour to client–nurse relationships and clients' well-being. *International Journal of Nursing Practice* 7(2):119–125.

Bolton J, Russell WJ (2001). Are nasal spectacles adequate for supplementary oxygen in patients after anaesthesia? *International Journal of Nursing Practice* 7(5):329–335.

Evans D, Hodgkinson B, Lambert L, Wood J (2001). Fall risk factors in the hospital setting: a systematic review. *International Journal of Nursing Practice* 7(1):38–45.

Kabeyama K, Miyoshi M (2001). Longitudinal study of the intensity of memorized labour pain. *International Journal of Nursing Practice* 7(1):46–53.

Tsay S, Halstead MT, McCrone S (2001). Predictors of coping efficacy, negative moods and post-traumatic stress syndrome following major trauma. *International Journal of Nursing Practice* 7(2):74–83.

Weiss SJ, Puntillo K (2001). Predictors of cardiac patients' psychophysiological responses to caregiving. *International Journal of Nursing Practice* 7(3):177–187.

Wengström Y, Häggmark C, Forsberg C (2001). Coping with radiation therapy: effects of a nursing intervention on coping ability for women with breast cancer. *International Journal of Nursing Practice* 7(1):8–15.

Oncology Nursing Forum

Badger TA, Braden CJ, Mishel MH (2001). Depression burden, self-help interventions, and side effect experience in women receiving treatment for breast cancer. *Oncology Nursing Forum* 28(3):567–574.

Foxall MJ, Barron CR, Houfek JF (2001). Ethnic influences on body awareness, trait anxiety, perceived risk, and breast and gynecologic cancer screening practices. *Oncology Nursing Forum* 28(4):727–738.

Lackey NR, Gates MF, Brown G (2001). African American women's experiences with the initial discovery, diagnosis, and treatment of breast cancer. *Oncology Nursing Forum* 28(3):519–527.

Lennie TA, Christman SK, Jadack RA (2001). Educational needs and altered eating habits following a total laryngectomy. *Oncology Nursing Forum* 28(4):667–674.

Maliski SL, Heilemann MV, McCorkle R (2001). Mastery of postprostatectomy incontinence and impotence: his work, her work, our work. *Oncology Nursing Forum* 28(6):985–992.

Meeske A, Ruccione K, Globe DR et al (2001). Posttraumatic stress, quality of life, and psychological distress in young adult survivors of childhood cancer. *Oncology Nursing Forum* 28(3):481–489.

Olsen DL, Raub W Jr, Bradley C et al (2001). The effect of aloe vera gel/mild soap versus mild soap alone in preventing skin reactions in patients undergoing radiation therapy. *Oncology Nursing Forum* 28(3):543–547.

Saleh US, Brockopp DY (2001). Quality of life one year following bone marrow transplantation: psychometric evaluation of the Quality of Life in Bone Marrow Transplant Survivors Tool. *Oncology Nursing Forum* 28(9):1457–1464.

Velji K, Fitch M (2001). The experience of women receiving brachytherapy for gynecologic cancer. *Oncology Nursing Forum* 28(4): 743–751.

Volker DL (2001). Oncology nurses' experiences with requests for assisted dying from terminally ill patients with cancer. *Oncology Nursing Forum* 28(1):39–49.

Rehabilitation Nursing

Akdolun N, Terakye G (2001). Sexual problems before and after myocardial infarction: patients' needs for information. *Rehabilitation Nursing* 26(4):152–158.

Baird KK, Pierce LL (2001). Adherence to cardiac therapy for men with coronary artery disease. *Rehabilitation Nursing* 26(6):233–237, 243, 251.

Burman ME (2001). Family caregiver expectations and management of the stroke trajectory. *Rehabilitation Nursing* 26(3):94–99, 121.

Chasens ER, Umlauf M, Valappil T et al (2001). Nocturnal problems in postpolio syndrome: sleep apnea symptoms and nocturia. *Rehabilitation Nursing* 26(2):66–71.

Gross JC, Faulkner EA, Goodrich SW et al (2001). A patient acuity and staffing tool for stroke rehabilitation inpatients based on the FIM instrument. *Rehabilitation Nursing* 26(3):108–113.

Holland B, Pokorny ME (2001). Slow stroke back massage: its effect on patients in a rehabilitation setting. *Rehabilitation Nursing* 26(5):182–186.

Karper WB, Hopewell R, Hodge M (2001). Perspectives: Exercise program effects on one woman with dermatomyositis. *Rehabilitation Nursing* 26(4):129–131, 158–159.

McSweeney JC, Crane PB (2001). An act of courage: women's decision-making processes regarding outpatient cardiac rehabilitation attendance ... including commentary by Bach CA. *Rehabilitation Nursing* 26(4):132–140, 163.

Pierce LL (2001). Caring and expressions of stability by urban family caregivers of persons with stroke within African American family systems. *Rehabilitation Nursing* 26(3):100–107, 116, 121.

Wilk C, Turkoski B (2001). Progressive muscle relaxation in cardiac rehabilitation: a pilot study ... including commentary by Miller ET. *Rehabilitation Nursing* 26(6):238–243.

Clinical journals regularly publish research on the care of adults. All these journals publish research within a confined specialty area. The research articles in *Australian Critical Care* are concerned with critical care usually seen in intensive care and trauma units. Most of the studies primarily target very specific and highly technical nursing interventions. The research articles published in *Heart and Lung: Journal of Acute and Critical Care* are divided between cardiovascular and pulmonary studies and use both quantitative and qualitative methodologies. Many are related to recognised areas of research priority (e.g. studies on health promotion, patients with chronic illnesses, and those targeted at carers of the chronically ill).

The *International Journal of Mental Health Nursing*, as you might expect, publishes studies on mental health issues. The *Australian Journal of Holistic Nursing* includes articles on the practice of natural therapies and holistic nursing in Australia and overseas. *Nursing Praxis in New Zealand* publishes articles with a view to developing practice. *AORN* has studies relevant to the perioperative experience. The *International Journal of Nursing Practice* seeks to advance the international understanding and development of nursing through its published works, both as a profession and as an academic discipline. *Oncology Nursing Forum* is a prolific source of research on cancer and cancer care. Many of the studies target and test highly specific nursing interventions (e.g. the role of protective clothing, use of routine and breakthrough analgesia, the effects of guided imagery, effects of nutritional supplements and catheter port cleansing). Others examine the larger picture of what it is like to have a diagnosis of cancer (e.g. the meaning of quality of life, life quality in women with breast cancer, anxiety while awaiting surgery).

Still others examine issues central to cancer patients such as fatigue, pain, side effects and quality of sleep. There are studies that address psychological, physical and sociocultural aspects of the cancer experience. Some studies examine screening activities such as Pap smears or breast self-examination or mammography. *Rehabilitation Nursing* studies target acute and long-term care issues and chronic illness or disability. The journals listed in Box 10-4 devote varying amounts of their journal space to research articles.

Other clinical journals stemming from Australia and New Zealand include: *ACCNS Journal for Community Nurses*; *ACORN, The Journal of Perioperative Nursing in Australia*; *Australasian Journal of Neuroscience*; *Australian Emergency Nursing Journal*; *Australian Journal of Midwifery*; *Australian Journal of Rural Health*; *JARNA*, the official journal of the Australasian Rehabilitation Nurses' Association; *Transplant Nurses Journal*. Although some of these journals publish fewer research articles, they still serve as useful resources.

Try a quick analysis of the clinical research titles using the following Student Challenge.

Student Challenge

Sorting Out Clinical Scan Results

1. Examine the results of the scan of clinical journals listed in Box 10-4.
2. What patterns do you see in the titles of the research?
3. Which of these articles might be relevant to the adult research priorities we discussed?
4. Can you determine which articles are qualitative and which are quantitative?
5. Can you distinguish the target of care, level of care, aspect of care, nursing specialty area and care setting from the titles?
6. Which studies seem to be research about specific nursing interventions?
7. Which studies do you need to see an abstract of to determine enough about the study to answer the questions raised in this challenge?

Summarising and using scan results

Several of the identified research articles have been selected to serve as examples of how research articles might be summarised and the findings used in clinical practice. A number of articles in both the research and clinical journals examined aspects of nursing care. They provide concrete data about the effectiveness of certain nursing interventions used in the care of adult populations. We will look at several of these articles in more depth.

The first article (Chan 2001) describes a within-subjects quasi-experiment to determine whether there was any difference in the intensity of injection-site pain and bruising when two different techniques for the administration of subcutaneous heparin were used. Thirty-four stroke patients were each given low-molecular-weight heparin by one of two injection modes for their morning dose, and then 12 hours later were given a second dose via the second injection technique. The technique was based on duration of injection. Using a tool called the vertical visual analogue scale, subjects rated the level of perceived site-pain intensity. Injection-site bruising was measured at predetermined intervals following each injection and a special tool used to measure the surface-area of bruise tracings. With the level of significance set at $p < 0.05$, the final data set of pain scores and bruise sizes was statistically analysed to determine the effects caused by injection duration. The results of the study indicated that the injection technique over 30 seconds caused significantly less intense site-pain and fewer and smaller bruises. Due to limitations of design, however, the author states that the generalisability of the results may be compromised. Clearly, the findings should be considered preliminary and follow-up studies conducted. Administering subcutaneous heparin is a task common to many nurses. Evidence of a less painful technique that produces less bruising should be of interest to nurses in a range of settings.

In a second study (Olsen et al 2001) the researchers set out to determine whether the use of mild soap and aloe vera gel as opposed to mild soap alone would have an ameliorating effect on the incidence of skin reactions in patients undergoing radiation therapy. The subjects consisted of a mix of Caucasians (74%) and African Americans (26%) with a mean age of 56 years. The setting was a radiation therapy outpatient clinic in a cancer centre attached to a major teaching hospital. The design of the study was a prospective, randomised, blinded clinical trial. On the first day of radiation therapy, as a prophylactic measure against radiation dermatitis, patients began cleansing the radiation area with mild, unscented soap. Those patients randomised into the experimental arm of the trial were instructed to liberally apply aloe vera gel to the area at various intervals throughout the day. The effects of the treatment were measured over time. The findings showed that at low cumulative dose levels, adding aloe vera made no difference. However, when the cumulative dose was high the median time prior to any skin changes in the aloe/soap arm was five weeks, compared to three weeks in the soap-only arm. The results suggest therefore that adding aloe vera to the soap regimen has a protective effect when the cumulative dose is increased over time. Oncology nurses would be aware that patients undergoing radiotherapy may be predisposed to skin problems and that the products used to treat radiation dermatitis are many and varied. This research throws light on an intervention that could prove a useful and cost-effective strategy to increase patient comfort. Nurses in the field may wish to consider its clinical significance.

The third quantitative study investigated the effect of music therapy in decreasing anxiety in ventilator-dependent patients (Wong et al 2001). The design of the study consisted of crossover repeated measures following random assignment and was carried out on 20 ventilator-dependent Chinese patients with a mean age of 58 years and mostly men (75%). Mean blood pressure and respiratory rate together with the Chinese version of the Spielberger State-Trait Anxiety Inventory were used to measure anxiety. The subjects were randomised to receive one of two treatments. The first consisted of 30 minutes of uninterrupted rest and then 30 minutes of music therapy or music therapy followed by an uninterrupted rest period. The relaxing music consisted of both Chinese and Western music chosen by the subjects from a given selection. The music was audible through audio cassette players and headphones.

Immediately before the intervention (or rest period) and at five-minute intervals throughout the intervention, physiological measurements were taken. Immediately before the intervention and after the intervention, the Chinese version of Spielberger's State-Trait Anxiety Inventory was completed. Following statistical analysis of the results, the indications are that anxiety is more effectively decreased by music therapy than by an uninterrupted rest period ($p < .01$). While analysis of variance with repeated measurements on blood pressure and respiratory rate showed no significant differences in the two conditions over time, at the end of the intervention (after 30 minutes) significant differences were observed between the two conditions, with music therapy being more effective than the rest period.

This study demonstrated that music therapy is a useful nursing intervention to decrease anxiety in ventilator-dependent patients, at least in Chinese patients. Depending on their appraisal of the research and consideration of its applicability to their own context and patient group, other critical care nurses may consider incorporating music therapy into the care of mechanically ventilated patients or perhaps replicating the study to more fully determine its effects. Music as therapy could be considered across a number of specialty fields.

We also examine several of the qualitative studies uncovered in the scanning process. The first study (Côté-Arsenault & Morrison-Beedy 2001) sought to describe women's experiences of pregnancy following a previous perinatal loss and the long-term effects of such a loss. This was a study informed by phenomenology and involved 21 women participating in three focus groups. The women differed in their obstetric and loss histories and the time since their losses ranged from 34 years to the preceding year. Colaizzi's procedural steps underpinned the data analysis. Results showed that perinatal loss was perceived as a life-altering event. In subsequent pregnancies women felt emotionally unsafe, afraid they would lose these babies too. The researchers discovered that despite the differences in the obstetric and loss histories and time since loss, the similarities expressed by the women in their responses to pregnancy far outweighed the differences. Six common themes emerged: (1) dealing with uncertainty; (2) wondering if the baby is healthy; (3) waiting to lose the baby; (4) holding back emotions; (5) acknowledging that loss happened and that it can happen again; and (6) changing self. The researchers concluded that in response to perinatal loss and subsequent pregnancy, women live through similar experiences with common concerns and that variations are not linked to the number or gestational age of the losses.

The results of this research are particularly useful to obstetric nurses and others who may care for pregnant women. Women's past losses need to be acknowledged and their concerns addressed during later pregnancies. Recognising the potentially lifelong effects that perinatal loss may have on a woman will assist the nurse to care more effectively for these individuals.

A second qualitative study (Bergman & Berterö 2001) sought to gain increased knowledge and understanding of the experience of coronary artery disease (CAD) and the way it affects an individual's life/lifestyle. The study took a hermeneutic approach to interpreting data gathered from eight people diagnosed with coronary artery disease. During an in-depth interview the participants were asked to talk about their life situation and the opportunities and obstacles they met in making lifestyle changes. Interviews were transcribed and analysed and three overarching spheres of interest emerged: (1) the causes of coronary artery disease; (2) difficulties in the work of rehabilitation, exacerbated by feelings of confusion, uncertainty and sadness; and (3) successful rehabilitation (appeared to be related to the personality of the individual patient and external supports). The conclusions drawn from this study are that while patients may comply with follow-up medical visits they are less successful in making recommended lifestyle changes. However, by working together with patients and providing more individualistic care, nurses can empower patients to make the necessary lifestyle changes and manage their self-care activities more effectively. This study will be useful to acute care and community nurses, who often play a significant role in supporting patients with coronary artery disease. The results of this study could be used as a baseline for generating new strategies aimed at empowering cardiac rehabilitation patients.

A third qualitative study (Thorpe & Barsky 2001) canvassed the voices of women on the process of healing through self-reflection and was part of a larger study that used survey technique to gather data on women's health, occupational and life experience. Eight women, all registered nurses, were selected through purposive sampling to participate in semi-structured interviews designed to be in-depth and personal. Major concepts stemming from the data drawn from the original questionnaire underpinned the interview schedule and included concepts such as health, stress and life cycle stage. Following analysis the emergent categories, themes and patterns were duly authenticated. The researchers discuss three themes stemming from the data (spirituality; being versus doing; and eustress versus distress) and state that self-reflection was clearly evident. In essence, the women used self-reflection to search for meaning in both their personal and professional lives, and through this process healing occurred. All the women spoke of the need to find balance in the business of work and family commitments that encompassed personal, professional, spiritual and social realms. If unchecked, the relentlessness of change and its demands could take a toll spiritually, emotionally, mentally and physically. Through self-reflection the women recognised the need to save some caring for themselves and that this was essential if they were to care for others.

Displaying perspectives in this way provides the opportunity for others to learn from and apply the knowledge gained to their own lives. Realisation of the usefulness of self-reflection may encourage nurses across a number of settings to learn more about the technique in order to facilitate self-healing in individuals and groups in their care. Importantly, the study signals the need for women and indeed nurses to self-reflect, to care for self and to nurture the important balance between work and leisure.

Now that you have seen several examples of how quantitative and qualitative studies might be considered for application in the care of adults, practise with some articles of your own by completing the following Student Challenge.

> **Student Challenge**
>
> Using Data from Journal Scans
>
> Use the articles that resulted from your journal scan.
>
> 1. Read the articles to determine what was studied, who was studied and what the study results were. Write a brief summary of each article. Use the articles cited earlier as examples.
> 2. Read the discussion sections of the articles and make a quick determination about how the results might be used in a clinical practice setting. Write out how the findings might be used and by whom.

Reading and Evaluating a Research Article on the Care of Adults

In this section we examine one quantitative research article on a clinical intervention in more depth. We again use our research reading strategy, research comprehension and research evaluation guidelines.

These exercises guide you through the critical reading, evaluation and visualisation of the selected research article. When you finish, print out your answers and our responses to the exercises. You should be feeling more confident about reading a research article and pulling out the key ideas.

Student Challenge

Surveying, Examining and Critically Reading an Adult Research Study

1. Log on to your CD-ROM and look for the 'Survey, examine and critically read' exercise in Chapter 10. Print out the reading strategy and the research article entitled 'Intradermal normal saline solution, self-selected music and insertion difficulty effects on intravenous insertion pain'.
2. Take your text, the article, the strategy and a notepad and pen, and find a conducive reading and study environment.
3. Survey the article using the strategy guidelines. Make notes of what you gleaned from your survey.
4. Now go back and read the article paragraph by paragraph and jot down the key idea in each paragraph. Note anything you don't understand.
5. When you have finished, consult references to clarify those things that are unclear.
6. When you have completed these steps, go back to the CD-ROM and complete the 'Survey, examine and critically read' exercise, the 'Study evaluation' exercise and the 'Application visualisation' exercise for Chapter 10.

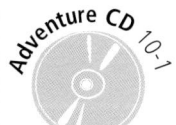
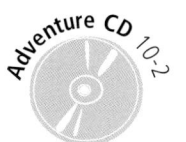

Resource Kit

Web Sources for Adult Research Priorities

The National Heart Foundation Australia

Diabetes Australia

The Cancer Council Australia

National Health and Medical Research Council: National Research Priorities

NH&MRC Submission Developing National Research Priorities: An Issues Paper

Australian Department of Health and Ageing: National Health Priority Areas

Department of Education, Science and Training—link to National Research Priorities

World Health Organization—run a search on the home page for Research Priorities

Health Research Council of New Zealand

National Institute for Nursing Research

Web Sources for Relevant Journal Tables of Contents and Abstracts

Australian Critical Care

Australian Journal of Holistic Nursing

> *International Journal of Mental Health Nursing*
>
> *Heart and Lung: Journal of Acute and Critical Care*
>
> *International Journal of Nursing Practice*
>
> *Oncology Nursing Forum*
>
> *Rehabilitation Nursing*
>
> ### Miscellaneous Web Resources
>
> Want to check out other nursing journals online? Check Evolve for a site that lists web links to 162 nursing journals. Many are in the process of making tables of contents available. Check the journals in Box 10-1 and see if any more of them are now scannable online.
>
> 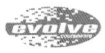 Visit the book's Evolve website at http://evolve.elsevier.com/AU/Borbasi/maze for further information.
>
> Check out the exercises on your CD-ROM.

References

Dodd MJ, Miaskowski C, Paul SM (2001). Symptom clusters and their effect on the functional status of patients with cancer. *Oncology Nursing Forum* 28(3):465–470.

Holley S, Borger D (2001). Energy for living with cancer: preliminary findings of a cancer rehabilitation group intervention study. *Oncology Nursing Forum* 28(9): 1393–1396.

Schwartz AL, Mori M, Gao R et al (2001). Exercise reduces daily fatigue in women with breast cancer receiving chemotherapy. *Medicine & Science in Sports & Exercise* 33(5):718–723.

http://evolve.elsevier.com/AU/Borbasi/maze

Learning Objectives

After reading this chapter and following critical reflection the student will be able to:

1. Identify clinical nursing journals that publish research articles relevant to older adults.
2. Discuss clinical and research priorities in the care of older adults.
3. Use research literature to clarify identified clinical practice problems for older adults.
4. Explore examples of research conducted in various areas of clinical practice with older adults.
5. Discuss the application of sample research results in clinical practice.
6. Apply the reading strategy to survey, examine, critically read and evaluate a sample research article on older adults.

Chapter Outline

What Research Resources Are Available for the Care of Older Adults?
What Approaches Can Be Used for Review of the Research Literature?
Addressing clinical and research priorities
Using issues that arise from clinical practice
Scanning available resources
What Current Research Is Available?
Nursing research journals
Clinical nursing journals
Summarising and using scan results
Reading and Evaluating a Research Article on the Care of Older Adults

Chapter 11
Reading and Using Research in the Care of Older Adults

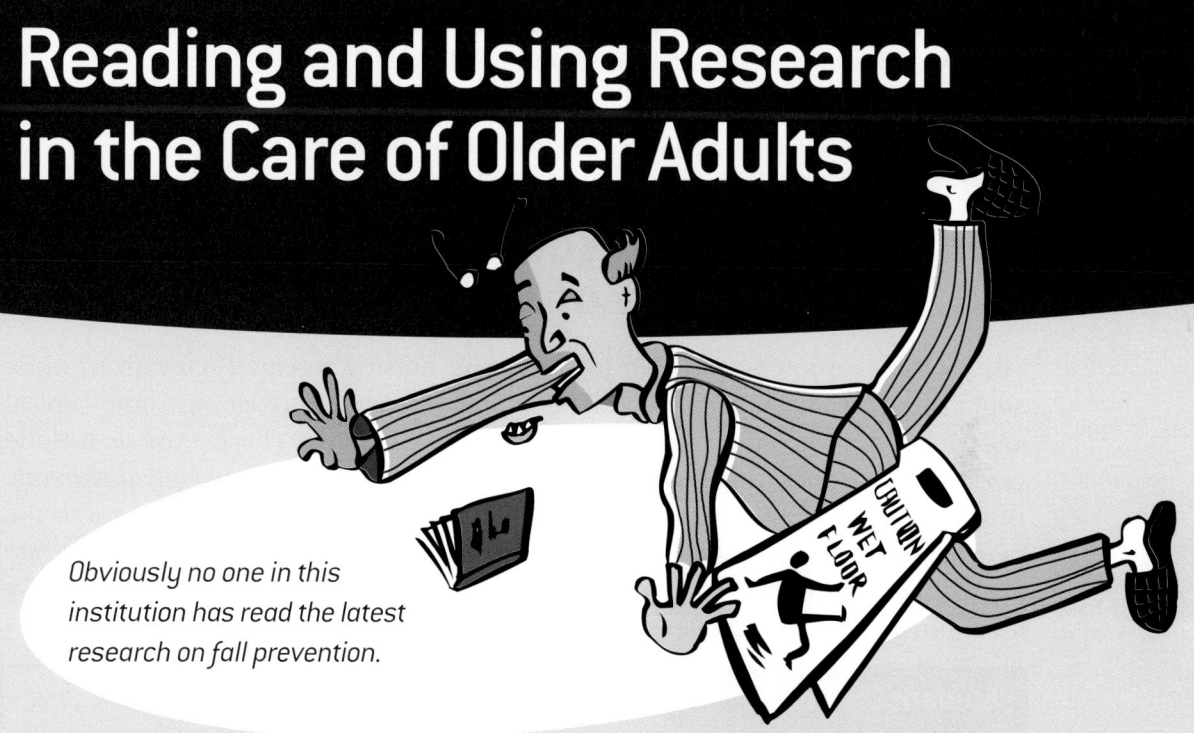

Obviously no one in this institution has read the latest research on fall prevention.

Student Quote

'I never connected with old people until I read a study [qualitative] that told it their way [from their perspective]. It really opened my eyes.'

Abstract

Several research sources publish articles pertinent to the care of older adults. Many of the research articles on older adults focus on the clinical specialty issues identified for adults and can be distinguished only by looking at the age of the sample. Other articles address specific clinical issues unique to the ageing population. These sources are used to demonstrate the research available on identified priorities for the ageing and sample problems and questions arising from clinical practice, and to examine a cross-section of current research about older adults. Samples of current studies are summarised, and clinical applications are discussed. The use of the research reading strategy is illustrated with one qualitative research article on an older adult population.

Section 3: Walking the Walk

In this chapter, we identify periodicals that contain nursing research on the care of older adults, target relevant research articles and preview sample selections of currently published research. Finally, we dissect a sample article using the reading strategy and evaluation criteria presented in Chapter 7.

> An older adult is defined as anyone 65 years of age or older.

What Research Resources Are Available for the Care of Older Adults?

Many of the resources available for reporting nursing research relevant to older adults are the same as those we identified for the adult population. Some clinical journals also focus on research relevant to the older adult. These journals include *Geriaction*, *Australian Journal on Ageing* and *Journal of Gerontological Nursing*. Box 11-1 contains a list of journals most likely to contain research relevant to the practice of nursing for older adults. As with adults, studies on the older adult are scattered across a wide range of journals other than those listed in Box 11-1. Try the following Student Challenge one last time.

Student Challenge
Perusing Specialty Journals
1. If any journals on the list in Box 11-1 are unfamiliar, take time to locate and scan two or three issues of each journal.
2. Locate a description of the journal's purpose and evaluate its readability.

BOX 11-1 Journals Containing Nursing Research Relevant to the Care of Older Adults

Nursing Research Journals
Australian Journal of Advanced Nursing
Journal of Advanced Nursing
Nursing Research
Research in Nursing & Health
Nursing Science Quarterly
Journal of Nursing Scholarship
International Journal of Nursing Studies
Western Journal of Nursing Research

Clinical Journals that Regularly Contain Research Articles About the Care of Older Adults
Geriaction
Australian Journal on Ageing
Australian Critical Care
Journal of Gerontological Nursing
International Journal of Mental Health Nursing
Heart and Lung: Journal of Acute and Critical Care
Nursing Praxis in New Zealand
AORN
International Journal of Nursing Practice
Oncology Nursing Forum
Rehabilitation Nursing

What Approaches Can Be Used for Review of the Research Literature?

We again explore our three strategies for use of the research literature as it pertains to older adults. We explore the relevant clinical and research priorities, identify some sample problems or questions that might arise from clinical practice with an ageing population, and we scan the research literature to get a feel for available research that might enhance clinical practice.

Addressing clinical and research priorities

Let's look at the care and research priorities relevant to the older adult. Important goals in the care of older adults are: slowing age-related changes such as visual or hearing impairment; loss of bone and muscle mass; maintaining functional independence in primary and secondary activities of daily living; coping with impairment, reduced function and disability; and death with dignity. We will review the pertinent Australian Department of Health and Ageing National Health Priorities as they relate to older people, and will explore the possibilities for nursing research visible in the aims and goals of organisations such as Geriaction. Other sources for research directions may be found by browsing through information on the web pages of various organisations such as The Continence Foundation of Australia, The National Heart Foundation Australia, Diabetes Australia, The Cancer Council Australia and the Australian Department of Health and Ageing—Ageing and Aged Care Division and Office for an Ageing Australia websites (see the Resource Kit at the end of this chapter for web addresses). Box 11-2 takes a more global view and

> **BOX 11-2** Elements of the United Nations Ageing Research Agenda
>
> Healthy ageing
> Biomedical issues
> Physical and mental functioning
> Care systems
> Quality of life
> Social participation and integration
> Policy process and evaluation
> Changing structures and functions of families (kin, primary groups and community)
> Economic security
> Macro societal change and development
>
> United Nations Research Agenda on Ageing for the 21st Century: Report of the Second Expert Consultative Meeting, New York, 10–12 November 1999. Online. Available: http://www.un.org/esa/socdev/ageing/ageraany.htm.

lists a number of key foci identified for ageing research by experts associated with the United Nations.

The healthcare goals and objectives for adults you discovered through taking the Student Challenge in Chapter 10 are also relevant to older adults. When you went to the Australian Department of Health and Ageing website (http://www.health.gov.au/pq/nhpa/index.htm#nhpa) you discovered that seven national health priority areas have been identified and endorsed. These include asthma, cancer control, cardiovascular health, diabetes mellitus, injury prevention and control, mental health, arthritis and musculoskeletal conditions. The main focus of course is on chronic disease and all have relevance to older adults as well as other members of the population.

The NH&MRC issues paper on Developing National Research Priorities (http://www.health.gov.au/nhmrc/research/general/devsub.pdf) has a section on research for healthy ageing and provision of effective care. As you saw in Chapter 10, the Australian Research Priorities include promoting and maintaining good health. One priority goal within this proposal is devoted to ageing well and ageing productively. In 2002 the NH&MRC funded strategic and priority-driven research in the areas of healthy ageing, chronic disease, mental health and palliative care, which included over a million dollars for research into better ways to care for the dying. More recently it has announced funding for grants that provide better understanding of healthy ageing (http://www.health.gov.au/nhmrc/media/2002rel/1_7mill.htm). In fact, at many of the websites of different organisations you can view the research projects that have been funded. These give you a good idea of priority areas. For example, The Centre for Ageing Studies (based in South Australia, http://www.cas.flinders.edu.au/about.html) has a keen interest in research on ageing. Visit the site and view the South Australian Network for Research on Ageing web page. You may like to check out their research directory at http://www.cas.flinders.edu.au/sanra/index.html and look at the research projects that are currently under way. Click on the Research Agenda link and look at the page(s) devoted to Priorities in Ageing Research—Identifying the Gaps. The New Zealand Positive Ageing strategy provides a platform for age-related research (http://www.msd.govt.nz/publications/docs/nzpositiveageingstrategy.pdf).

As you can see, there is currently a great deal of interest in ageing research.

Try the following Student Challenges to discover the very latest national and international research priorities for the older adult.

Student Challenge

Checking Research Priorities for Older Adults

1. Access the United Nations website and see if you can find the Report of the Second World Assembly on Ageing held in Madrid 8–12 April 2002. This is a comprehensive document on ageing and provides a framework for international research initiatives.

2. Now come closer to home. Go to the Australian Department of Health and Ageing website. As you saw in Chapter 10, this department is responsible for a range of policy and program responses to enhance the health and well-being of Australians.

   a. Do a search and access their Office for an Ageing Australia—Ageing and Aged Care Division internet site.

   b. Go to their Research and Policy pages. Locate the Healthy Ageing discussion paper. This paper looks at issues surrounding health promotion and illness prevention and strategies from a population health perspective. Health goals and objectives for older people outlined in that document include: maintenance of physical and mental health, performance of physical activity, prevention of falls and injury, maintenance of adequate nutrition, early detection of sensory loss, management of incontinence, evaluation of alcohol and other drug usage, and the conduct of further research and data collection.

   c. You may also like to look at the other publications on this website, including the National Strategy for an Ageing Australia Background Paper.

3. Compare the focal points related to ageing in these documents to those in Box 11-2. Note the similarities and differences.

4. Check to see if any research priorities for the older adult have been reported by specialty journals after 2001. (Hint: Run a CINAHL search using the key words 'nursing research priorities'.)

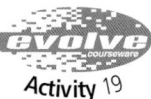

Activity 19

> **5** Choose one of the research priorities previously listed or that you have uncovered in your search. Run a literature search for the years 2001 to the present and see what nursing research has been conducted in your selected area.

Using issues that arise from clinical practice

In this section we examine another example of a clinical question that might arise during clinical practice, explore the search process and examine the search results. When we look at problems arising in our practice with older adults, we need first to ask what function age plays in the identified problem. Is age a primary focus (i.e. a major factor in the cause of the problem) or is the problem one that could occur at any age? If the answer is the latter, then ask whether you are focusing on how the problem uniquely affects the older adult. Remember the other parameters we've used to help define problems (i.e. the target of care, level of care, aspect of care and care setting).

We work in a residential care setting for the elderly. There has been increased concern regarding several residents who have fallen lately. We are getting ready to adopt a risk factors checklist. We have been asked to come up with additional ideas to help decrease the number of falls. We head for the literature with an interest in the current research available on the subject of falls and how they might be prevented or reduced. We do a CINAHL search, entering the key word 'falls'. This sends us to a mapping display with two subject headings. We choose 'accidental falls' and tick the Explode box. We are then given the option of 12 subheadings under accidental falls. Because we are unsure what might be useful, we tick the box to include all the headings. We now decide to place several limits on the search by clicking on the 'Limit' heading at the top of the search screen. We then limit the search to Australian and New Zealand journals for the years 1999 to 2001 that reported research on falls for those aged 65 to 79. We get a total of 22 articles from the search. We later run a second search to include those aged 80 and above. It yields no additional studies. So we still have a total of 22 studies to look at.

We pull the abstracts for all 22 articles. Some articles are quickly eliminated because falls were not a primary focus of the study, others because they were testing reliability and validity of instruments, and still others because they were investigating quite different cohorts of people to those found in residential aged care or they were not research studies. Two articles are in fact systematic reviews. One of these analysed nine randomised controlled trials that seemed to suggest that regular exercise may be one way to prevent falls but went on to say that the evidence as yet is inconclusive. The other examined fall risk factors in the hospital setting. This looks promising as the information might well translate to the residential setting, and as it is available in full text we print it immediately. This leaves us with four articles. All of these examined various risk factors for falls. One looked at the role of bedrails in fall prevention; two involved retrospective chart audits to determine risk factors for falling, and the last one examined the efficacy of education to raise staff awareness in order to minimise risk. There are no qualitative studies in this selection of articles. All these studies provide helpful information.

One risk factor article (van Leeuwen et al 2001) challenged the role of bedrails in the management of aged people and particularly those who are confused or 'nonrational'. Analysing retrospective accounts of 419 patient falls drawn from the records of a metropolitan acute care service provider, the audit identified 136 falls from bed. Of particular note was the fact that when the bedrails/cotsides were up (seemingly to protect the patient) the incidence of falls was equal to or higher than when the bedrails were not raised. Moreover it was discovered that patients deemed in a 'nonrational' state at the time of falling were significantly more likely to have fallen when attempting to get out of a bed that had raised cotsides. The position of the bedrails and the severity of injury did not appear to be correlated, but the fact that one patient died as a result of falling over elevated bedrails was deemed particularly significant to clinical practice. As our residents require hospitalisation at times this research finding is deemed important.

Another group of researchers (Barr, Brown & Perry 1999) studied an elderly rehabilitation client group to determine risk factors associated with falls. Conducting a retrospective chart analysis, the group evaluated the records of 87 clients who had fallen in the unit over four years. The same number of individuals who had not fallen during their rehabilitation were randomly selected and used as a comparison group. Factors associated with falling were statistically analysed and from that a model of risk developed. It was discovered that most at risk of falling were older people who were confused, had a primary diagnosis of stroke, a lower limb amputation or sleep disturbances. Some of these factors are applicable to the residents in our aged care home.

In the first instance we decide to use these two articles for discussion by the facility's journal club as this may help in advancing ideas for a staff training program. In addition we make a note to retrieve the full systematic review on falls in the hospital setting from the Joanna Briggs Institute for Evidence Based Nursing and Midwifery (Evans et al 2001). Now try the following Student Challenge.

> **Student Challenge**
>
> Chasing the Challenges of Ageing
>
> 1. Review your experiences in caring for older adults and think about a situation you wish to explore in the current research literature.
> 2. Identify appropriate search parameters for the subject material and conduct a library search for the years 2001 to present. What did you find?
> 3. If your search was fruitful, retrieve one or two promising articles.
> 4. Review the articles. How might the results of the studies be helpful in clinical practice?

Scanning available resources

Let's explore what was available in the research literature by using our third strategy and scanning the tables of contents and abstracts of the research and clinical specialty journals listed in Box 11-1.

> **Student Challenge**
>
> Scanning Relevant Journals
>
> Select one research journal and one clinical journal from those listed in Box 11-1 that are available in your library.
>
> 1. Scan the 2001 table of contents for each of these journals and note those research articles that seem relevant to the care of older adults.
> 2. Read the abstracts for the selected articles. Weed out any articles that are not clinically relevant. How long did this take you? Are you getting more proficient?
>
> Save these articles. You will use them again in the next Student Challenge.

What Current Research Is Available?

The following are specific examples of pertinent research articles for the care of older adults that we found by scanning the 2001 tables of contents of some of the research and clinical journals listed in Box 11-1. Selected articles are briefly summarised and clinical implications are discussed.

Nursing research journals

The articles found by scanning the tables of contents of selected research journals include the article titles listed in Box 11-3.

BOX 11-3 Relevant Titles for the Ageing in Research Journals

Australian Journal of Advanced Nursing

Kermode S, MacLean D (2001). A study of the relationship between quality of life, health and self-esteem. *Australian Journal of Advanced Nursing* 19(2):33–40.

Santamaria N, Daly S, Addicott R et al (2001). The development, validity and reliability of the hospital in the home dependency scale (HDS). *Australian Journal of Advanced Nursing* 18(4):8–14.

van Leeuwen M, Bennett L, West S et al (2001). Patient falls from bed and the role of bedrails in the acute care setting. *Australian Journal of Advanced Nursing* 19(2):8–13.

Journal of Advanced Nursing

Achterberg WP, Holtkamp CCM, Kerkstra A et al (2001). Improvements in the quality of co-ordination of nursing care following implementation of the Resident Assessment Instrument in Dutch nursing homes. *Journal of Advanced Nursing* 35(2):268–275.

Andersson I, Sidenvall B (2001). Case studies of food shopping, cooking and eating habits in older women with Parkinson's disease. *Journal of Advanced Nursing* 35(1):69–78.

Bull MJ, Roberts J (2001). Components of a proper hospital discharge for elders. *Journal of Advanced Nursing* 35(4):571–581.

Costello J (2001). Nursing older dying patients: findings from an ethnographic study of death and dying in elderly care wards. *Journal of Advanced Nursing* 35(1):59–68.

de Veer A, Kerkstra A (2001). Feeling at home in nursing homes. *Journal of Advanced Nursing* 35(3):427–434.

Faulkner M (2001). A measure of patient empowerment in hospital environments catering for older people. *Journal of Advanced Nursing* 34(5):676–686.

Graneheim U, Norberg A, Jansson L (2001). Interaction relating to privacy, identity, autonomy and security: An observation study focusing on a woman with dementia and 'behavioural disturbances', and on her care providers. *Journal of Advanced Nursing* 36(2):256–265.

Hendriksen H, Harrison R (2001). Occupational therapy in accident and emergency departments: a randomized controlled trial. *Journal of Advanced Nursing* 36(6):727–732.

Hsu H, Gallinagh R (2001). The relationships between health beliefs and utilization of free health examinations in older people living in a community setting in Taiwan. *Journal of Advanced Nursing* 35(6):864–873.

Jansson W, Nordberg G, Grafstrom M (2001). Patterns of elderly spousal caregiving in dementia care: an observational study. *Journal of Advanced Nursing* 34(6):804–812.

Jonsdottir H, Jonsdottir G, Steingrimsdottir E et al (2001). Group reminiscence among people with end-stage chronic lung diseases. *Journal of Advanced Nursing* 35(1):79–87.

Laakso S, Routasalo P (2001). Changing to primary nursing in a nursing home in Finland: experiences of residents, their family members and nurses. *Journal of Advanced Nursing* 33(4):475–483.

McGarry J, Arthur A (2001). Informal caring in late life: a qualitative study of the experiences of older carers. *Journal of Advanced Nursing* 33(2):182–189.

Marshall MJ, Hutchinson SA (2001). A critique of research on the use of activities with persons with Alzheimer's disease: a systematic literature review. *Journal of Advanced Nursing* 35(4):488–496.

May J, Ellis-Hill C, Payne S (2001). Gatekeeping and legitimization: how informal carers' relationship with health care workers is revealed in their everyday interactions. *Journal of Advanced Nursing* 36(3):364–375.

Walker E, Dewar BJ (2001). How do we facilitate carers' involvement in decision making? *Journal of Advanced Nursing* 34(3):329–337.

Waters K, Allsopp D, Davidson I et al (2001). Sources of support for older people after discharge from hospital: 10 years on. *Journal of Advanced Nursing* 33(5):575–582.

Westergren A, Ohlsson O, Hallberg IR (2001). Eating difficulties, complications and nursing interventions during a period of three months after a stroke. *Journal of Advanced Nursing* 35(3):416–426.

Yoon SL, Horne CH (2001). Herbal products and conventional medicines used by community-residing older women. *Journal of Advanced Nursing* 33(1):51–59.

Nursing Research

DiMattio MJK (2001). Brief report: recruitment and retention of community-dwelling, aging women in nursing studies. *Nursing Research* 50(6):369–373.

Given B, Given C, Azzouz F et al (2001). Physical functioning of elderly cancer patients prior to diagnosis and following initial treatment. *Nursing Research* 50(4):222–232.

Neumark DE, Stommel M, Given CW et al (2001). Brief report: research design and subject characteristics predicting nonparticipation in a panel survey of older families with cancer. *Nursing Research* 50(6):363–368.

Powers BA (2001). Ethnographic analysis of everyday ethics in the care of nursing home residents with dementia: a taxonomy. *Nursing Research* 50(6):332–339.

Resnick B, Zimmerman S, Orwig D et al (2001). Model testing for reliability and validity of the Outcome Expectations for Exercise Scale. *Nursing Research* 50(5):293–299.

Nursing Science Quarterly

Baumann SL, Carroll KA, Damgaard GA et al (2001). An international human becoming hermeneutic study of Tom Hegg's A Cup of Christmas Tea. *Nursing Science Quarterly* 14(4):316–321.

Parse RR (2001). The lived experience of contentment: a study using the Parse research method. Nursing Science Quarterly 14(4):330–338. Adapted with permission from Parse RR & Sudbury MA (2001). Qualitative inquiry: the path of sciencing. *Nursing Science Quarterly* 14(4):183–203.

Soderhamn O, Cliffordson C (2001). The structure of self-care in a group of elderly people. *Nursing Science Quarterly* 14(1):55–58.

Journal of Nursing Scholarship

Aroian KJ, Khatutsky G, Tran TV et al (2001). Health and social service utilization among elderly immigrants from the former Soviet Union. *Journal of Nursing Scholarship* 33(3):265–271.

Asahara K, Momose Y, Murashima S et al (2001). The relationship of social norms to use of services and caregiver burden in Japan. *Journal of Nursing Scholarship* 33(4):375–380.

Research in Nursing & Health

Lee HS, Brennan PF, Daly BJ (2001). Relationship of empathy to appraisal, depression, life satisfaction, and physical health in informal caregivers of older adults. *Research in Nursing & Health* 24(1):44–56.

McDonald DD, Freeland M, Thomas G et al (2001). Testing a preoperative pain management intervention for elders. *Research in Nursing & Health* 24(5):402–409.

Resnick B (2001). Testing a model of exercise behavior in older adults. *Research in Nursing & Health* 24(2):83–92.

Western Journal of Nursing Research

Algase DL, Beattie ERA, Therrien B (2001). Impact of cognitive impairment on wandering behavior. *Western Journal of Nursing Research* 23(3):283–295.

Hawranik PG, Strain PA (2001). Cognitive impairment, disruptive behaviors, and home care utilization. *Western Journal of Nursing Research* 23(2):148–162.

Zauszniewski JA, Chung C, Krafcik K (2001). Social cognitive factors predicting the health of elders. *Western Journal of Nursing Research* 23(5):490–503.

International Journal of Nursing Studies

Blomqvist K, Hallberg IR (2001). Recognising pain in older adults living in sheltered accommodation: the views of nurses and older adults. *International Journal of Nursing Studies* 38(3):305–318.

> Edberg A, Hallberg IR (2001). Actions seen as demanding in patients with severe dementia during one year of intervention: comparison with controls. *International Journal of Nursing Studies* 38(3):271–285.
>
> Holtkamp CCM, Kerkstra A, Ooms ME et al (2001). Effects of the implementation of the Resident Assessment Instrument on gaps between perceived needs and nursing care supply for nursing home residents in the Netherlands. *International Journal of Nursing Studies* 38(6):619–628.
>
> Richter J, Eisemann MR (2001). Attitudinal patterns determining decision-making in severely ill elderly patients: a cross-cultural comparison between nurses from Sweden and Germany. *International Journal of Nursing Studies* 38(4):381–388.
>
> Salazar Gonzalez BC, Jirovec MM (2001). Elderly Mexican women's perceptions of exercise and conflicting role responsibilities. *International Journal of Nursing Studies* 38(1):45–49.
>
> Wang JJ, Snyder M, Kaas M (2001). Stress, loneliness, and depression in Taiwanese rural community-dwelling elders. *International Journal of Nursing Studies* 38(3):339–347.

The scan produced more than 40 articles on the older adult population. The articles comprise a mix of quantitative method including randomised control trial, retrospective chart audit, structured interview and survey method, as well as qualitative work using interview and observation in order to explore caregiver, older person and staff experiences. An examination of the titles of the articles listed in Box 11-3 reveals several patterns. A number of the articles have as their target population older people in the hospital setting, while others report research conducted overseas on elderly cohorts. Issues of primary importance in an older population are clearly evident by the article topics: nutritional needs, adequate support and quality of care, preservation of personal integrity and maintaining functional status. Nursing issues such as discharge planning, establishing successful relationships with carers, providing therapeutic activity for older people with cognitive deficits, end of life care, medication management, pain control and exploring different models of service delivery are also addressed.

Clinical nursing journals

The articles found by scanning the tables of contents of selected clinical journals yielded several relevant research articles, listed in Box 11-4.

BOX 11-4 Relevant Research Article Titles for Older Adults in Clinical Journals

Australian Critical Care
Boyle M, Green M (2001). Pressure sores in intensive care: defining their incidence and associated factors and assessing the utility of two pressure sore risk assessment tools. *Australian Critical Care* 14(1):24–30.

Australian Journal on Ageing
Bramston P, Tomasevic V (2001). Health locus of control, depression and quality of life in people who are elderly. *Australian Journal on Ageing* 20(4):192–195.

Chan FHW, Pei CKW, Chiu KC et al (2001). Strategies against polypharmacy and inappropriate medication—are they effective? *Australian Journal on Ageing* 20(2):85–89.

Cripps D (2001). Rights focused advocacy and elder abuse. *Australian Journal on Ageing* 20(1):17–22.

Hall SE, Williams JA, Criddle RA (2001). A prospective study of falls following hip fracture in community dwelling older adults. *Australian Journal on Ageing* 20(2):73–78.

Harris A, Gospodarevskaya E, Callaghan J et al (2001). The cost effectiveness of a pharmacist reviewing medication among the elderly in the community. *Australian Journal on Ageing* 20(4):179–186.

Hasan S, Byles JE, Mishra G et al (2001). Use of sleeping medication and quality of life among older women who report sleeping difficulty. *Australian Journal on Ageing* 20(1):29–35.

Leong J, Madjar I, Fiveash B (2001). Needs of family carers of elderly people with dementia living in the community. *Australian Journal on Ageing* 20(3):133–138.

Livermore P, Bunt R, Biscan K (2001). Elder abuse among clients and carers referred to the Central Coast ACAT: a descriptive analysis. *Australian Journal on Ageing* 20(1):41–47.

Journal of Gerontological Nursing
Armer JM, Conn VS (2001). Exploration of spirituality & health among diverse rural elderly individuals. *Journal of Gerontological Nursing* 27(6):28–37.

Campbell J, Aday RH (2001). Healthy People 2010: Benefits of a nurse-managed wellness program: a senior center model: using community-based sites for older adult intervention and self-care activities may promote an ability to maintain an independent lifestyle. *Journal of Gerontological Nursing* 27(3):34–43.

Crogan NL, Shultz JA, Adams CE et al (2001). Barriers to nutrition care for nursing home residents. *Journal of Gerontological Nursing* 27(12):25–31.

Dunn KS (2001). The effects of physical restraints on fall rates in older adults who are institutionalised. *Journal of Gerontological Nursing* 27(10):40–48.

Fitzsimmons S (2001). Interdisciplinary care: Easy Rider wheelchair biking, a nursing-recreation therapy clinical trail for the treatment of depression. *Journal of Gerontological Nursing* 27(5):14–23.

Forbes S (2001). This is heaven's waiting room: end of life in one nursing home. *Journal of Gerontological Nursing* 27(11):37–45.

Gueldner SH, Smith CA, Neal M et al (2001). Patterns of telephone use among nursing home residents. *Journal of Gerontological Nursing* 27(5):35–41.

Harrison B, Booth D, Algase D (2001). Studying fall risk factors among nursing home residents who fell. *Journal of Gerontological Nursing* 27(10):26–34.

Hawk C, Byrd L, Killinger LZ (2001). Interdisciplinary care: Evaluation of a geriatrics course emphasizing interdisciplinary issues for chiropractic students. *Journal of Gerontological Nursing* 27(7):6–12.

O'Rourke DJ, Klaasen KS, Sloan JA (2001). Redesigning nighttime care for personal care residents. *Journal of Gerontological Nursing* 27(7):30–37.

Patrick L, Blodgett A (2001). Assessment. Selecting patients for falls-prevention protocols: an evidence-based approach on a geriatric rehabilitation unit. *Journal of Gerontological Nursing* 27(10):19–25.

Richards KC, Sullivan SC, Phillips RL et al (2001). The effect of individualized activities on the sleep of nursing home residents who are cognitively impaired: a pilot study. *Journal of Gerontological Nursing* 27(9):30–37.

Santo-Novak DA, Duncan JW, Grissom KR et al (2001). MSHAKE: a tool for measuring staff knowledge related to geriatric mental health. *Journal of Gerontological Nursing* 27(2):29–35.

Sullivan-Marx EM (2001). Achieving restraint-free care of acutely confused older adults. *Journal of Gerontological Nursing* 28(4):56–61.

Tremethick MJ (2001). Alone in a crowd: a study of social networks in home health and assisted living. *Journal of Gerontological Nursing* 27(5):42–47.

Turner JT, Lee V, Fletcher K et al (2001). Measuring quality of care with an inpatient elderly population: the Geriatric Resource Nurse Model. *Journal of Gerontological Nursing* 27(3):8–18.

van Wynen EA (2001). Healthy People 2010: A key to successful aging: learning-style patterns of older adults. *Journal of Gerontological Nursing* 27(9):6–15.

Wakefield B, Johnson JA (2001). Acute confusion in terminally ill hospitalized patients. *Journal of Gerontological Nursing* 28(4):49–55.

Wolfsen CR, Barker JC, Mitteness LS (2001). Healthy People 2010: Smoking and health views of elderly nursing home residents. *Journal of Gerontological Nursing* 27(8):6–12.

American Journal of Operating Room Nurses (AORN)

Deaton C, Kurtz S, Weintraub WS (2001). A collaborative program for cardiovascular patient follow-up. *American Journal of Operating Room Nurses* 74(1):22–23, 25–28, 30–31.

Scott EM, Leaper DJ, Clark M et al (2001). Effects of warming therapy on pressure ulcers—a randomized trial. *American Journal of Operating Room Nurses* 73(5):921–933, 937–938.

Tappen RM, Muzic J, Kennedy P (2001). Elder care: Preoperative assessment and discharge planning for older adults undergoing ambulatory surgery. *American Journal of Operating Room Nurses* 73(2):464, 467, 469–470.

International Journal of Nursing Practice

Allen KE, Wellard SJ (2001). Older women's experiences with sternotomy. *International Journal of Nursing Practice* 7(4):274–279.

Fagerberg I, Kihlgren (2001). Registered nurses' experiences of caring for the elderly in different health-care areas. *International Journal of Nursing Practice* 7(4):229–236.

Ragneskog H, Asplund K, Kihlgren M et al (2001). Individualized music played for agitated patients with dementia: analysis of video recorded sessions. *International Journal of Nursing Practice* 7(3):146–155.

Soderhamn U, Soderhamn O (2001). Developing and testing the Nutritional Form for the Elderly. *International Journal of Nursing Practice* 7(5):336–341.

Geriaction

Tan L, Fleming A, Ledwidge H (2001). The caregiving burden of relatives with dementia: experiences of Chinese–Australian families. *Geriaction* 19(1):10–16.

Oncology Nursing Forum

Galbraith ME, Ramirez JM, Pedro LW (2001). Quality of life, health outcomes and identity for patients with prostate cancer in five different treatment groups. *Oncology Nursing Forum* 28(3):551–560.

Hermann CP (2001). Spiritual needs of dying patients: a qualitative study. *Oncology Nursing Forum* 28(1):67–72.

Rehabilitation Nursing

Bays CL (2001). Older adults' descriptions of hope after a stroke. *Rehabilitation Nursing* 26(1):18–20, 23–27.

Borrie MJ, Campbell K, Arcese ZA et al (2001). Urinary retention in patients in a geriatric rehabilitation unit: prevalence, risk factors, and validity of bladder scan evaluation. *Rehabilitation Nursing* 26(5):187–191.

Several clinical journals regularly publish research on the care of older adults. The *Journal of Gerontological Nursing* publishes articles in the area of gerontological nursing, and many of these articles are research studies. Over 30 relevant articles surfaced, many of which were found in the *Journal of Gerontological Nursing* and the *Australian Journal on Ageing*. As expected, the articles in the specialty journals focus on specialty topics (e.g. cancer, cardiovascular or mental health). However, themes are once again evident as we review the titles. Elder issues such as self-care, quality of life and pain are evident. Diseases and conditions common to the older adult such as dementia, cancer and stroke are addressed. Nursing intervention issues such as falls, use of restraints, activity patterns and general nursing interventions are apparent. Articles relating to conditions to which older persons may be more prone are also included (e.g. pressure sores, cardiac disease). There is further reference to caregivers and articles on the emerging problem of elder abuse. What other trends or patterns do you see when scanning the titles in Box 11-4?

Summarising and using scan results

We have selected several of the identified research articles to serve as examples of how research articles might be summarised and the findings used in clinical practice. Several articles in both the research and clinical journals examined aspects of nursing care. They provide concrete data about the effectiveness of certain nursing interventions used in the care of older adult populations. We look at several of these articles in more depth.

One study by Yoon & Horne (2001) looked at the use of complementary medicine, specifically herbal products, and the potential for interaction between the use of herbs and conventional medicine. This is an area of emerging importance to healthcare providers as consumers increasingly turn to alternative remedies for relief of symptoms, and yet traditionally little research has been conducted in this area. This study examined a random sample of older women, some of whom used herbs for medicinal purposes and some who did not. The subjects were asked to participate in a structured interview during which a questionnaire was completed that ascertained demographic details, the use of conventional medicine and herbal products, and health status. The research showed that 45 per cent of the women had used herbal medicine in the preceding year and that on average each woman had used 2.5 herbal products during that time, mainly to prevent health problems but also to treat illness and at times for both purposes. The researchers found no significant difference in the demographic characteristics or perceived health status of those women who used herbal products compared with those who did not use them. Although herb users reported more concern with memory loss, this was found to be no more or less serious than that perceived by the non-using group. The study points to the need for health professionals to be knowledgeable about the effects of alternative medicine in order to more fully inform consumers about the relative merits or drawbacks of its use. Given the propensity for older people to use a variety of medications and the increasing interest in nontraditional remedies, this study provides a backdrop for further investigation.

Another study (Given et al 2001) using quantitative data collection techniques examined the physical functioning of older cancer patients both prior to diagnosis and following preliminary treatment for the disease. The researchers interviewed a number of patients with newly diagnosed breast, colon, lung or prostate cancer, and after controlling for certain variables looked at whether the site and stage of cancer predicted functional capacity prior to diagnosis. In addition they examined how well certain factors such as age, comorbidity, stage, treatment and symptom clusters explained changes in physical capacity both before and after diagnosis. Instruments included the SF-36 questionnaire, patient report and audit of patient records. Their findings showed that prior to diagnosis the physical functioning of their cancer patients was better than the average US population and that the site and stage of the tumour had no effect on physical functioning. Following treatment, however, those subjects with more extensive treatments suffered greater loss of functioning. The symptom cluster of pain, fatigue and insomnia played a significant role in loss of physical function and pointed to the need for health professionals to manage those symptoms early in the course of treatment. The study has implications for the role of nurses in optimising recovery of patients following treatment for cancer.

Australian studies include one by Hall, Williams & Criddle (2001), who followed a cohort of older people living in the community who had experienced hip fractures, and compared their incidence of subsequent falls, trips and stumbles and the circumstances surrounding such events, to a group of matched controls (who had not previously suffered hip fracture). Telephone interviews using a number of previously tested measurement tools demonstrated that the hip fracture cohort were no more likely to fall than those individuals in the control group. However, it was found that the hip fracture group were less active and when they did fall were likely to sustain more serious injury. Livermore, Bunt & Biscan (2001) took a retrospective and prospective approach to identify the prevalence and types of elder abuse in one geographical area in New South Wales. The findings confirm the issue as a cause for concern, with a prevalence of 5.4 per cent in their sample population. Differences were found between cases where the older person was abused and those in which the carer was abused. Psychological abuse was the most common form of abuse. The researchers call for an urgent and coordinated response to the issue of elder abuse, which would of course include health professionals.

Other useful quantitative studies looked at issues such as preoperative education for older people in order to better manage their postoperative pain (McDonald et al 2001), cognitive impairment as a predictor of wandering behaviour (Algase, Beattie & Therrien 2001) and a study that tested factors shown to influence exercise in older persons (Resnick 2001).

Several qualitative investigations were conducted on elders and elder care experiences. An ethnographic research design used by Costello (2001) to explore the care provided to dying patients on three elderly care wards focused specifically on management of care for the dying. Through a process of observation and interview Costello collected data which he later analysed to demonstrate that the model of care he had witnessed was shaped by a lack of 'emotional attachment' to the patient and poor communication about the subject of death and dying. The study calls for greater communication about terminal illness and more effective approaches by health professionals to deal with the subject. The increasing focus on carers in the community is highlighted in a qualitative study by McGarry & Arthur (2001), who carried out a number of personal interviews to gather data about the experience of informal carers aged 75 years and over. Emergent themes from their data were categorised under four headings which included aspects such as the relationship between carer and caree, support networks, professional services and the demands of the role. Implications for practice stemming from this work include the fact that this older carer group is especially vulnerable, and need to be identified quickly and provided with adequate support in their role.

Other interesting qualitative studies explored the ethics embedded in the ordinary care of patients with dementia in aged care homes (Powers 2001), the facilitation of carers' involvement in decision making (Walker & Dewar 2001) and the experience of chronic illness in an aged care facility (Forbes 2001). Australian studies include one by Tan, Fleming & Ledwidge (2001), who examined the experience of Chinese–Australian families in caring for relatives with dementia.

Now complete the following Student Challenge.

Student Challenge

Using Data from Journal Scans

Use the articles that resulted from your journal scan.

1. Read the articles to determine what was studied, who was studied and what the study results were. Write a brief summary of each article. Use the previously cited articles as examples.
2. Read the discussion sections of the articles and make a quick determination of how the results might be used in a clinical practice setting. Write out how the findings might be used and by whom.

Reading and Evaluating a Research Article on the Care of Older Adults

In this section we examine one qualitative research article on a clinical intervention in more depth. We again use our research reading strategy, research comprehension and research evaluation guidelines.

The following CD-ROM exercise guides you through the critical reading, evaluation and visualisation of the selected research article. When you finish, print out your answers and our responses to the exercises. You should be feeling pretty confident about your ability to read and summarise a research article by now.

Student Challenge

Surveying, Examining and Critically Reading an Older Adult Research Study

1. Log on to your CD-ROM and look for the 'Survey, examine and critically read' exercise in Chapter 11. Print out the reading strategy and the research article entitled '"Getting up from here": frail older women's experiences after falling'.
2. Take your text, the article, the strategy and a notepad and pen, and find a conducive reading and study environment.
3. Survey the article using the strategy guidelines. Make notes of what you gleaned from your survey.
4. Now go back and read the article paragraph by paragraph and jot down the key idea in each paragraph. Note anything you don't understand.
5. When you have finished, consult references to clarify those things that are unclear.
6. When you have completed these steps, go back to the CD-ROM and complete the 'Survey, examine and critically read' exercise, the 'Study evaluation' exercise and the 'Application visualisation' exercise for Chapter 11.

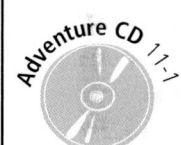
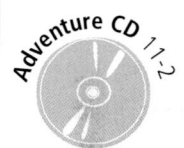
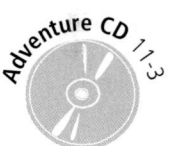

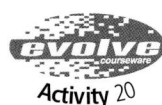

Activity 20

> ### Resource Kit
>
> **Web Sources for Older Adult Research Priorities**
>
> Geriaction
>
> The Continence Foundation of Australia
>
> The National Heart Foundation Australia
>
> Diabetes Australia
>
> The Cancer Council Australia
>
> The Australian Department of Health and Ageing—Ageing and Aged Care Division
>
> Office for an Ageing Australia
>
> US National Institute for Nursing Research
>
> **Web Sources for Relevant Journal Tables of Contents and Abstracts**
>
> *Australasian Journal on Ageing*
>
> *Journal of Gerontological Nursing*
>
> *Nursing Research*
>
> *Research in Nursing & Health*
>
> **Miscellaneous Web Resources**
>
> Council on the Ageing
>
> Go to Evolve and link to the 162-journal site to see if any journals are relevant to care of the older adult.
>
> 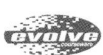 Visit the book's Evolve website at http://evolve.elsevier.com/AU/Borbasi/maze for further information.

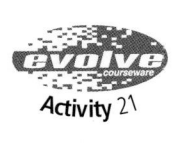

Activity 21

References

Barr J, Brown P, Perry G (1999). Risk factors associated with falls in the elderly rehabilitation client. *Australian Journal on Ageing* 18(1):27–31.

Evans D, Hodgkinson B, Lambert L et al (2001). Fall risk factors in the hospital setting: a systematic review. *International Journal of Nursing Practice* 7(1):38–45.

van Leeuwen M, Bennett L, West S et al (2001). Patient falls from bed and the role of bedrails in the acute care setting. *Australian Journal of Advanced Nursing* 19(2):8–13.

http://evolve.elsevier.com/AU/Borbasi/maze

Learning Objectives

After reading this chapter and following critical reflection, the student will be able to:

1. Discuss research utilisation and its importance to practice development.
2. Demonstrate an understanding of the main arguments about evidence-based nursing.
3. Explain the major barriers affecting translation of research findings into practice.
4. Describe the responsibilities of researchers, clinicians, administrators/nurse managers and educators in the use of research.
5. Review approaches for exploration of the research literature.
6. Describe the criteria for determining whether research findings are useable.
7. Discuss strategies to promote development and retention of research utilisation skills.

Chapter Outline

What Is Research Utilisation?
Evidence-based nursing
Barriers to research utilisation
Who Is Involved in Research Utilisation?
Client/patient
Researcher
Clinician
Administrator/nurse manager
Nurse educator
How Is Research Used in Practice?
Approaches to research utilisation
Criteria for research utilisation
Relevance
Merit and applicability
Implementation
Strategies to strengthen your utilisation potential
Maintain ties with library resources
Exploit additional research learning opportunities
Plan for timely perusal of research literature
Assess your clinical environment
Get other nurses involved
Explore institutional research support systems

Chapter 12
Use It or Lose It: Putting Research Into Action

Whadda ya mean this is not what you meant by putting research into practice?

Student Quote

'I've been a nurse for a while, but I never thought of research as being part of my responsibilities before.'

Abstract

Research utilisation is the mechanism used to translate research into practice. The utilisation approach may be formal (practice development or procedural changes) or informal (individual enactment). One type of research utilisation is evidence-based nursing, which may also be formal or informal. Though there are many barriers to research utilisation, all nurses share responsibility for practice development through the enacting of different roles (researcher, clinician, manager etc). The goal is for the practising nurse to be a research consumer who uses relevant research findings to define and enhance his or her clinical practice. This can be done by using a variety of approaches, criteria and strategies to find, read, evaluate and implement research findings.

> **Key Terms**
>
> **Utilisation Explanations**
>
> **conceptual utilisation** Using research findings to broaden or alter thinking or perspectives without any particular specified change in behaviour or nursing intervention approach.
>
> **replication** Conduct of additional research studies on an identified problem to determine whether consistent results can be achieved.
>
> **research utilisation** The process of translating research findings into practice. This process is sometimes called evidence-based practice (EBP).
>
> **utilisation criteria** Criteria used to evaluate whether research findings can be adapted for use in the clinical arena.

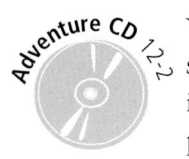

You should now be feeling more at ease with your ability to find and read research studies. This ability will continue to develop if you use it regularly. The next step is to incorporate research results into your clinical practice. Research-based care promotes a practice environment in which you use research findings and critical thinking skills to make informed patient care decisions. When you use research findings as a foundation for nursing care, you become a true research consumer. As a research consumer, you have another tool that allows you to regularly evaluate, update and improve your nursing care. This chapter is designed to assist you in integrating your new skills into the regular conduct of your clinical practice. This is the final step needed to become a research consumer.

What Is Research Utilisation?

Research utilisation is the mechanism used to translate the knowledge that has been generated by research into clinical practice. Estabrooks (1998, p 19) puts it very simply when she states that research utilisation is a way of closing the 'gap between what is known and what is done'. It may be viewed as an informal or a formal process. For example, you might read a study, think the findings are useful, and decide you would like to try them out with your next patient. This is an informal approach to research utilisation. Most individually instituted research utilisations are informal in nature. To achieve a more broad or formal uptake of research findings many healthcare facilities have implemented clinical practice or research utilisation committees, who have an interest in promoting and facilitating practice change and development. These committees are an avenue for formalising practice change. Research utilisation efforts that are systematically introduced within an organisation or institution are formal.

A research or evidence-based intervention protocol that replaces the previous protocol in an institution's procedure manual is a formal approach to research utilisation.

When we first begin to read and attempt to integrate research findings into practice, most of our utilisation efforts tend to be informal. However, the ultimate goal is to formalise research utilisation in order to promote research-based policies, procedures and clinical practice guidelines. Ultimately, only when research findings are used in a systematic and structured way will we ensure the promotion of consistent, cost-effective and high-quality nursing care.

Evidence-based nursing

Australian nurses have attempted to increase the utilisation of research findings through evidence-based nursing. This process involves a rigorous analysis and systematic review of all evidence about a particular nursing issue or concern. When conducting a systematic review all available evidence is taken into account. The evidence is ranked (level 1–5), with the randomised control trial (RCT) being considered the gold standard. A systematic review and meta-analysis of all available RCTs is considered best available evidence (for levels of evidence see evidence-based practice sites, e.g. Bandolier Library). Rolfe (1999) problematises the notion of evidence-based nursing in his critique of what counts as evidence. He suggests that having the RCT as the gold standard is problematic for nursing, and urges us to think in new and different ways about what counts as evidence. Parker (2002) posits evidence-based nursing as a means for nurses to speak of and justify significant aspects of their practice.

When applying evidence-based nursing in practice it is essential to consider the critical role of context in shaping clinical strategies. The needs and particular situation of an individual patient and the skilled judgment of the attending nurse will ultimately determine the clinical intervention used. What evidence-based nursing does is to make available the most current and rigorous evidence to assist nurses in guiding individualised and contextualised research-based care decisions.

Barriers to research utilisation

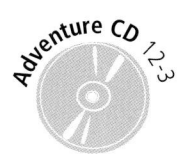

Although reading a research report can give you greater insight into an issue, thus informing your ideas and your practice (conceptual utilisation; Estabrooks 1999), the actual translation of research into practice is far more complex. There are many barriers to practice development through use of research findings. These barriers include: resistance to change, insufficient time and resources to implement changes to practice, lack of supportive infrastructure, lack of research skills including an inability to critique, lack of professional autonomy to effect change, and inability to access and engage with research findings (Nolan et al 1998). In addition, any practice change brings with it considerable cost in terms of staff education, new equipment and organisational constraints. Nagy et al (2001) undertook a survey of Australian nurses and identified lack of confidence in accessing and evaluating research, the belief that research is irrelevant, and lack of time as the major barriers to the application of research findings in practice.

Who Is Involved in Research Utilisation?

All nurses share responsibility for the utilisation of clinical research findings. However, the responsibilities vary with the role or position of the nurse. We will now look at some of the differences for the researcher, the clinician, the administrator/nurse manager, the educator and the client.

Client/patient

As consumers, clients have a set of expectations about their care, and are increasingly well-informed about treatment options and their right to access the best available treatment. Pressure from clients to have more effective and efficient treatments acts as an impetus for health-related research activities. Often it is an unmet need of clients/patients or poor client/patient outcomes that generates research projects. Therefore there is pressure from clients to receive the best available treatment based on evidence.

Researcher

Researchers conduct the research that will ultimately form the foundation for clinical practice, and so it must be high-quality, rigorous, scientifically grounded, ethical and built on previous knowledge. Researchers have several responsibilities. First, they must choose research topics that address identified priorities and critically defined problem areas in the clinical arena. Collaboration with clinicians can keep researchers in better touch with clinical issues and can assist in more relevant and timely problem identification. Sometimes researchers and clinicians form collaborative alliances to jointly conduct research and this will be apparent from the credentials of the authors of published research papers.

Research is often replicated to provide a broader base for clinical utilisation and to ensure that the results can be achieved again and again (reliability). In order to be accepted as part of the knowledge base that informs the discipline of nursing, research reports must be disseminated (communicated) in peer-reviewed clinical nursing journals that are widely read by clinicians and administrators and at nursing conferences attended by clinicians and administrators. The peer review process ensures that the article has been scrutinised by two or more well-qualified reviewers and has been accepted as rigorous, ethical and relevant to practice. The study should be presented in a clear, organised and easily read format. The design and results should be easily understood by any intelligent reader. Clinical implications should be clearly spelled out, with concrete examples given. The researcher should identify the study's limitations and fully discuss the generalisability and transferability of the results.

Clinician

Clinicians are the front line in research utilisation. If they do not regularly read, evaluate and incorporate research results into their daily practice regimens, then the work of the researcher and the outcomes of the research are lost. Thus clinicians bear many responsibilities for research utilisation. First, they must regularly search and read the available research literature. They also need to avail themselves of ongoing educational opportunities that boost research utilisation skills. These include attendance at professional and clinical conferences where research papers and presentations are featured. Applicable research findings should be noted, shared with colleagues, and considered for integration into clinical practice. Clinicians need to be attuned to problems and questions that arise in the clinical area that might be addressed by research. Relationships with researchers should be cultivated and administrative support mechanisms explored. Clinicians should exploit opportunities to be involved in clinical research projects and formal research utilisation projects.

Research utilisation is a part of clinical lifelong learning and a means to ensure continuing professional competence. Activities based around research utilisation should be recorded in your professional portfolio. The portfolio is a useful and current source of evidence about your research activities that can be viewed by registering authorities or employers as well as providing you with a record of your professional development.

Administrator/nurse manager

Administrators and nurse managers are key players in formalising research utilisation in the clinical area. They play a pivotal role in ensuring that research utilisation is a systematic process used to promote the delivery of consistently effective and scientifically grounded nursing care. As such, administrators and nurse managers must foster a climate that supports and rewards the use of research in practice. This includes provision of adequate resources and personnel and a positive emotional climate, as well as providing formalised mechanisms for the promotion of research utilisation. Such mechanisms might include an institutional research utilisation committee with regular review of current clinical research, regular review and revision of institution policies, and procedures and prevailing practices that reflect the use of research literature. Mechanisms should also be in place to conceive, carry out and evaluate formal utilisation projects and clinical protocols. Administrators/nurse managers should foster relationships with researchers and encourage the conduct of research in the institution. In some areas this desire to foster relationships between clinicians and the education sector has facilitated the evolution of Clinical Professors of Nursing. These positions are generally held by doctorally prepared and clinically experienced nursing researchers. Finally, administrators/nurse managers have a responsibility to systematically evaluate and reward clinicians for research utilisation and clinical innovation.

Nurse educator

Educators are responsible for ensuring that other nurses (researcher, clinician, administrator/nurse manager) are adequately prepared for their roles in the research utilisation process. This could include arranging research events and colloquia, and designing course offerings and learning packages at all levels (undergraduate, graduate, continuing education) that articulate effective approaches and strategies to research utilisation. Because the level of focus for this text is undergraduate education, we will use undergraduate students as an illustrative example.

Undergraduate students require ample opportunity to develop and practise the requisite skills for use of research results in the clinical practice arena. If students are to incorporate research into their practice as graduates, it is necessary to cultivate such utilisation as a habit. Nurse educators and academics are also responsible for incorporating current relevant research results into their clinical and classroom teaching. This incorporation should be openly articulated and demonstrated to students. In this way, teachers serve as role models for students. Teachers must require that students demonstrate the use of relevant research in the preparation of clinical care plans and in the nursing care given. Research findings and their utilisation should be included as expected discussion in clinical practice conferences.

Student Challenge

Exploring Roles and Responsibilities

Let's explore how serious your clinical institution is about research in nursing. If you are currently employed, use that institution for the exercise. If not, do this when you are at your next clinical placement.

1. Ask some of your colleagues in the ward whether the institution supports nursing research (e.g. Is the institution involved in nursing research? In research utilisation projects/protocols?).
2. Is there a Clinical Professor of Nursing or a Practice Development Unit attached to the facility?
3. Does the facility have a formal relationship with a university School of Nursing that helps to facilitate nursing research?
4. Does the facility provide access to internet databases to assist nurses in the collection of research evidence to support practice (e.g. DHS Victoria's Clinicians' Health Channel)?

> 5 Does the facility include a research utilisation committee?
> 6 Does the facility have a formal relationship with an evidence-based practice organisation such as the Joanna Briggs Institute of Evidence Based Nursing or the Cochrane Collaboration?
> 7 Are clinicians evaluated and rewarded for utilising nursing research in their practice?
> 8 Is support readily available (e.g. research and clinical journals in library, nursing research department or committee, nurse researcher on staff, time and funding to attend clinical and research conferences, in-services on research utilisation, journal clubs)?

How Is Research Used in Practice?

Helping you as a research consumer to translate research into practice is the ultimate goal of this book. Although organisations can use many formal strategies and processes, the focus here is on you—the individual consumer—and how you can incorporate what you read into your real-world practice of nursing. This section examines three basic approaches to searching the research literature, discusses criteria to judge the use of various research findings, and then illustrates strategies you can use to enhance your ability to integrate research findings into your practice.

Approaches to research utilisation

In Chapters 8 to 11 we used three approaches in exploring the research literature for use in the clinical area. These three approaches form the backbone of research utilisation. They are as follows:

1. Identification and review of the clinical and research priorities in a defined area of clinical practice
2. Identification of problems routinely confronted in clinical practice
3. Identification of useful research findings through scanning pertinent published research resources.

All three approaches are valuable. We examined several sources for clinical and research priorities: the public policy arena (e.g. NH&MRC Strategic and Priority Driven Research objectives, the Commonwealth Department of Health and Ageing, the National Institute of Nursing Research (NINR, United States), the World Health Organization global nursing research priorities), research and educational bodies, and professional clinical specialty organisations. Timely review of these priorities keeps you on top of what is happening in your practice area and alerts you to what is viewed as important at a national level.

The second approach to identifying problems in your clinical practice requires you to actively engage in questioning what you do and why you do it. In fact, finding and raising questions that are answerable through research is possible at every point in the nursing process. Research can help you focus on better ways to collect and use data. For example, you might find alternative collection formats that improve data accuracy; or you might discover what data should be collected about certain types of clients with certain types of problems in various clinical settings. Research can also make planning more effective. It can look at a patient problem, identify which nursing actions are needed, when they are needed, and who is most likely to benefit. We have seen how helpful research is in testing the effectiveness of nursing interventions.

The third approach of scanning the available current literature may be the most valuable approach for novice clinical nurses and research consumers. The literature keeps you in contact with the relevant research being conducted in your area of clinical practice. As you read these studies and struggle with how you might use the findings in your own clinical area, it should trigger additional questions in your mind about your practice. This then feeds back into approach number 2 and helps you identify additional clinical questions and problems.

Criteria for research utilisation

After you have located and surveyed a research study, you must determine whether it is relevant to your clinical area, whether the results have merit and are applicable to your area and your patients. You must also determine how to implement any relevant and applicable results. We have addressed these **utilisation criteria** in a number of places in this book. However, we will now group and identify the criteria for deciding whether to use research findings in your clinical setting.

Relevance

The first issue you must address is relevance. You are trying to determine whether the findings from a particular research study are useful or helpful to your clinical practice. You begin to address this issue when you first evaluate the title of a research study and make a decision about whether to call up the abstract. You make further judgments about relevance when you evaluate the abstract and decide whether to survey the article itself. Your final evaluation of relevance comes when you determine whether the stated findings of the study apply to your clinical situation. To determine relevance you might ask yourself the series of questions that appear in Box 12-1. An answer of 'no' to any of the proposed questions calls the relevance of the study into question for your particular situation.

BOX 12-1 Criteria for Determining Clinical Relevance

- Is the study a clinical study?
- Are the sample/participants in the study similar to patients you work with in clinical settings?
- Is the setting used in the study similar to the setting you work in?
- Is the problem being studied one you have seen in your clinical area?
- Do the study findings address issues that nursing has the power to change? Do they affect the activities of daily living? Do they have ramifications for patient comfort and well-being?
- Are the study findings helpful to your clinical routine?
- Do they add to your knowledge base?

Merit and applicability

The second issue you want to address concerns the merit and applicability of the study. Here you are trying to decide whether the study results are accurate, believable and meaningful, and whether they can be applied to your clinical setting. When you evaluated the studies in Chapters 7 to 11 using Step 4 of your reading strategy, you were examining merit. You were asking how well the researcher used the research process and whether the study was a good study. As stated in Chapter 7, you do not yet have the skills to address the theoretical and methodological merits of a study, but you can make beginning judgments about the quality of a study. To help determine the study's merit you might ask yourself the questions in Box 12-2.

BOX 12-2 Criteria for Determining Clinical Merit

- Are key elements of the study easily identified?
- Are the steps of the research process followed?
- Are ideas concisely and comprehensively identified?
- Are sampling methods clearly described? Are they appropriate to the study?
- Do the results make sense?
- Do quantitative studies use reliable and valid instruments?
- Do qualitative studies address issues of auditability, transferability and credibility of data?
- In qualitative studies, does the final picture of the phenomena under study flow logically from the data?
- In quantitative studies, does the discussion section clearly identify who the results could be applied to? Are the findings clearly tied to existing knowledge?
- Have other studies been done that address the identified problem (i.e. are there replications, meta-analysis or evidence in the literature of similar findings)?

If the answer to any of the questions is 'no,' then the merit might need further consideration. Merit is particularly important if you are considering using the study findings to alter an existing nursing intervention. If you wish to use the study results to support a formal change in intervention protocols, proof of merit is crucial, and you may need a resource person with research critiquing skills to evaluate the study from a theoretical and methodological point of view.

Implementation

The third issue to be addressed is whether the findings from a particular study can be effectively implemented in your practice setting. This involves looking at such issues as importance, feasibility, cost, risk versus benefit and patient preference. To help determine the study's potential for implementation, try asking the questions listed in Box 12-3. Assessing implementation is important for utilisation that requires a change in the prevailing procedures or policies in an institution.

> **BOX 12-3** Criteria for Determining Implementation Possibilities
>
> - Who will be affected and in what numbers?
> - What are the advantages of implementation?
> - What are the risks of implementation?
> - What are the risks of no implementation?
> - Do the advantages outweigh the risks?
> - How complex is the change (e.g. a simple intervention, or a lengthy protocol that requires extensive retraining of personnel)?
> - How much will it cost (e.g. needed staff training, equipment, supplies)?
> - Who will be affected by the change besides nursing (e.g. physicians, pharmacy, housekeeping, billing, patient services)?
> - What are the tangible observable outcomes of the utilisation? (e.g. Will it save money? Make the staff function better? Decrease patient complications?)

These criteria usually become important if you are trying to persuade people to make changes. These are the kinds of questions hospital managers or utilisation committees are likely to evaluate before deciding to try out an intervention or care protocol that changes standing policies, procedures or practices. If you are integrating study results as part of your nursing knowledge base and do not intend to initiate practice change, an implementation review is unnecessary. If you decide to informally try a research-based intervention in your practice and this intervention fits within the standard practices of the institution (i.e. it violates no protocol or procedure guideline) and requires no resource expenditures or risk to the patient, an implementation review may be unnecessary. You will need to check on your institution's policy. Examples of this informal implementation might include

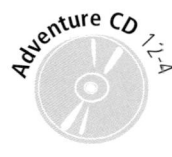

expanding the questions asked about assessing a certain patient problem such as pain, or using music as a distraction technique during a painful procedure.

Strategies to strengthen your utilisation potential

You can cultivate many practical ideas and strategies to ensure that the knowledge generated from research becomes a part of your clinical practice. We examine some of these in the following sections.

Maintain ties with library resources

Upon graduation many students lose touch with the library. This may be because they move, or simply because they associate the library with being in school. Don't let this happen to you.

1. Continue using your academic library. Most universities extend library privileges to their alumni. Take advantage of this perk.
2. If your school library is not accessible, explore other library resources in your community that carry nursing materials. Examples could be public libraries, colleges of nursing and other nursing organisations such as Sigma Theta Tau.
3. Explore the library resources available in your employing institution. Most health facilities have a library and carry a number of nursing journals. If there are journals you want to access that are not available find out how you can make requests to extend the collection.
4. Remember to maximise your use of electronic resources. Use your home computer to log on to the internet and to do literature searches and read journals online. You can also regularly log on to evidence-based sites such as the Cochrane and NHS DARE databases and the Joanna Briggs Institute to keep appraised of the latest systematic reviews.
5. Subscribe to key nursing journals that regularly publish articles relevant to your clinical area (particularly research articles). You might choose one clinical research journal and one or two clinical specialty journals.

Exploit additional research learning opportunities

Look beyond your formal education for experiences to reinforce and enhance your research consumer skills.

1. Maintain your membership of professional associations, including clinical specialty associations. Subscriptions to certain journals are often provided as a part of the membership package.
2. Attend professional conferences and take advantage of research presentations and research poster sessions. Talk to the researchers, ask them about how they see their results being used in the world of nursing practice.
3. Take advantage of research opportunities that come your way. Volunteer to be involved in research projects in your institution. Make yourself known and

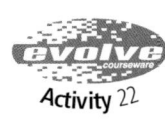
Activity 22

express your interest in research to the Clinical Professor of Nursing if your facility has one.
4   Pay attention to journal articles that describe research utilisation projects or highlight the application of research findings to solve a specified clinical problem.
5   Avail yourself of journals that focus on the use of research findings in practice and the synthesis of research knowledge. (Check out the Resource Kit for journal listings.)
6   Attend continuing education on evidence-based practice and practice development initiatives.

Plan for timely perusal of research literature

You have learned and practised a valuable strategy for scanning available research in various clinical areas. Make this scanning process a habit.
1   Make a list of journals that regularly contain research articles relevant to your clinical area.
2   Perform an electronic search of these journals at least twice a year. Schedule time in your calendar. When you find relevant studies, retrieve them.
3   Read the articles using your systematic reading strategy.
4   Critically read and evaluate the studies.
5   Deliberately determine how you will use the findings in your practice.

Assess your clinical environment

Be aware of what is happening in your practice environment. Ask questions about standard procedures and practices. Why is it done this way? What is the rationale? Is it based on a scientific foundation or is it just because it's always been done that way?
1   Identify gaps, inefficiencies and problems in clinical practice.
2   Review the literature for research-based solutions or for findings to enhance your knowledge base or supply rationales for nursing decisions.

Get other nurses involved

Do not keep your new consumer skills a secret.
1   Share your research discoveries with your co-workers and your supervisors. Let them know what you find in the literature.
2   Get other nurses involved in reading and interpreting research articles.
3   Start a journal club where a group of nurses share their insights on research articles. (Check the Resource Kit for more information.)
4   Bring examples of research utilisation projects that have been tried in other institutions and ask about trying them in your setting.

Explore institutional research support systems

It is much easier to use research findings in the clinical area if you work in an institution that values and rewards such behaviour.

1. Ask questions about the institution's commitment to research-based nursing practice before you are employed. (e.g. Do they have a research utilisation committee? Are nurses evaluated for use of research in their practice? Is nursing research occurring in the institution? Are the nurses in the facility encouraged to participate? What nursing resources are available in the library? Is there access to a Clinical Professor of Nursing, Practice Development Nurse or a Nursing Development Unit? Does the facility offer support for nurses wishing to do honours or a research higher degree?)
2. If possible choose an employing institution that demonstrates its value for the implementation of nursing research. (Hint: They are likely to be progressive in other areas of nursing as well.)
3. If support for utilisation of nursing research is lagging, investigate what you might do to contribute to increasing it. (Hint: Enthusiastic sharing with your co-workers and supervisor can often spark a wave of interest.)
4. The use of the approaches, criteria and strategies that have been discussed to enhance research utilisation will help you grow, develop and mature in the clinical practice arena. As you keep expanding your knowledge base and insist on using a scientifically based foundation for practice, you will ensure that you are providing your patients with the best nursing care possible.

Now go forth and become research consumers!

Resource Kit

Useful Resources for Evidence-based Practice Information

Cochrane Library

Australasian Cochrane Centre

University of York, NHS Centre for Reviews and Dissemination

Joanna Briggs Institute

Centre for Evidence Based Nursing AOTEAROA (New Zealand)

Agency for Healthcare Research and Quality

Journal Clubs

A journal club provides a way to receive support and confirmation of newly developing research consumer skills. It allows you to critically read and explore various research articles with a group of your peers. If you are interested in starting such a club and need guidance, check out the following articles:

- Letterie GS, Morgenstern LS (2000). The journal club. Teaching critical evaluation of clinical literature in an evidence-based environment. *Journal of Reproductive Medicine* 45(4):299–304.
- Mazuryk M, Daeninck P, Neumann CM et al (2002). Daily journal club: an education tool in palliative care. *Palliative Medicine* 16(1):57–61.
- Speers AT (1999). An introduction to nursing research through an OR nursing journal club. *AORN Journal* 69(6):1232.

More Journals

Several journals provide examples of research that has been translated into practice or describes research utilisation projects. You have been introduced to many of them in the lists of clinical journals that report research studies presented in Chapters 8 to 11. Check out your specialty area for journals that report on use of nursing research and give clinical examples of application of research findings. Don't forget journals such as *Evidence Based Nursing* (available in print and online) that provide critique of single research studies together with synopses written by experts regarding the clinical applicability of each study. These journals save you time because much of the critical appraisal and consideration of application to practice has been done, although of course you will still need to consider the research in light of your own patients and context.

And More Journals

Remember the two electronic journals that provide resources for translating research into practice. You might want to check them out on the internet.

- *Research for Nursing Practice* publishes examples of research that has been carried out in nursing practice settings.
- The *Online Journal of Knowledge Synthesis for Nursing* is sponsored by Sigma Theta Tau and provides critical reviews of research literature on a topic and implications for practice.

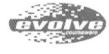 Visit the book's Evolve website at http://evolve.elsevier.com/AU/Borbasi/maze for further information.

 Check out the puzzles, mazes and games on your CD-ROM.

References

Bandolier Library. Online. Available: http://www.jr2.ox.ac.uk/bandolier/band6/b6-5.html.

Estabrooks CA (1998). Will evidence-based nursing practice make practice perfect? *Canadian Journal of Nursing Research* 30(1):15–36.

Estabrooks CA (1999). The conceptual structure of research utilization. *Research in Nursing & Health* 22(3):203.

Nagy S, Lumby J, McKinley S et al (2001). Nurses' beliefs about the conditions that hinder or support evidence-based nursing. *International Journal of Nursing Practice* 7:314–321.

Nolan M, Morgan L, Curran M et al (1998). Evidence based care: can we overcome the barriers? *British Journal of Nursing* 7(20):1273–1278.

Parker J (2002). Evidence-based nursing: a defence. Editorial. *Nursing Inquiry* 9(3):139–140.

Rolfe G (1999). Insufficient evidence: the problems of evidence based nursing. *Nurse Education Today* 19:433–442.

Glossary

abstract Summary of the essential characteristics of something more extensive (e.g. a summary of a research article).

abstracts Special indexes that include citations and summaries of articles.

accuracy Conformity to existing facts and the truth as we know it.

adequacy The scope and depth of information presented for a specific audience.

advance organisers Preselected mental landmarks that serve to organise materials as you read. They are often provided by bold headings, outlines and so on.

applied research Research directed at solving a practical problem.

archive Collection of older materials that have some historical value.

audit trails (decision trails) Validity check used in qualitative research to ensure that adequate documentation is available about the process of data collection and analysis.

authority Knowledge gleaned from the expertise of others.

balance Presentation of competing points of view.

basic (pure) research Research done to establish or extend concepts or theories.

basic social process Social or psychological process identified as enduring over time regardless of environmental conditions (e.g. stages of death and dying).

bias Any influence that may alter the outcomes of a research study.

biophysical instrument Instrument used to measure physiological characteristics of a subject (e.g. glucometer).

book (monograph) A volume about a single subject or related subjects published once (later editions may update material).

bookmark A way to mark and easily access a favourite or easily used website in Netscape Navigator (referred to as 'Favorites' in Internet Explorer).

bracketing Process used in some forms of phenomenology to identify and set aside personal beliefs about the phenomenon under study.

browser Program that opens and displays pages on the world wide web.

call number (classification number) Number or letter-and-number combination assigned to each book and/or journal to indicate where it is shelved in a library.

case study In-depth research study of an individual unit (e.g. a person, family, group or other identified social unit). A case study generally uses both qualitative and quantitative data.

catalogue List of all books owned by the library with a citation and call number (location details) for each book.

CD-ROM Compact disc containing one or more electronic databases, programs or images.

circulating Describes materials that may be checked out of the library.

citation Bibliographic information about books or journals (e.g. author, title, source, date of publication).

clinical nursing research Nursing research that has a direct impact on nursing interventions with clients.

closed reserve (special reserve) Materials that cannot be checked out of the library.

cluster sample Multistage probability sampling where larger clusters (groups) are randomly selected first and then smaller clusters (e.g. patients) are randomly chosen.

coding Process by which data are categorised and conceptualised. It is most often seen in studies using a grounded theory approach.

collection All materials owned by a library.

collective case study Series of case studies that examine similar patterns about identified phenomena.

comprehension The ability to perceive and understand concepts or ideas.

concept Mental picture of an object or phenomenon. Concepts may be concrete or abstract.

conceptual definition Statement attaching a specified meaning to a word (e.g. what the word means for a particular research study).

conceptual framework Loosely related collection of concepts that have not yet been tested.

conceptual utilisation (indirect) The use of research findings to broaden or alter thinking or perspectives without any particular specified change in behaviour or nursing intervention approach.

constant Characteristic that does not vary for a particular research study.

constant comparative method Method of analysis used in grounded theory where categories of meaning are derived by comparing collected data incidents to one another until concepts emerge.

construct validity Validity that is assessed using a combination of logic and statistical measures.

content validity Validity that is assessed by a logical evaluation and judgment of whether the instrument reflects the content of the concept.

control Mechanisms used by the researcher to reduce the influence of extraneous variables.

control group The group of subjects in an experimental study that do not receive the treatment.

convenience (accidental) sample Non-probability sample that selects the most convenient subjects at hand.

credibility Steps taken to make certain of accuracy, authenticity and validity of data.

criterion (concurrent/predictive) validity Validity that is assessed using statistical measures.

critical approaches Approaches that endeavour to produce research findings to generate change of some sort. When referring to this concept of change, authors often state that their research has transformative or emancipatory potential (that is, the potential to be a catalyst for change).

critical case sampling Selection of subjects identified as demonstrating what has been identified by the researcher as a 'critical incident' during data collection.

critically read Step 3 of the research reading strategy. Designed to focus on key steps in the research process.

cross-sectional study Quantitative research in which data are collected at one point in time.

currency The immediacy of presented information.

data Measurable bits of information collected for the purpose of analysis.

database Collection of related information such as a catalogue, index or abstract.

data collection The gathering of information necessary to address the research problem.

data immersion Repeated engagement with primary data to become familiar with its content, feeling and tone. This can mean listening and re-listening to audiotaped data, reading and rereading text.

deductive reasoning Logical system of thinking that starts with the whole and breaks it down into its component parts.

dependent variable Variable that is affected by the action of the independent variable.

descriptive statistics Statistics used to describe and summarise data.

descriptive study Research that describes the concepts under study.

dichotomy Division into two parts.

dissertation (thesis) Research paper written by a graduate student as part of the degree requirement.

download Transfer a file from the internet to a computer.

effective reading rate The number of words that can be read in a minute while maintaining a high level of comprehension.

electronic database Database accessed for a search by computer.

email Electronic mail; postage-free messages that are sent via the internet from one computer to another.

empirical Describes data generated through objective means.

epistemology The philosophical theory of knowledge.

equivalence Assessment of reliability by correlating two different forms of the same instrument (parallel forms) or the scores of two or more raters (interrater reliability).

ethics committee Committee responsible for review of research proposals to ensure that human subjects are protected from harm.

ethnography Qualitative research design that focuses on the world view of an identified cultural group.

evaluate Step 4 of the research reading strategy. Designed to judge the quality of the article.

examine Step 2 of the research reading strategy. Designed to identify key ideas and sort out the meaning of the article.

experimental design Research design characterised by three factors: manipulation, use of a control group, and random assignment.

experimental research Quantitative research in which one concept (independent variable) is manipulated to determine whether another concept (dependent variable) is affected.

explanatory study Quantitative research that attempts to uncover why certain concepts occur and/or how they interact.

exploratory study Research that explores the dimensions of concept(s) under study.

extraneous variable Variable that interferes with the relationship of the independent and dependent variables in a specified study.

extreme (deviant) sampling Selection of subjects who exemplify the phenomena to be studied.

field Natural setting where investigation and data collection take place in a qualitative study.

field notes Written accounts of what a researcher sees, hears, experiences and thinks during the course of data collection in a qualitative study.

file attachment File that is added to an email message.

file transfer protocol (FTP) Program that allows you to transfer files from the internet to your computer.

findings Results of the statistical analysis of study data.

frequency The number of times that scores or categories of a variable occur.

frequency distribution Ordered graphic display or plot of the frequencies for an interval or ration level variable.

generalisation The ability to apply study results from the sample to the population.

grounded theory Qualitative research that develops theoretical propositions about identified social–psychological processes from collected data.

hegemony Dominance, usually of one group over another.

historical method Qualitative analysis of historical events to draw additional insights or inferences about how past events affect the present.

holdings The specific volumes or issues of periodicals owned by the library.

holism Belief that for any aspect of life to be fully understood, the associated factors and context must also be recognised and understood.

home page The first or base page for a website. It often serves as a map, directing you to places of interest on the site.

hypertext Electronic document format that permits links to other web pages or other related websites. The link is underlined and can be accessed by a mouse click on the link.

hypertext markup language (HTML) The codes and instructions used to control the appearance and function of a website. It inserts links, graphics and other multimedia objects on the web page.

hypertext transfer protocol (HTTP) (1) The language used to transfer web pages over an internet connection. (2) The first letters in a URL for a site on the world wide web.

hypothesis Statement of predicted relationship or difference between two or more variables. A hypothesis contains at least one independent and one dependent variable.

implication Inference drawn about the results of a research study.

independent variable Variable that causes a change in the dependent variable.

index List of periodical citations arranged by subject or author. Indexes are usually organised around a specific subject area or field of study.

inductive reasoning Logical system of thinking that begins with the component parts and builds them into a whole.

inferential statistics Statistics used to study relationships or differences among variables in a sample and infer the results back to the population.

information literacy The ability to recognise the need for information, and to identify, locate, access, evaluate and apply the needed information (Australian Library and Information Association).

information-rich sample Sample that provides a powerful picture of the phenomena under study in qualitative research.

informed consent Agreement by a research subject to voluntarily participate in a study after being fully informed about the study and the inherent risks and benefits of participation.

institutional ethics committee (IEC) Committee responsible for review of research proposals to ensure that human subjects are protected from harm.

instrument Device or technique used to collect data in a research study (e.g. biophysical instruments such as glucometers, psychological instruments such as questionnaires or interviews, behavioural instruments such as observation).

instrumental utilisation (direct) Concrete application of research findings to institute new nursing interventions or alter or delete existing interventions.

intensity sampling Selection of subjects who are experiential experts or authorities on a selected phenomenon.

interlibrary loan Library service that allows books and copies of articles to be borrowed from other libraries.

internal consistency Assessment of reliability using correlation statistics to measure whether the subparts of an instrument all measure the same thing.

internet service provider (ISP) Company that provides a connection to the internet (e.g. Telstra BigPond, Ozemail).

interval Level of measurement where categories of a variable are made up of 'real' numbers that allow us to order the numbers and to know the distance between those numbers.

interview Instrument used to collect self-reported psychological data using oral question-and-answer format. The interview may be structured or unstructured.

intuition Insight into the whole of a situation without possessing readily supportable or confirming data.

journal (periodical) Published collection of articles, usually of a scholarly nature.

knowledge Essential information about the world around us that allows us to function more effectively.

kurtosis The height of the distribution curve.

limitations Identified problems or weaknesses in a research study.

listserver (listserv) Electronic mailing list.

literature review Critical summary of available theoretical and research literature on the selected research topic. It places the research problem for a particular study in the context of what is currently known about the topic.

lived experience Some dimension of daily experience for a particular set of individuals.

log off Disconnect from the internet.

log on Connect to the internet.

longitudinal study Quantitative study that collects data at several points over a period of time.

manipulation Intervention or treatment introduced by the researcher in an experimental study.

maximum variety sampling The deliberate selection of subjects who are different, who come from different backgrounds, for the purpose of observing commonalties of experience.

mean The average of all the scores.

measurement Set of rules used to assign numbers to variables.

measures of central tendency Statistical tests that describe how data for a variable tend to cluster together in a distribution (e.g. mode, median, mean).

measures of dispersion Statistical tests that describe how data for a variable tend to spread out in a distribution (e.g. range, variance, standard deviation).

measures of shape Statistical tests that describe the shape of the distribution for a variable (e.g. skewness, kurtosis).

median The middle value in a frequency distribution of numbers.

member checks Validity measures used in qualitative research. They are made by having study participants review the material once it has been analysed and interpreted.

meta-analysis Specialised statistical technique that combines and examines the statistical outcomes of several similar research studies.

microfiche Materials that have been reduced and placed on photographic film (e.g. microform, microfilm).

mode The numerical value that occurs most often for a particular variable.

navigate Move from site to site on the internet.

newsgroup Discussion via posting messages on an electronic bulletin board.

nominal Level of measurement where a variable is broken into two or more categories and assigned arbitrary numbers.

noncirculating Describes materials that cannot be checked out of the library.

nonexperimental design Research design for which there is no treatment or manipulation of the independent variable.

nonexperimental research Quantitative research where concepts are not manipulated but are examined as they occur naturally.

nonparticipant observation Observation method where the researcher is a bystander or passive participant in the activities being observed.

nonprobability sampling Selection of a sample using non-random techniques.

nursing research Research usually conducted by nurses to generate knowledge that informs and develops the discipline and practice of nursing.

observation Data collection method using the researcher as the instrument to gather behavioural data from subjects by watching and/or interacting with them. May be structured or unstructured and participant or nonparticipant.

online (1) Computerised materials that are accessed by other computers (e.g. a computer network). (2) Having an active connection to the internet.

online service Commercial networks (e.g. AOL, Telstra.com) provide a wide range of online services, including access to the internet, news, games, travel information and so on.

operational definition Specifies how a variable is to be measured.

ordinal Level of measurement that reflects a rank order among the categories of a variable.

paradigm Set of philosophical assumptions that underpin one's approach to inquiry.

participant observation Method of observation in which the researcher is an active part of the activities or behaviours engaged in by the participants being observed.

periodical Journal or magazine.

personal experience Knowledge derived from the cumulative experiences of living.

persuasive utilisation (symbolic) Use of research findings as a tool to advocate for a certain practice or intervention.

phenomenology The study of lived experience. Its purpose is to understand and attribute meaning to the phenomenon of interest.

population All known subjects that possess a common characteristic of interest to a researcher.

predictive study Quantitative research that attempts to predict the occurrence of explained events.

presentation Manner in which information is displayed.

probability (random) sampling Selection of a sample using techniques to ensure that each subject in the population has an equal chance of being selected.

probes Questions used to elicit more detailed information from a respondent when using an unstructured interview approach.

problem statement Interrogative or declarative statement that describes the purpose of a research study, identifies key concepts and sets study limits.

prospective study Quantitative research that collects data as the events occur.

purposive sample Nonprobability sample in which subjects are handpicked by the researcher based on a set of defined criteria.

qualitative (categorical) variable Variable that changes in terms of the presence or absence of a specified trait.

qualitative research An objective way to study the subjective human experience using nonstatistical methods of analysis.

quantitative (continuous) variable Variable that changes in terms of amount or degree (e.g. income, height, weight).

quantitative research Systematic process used to gather and statistically analyse information that has been measured by an instrument and converted to numerical data.

quasi-experimental design Type of experimental design in which there is neither a control group nor random assignment.

questionnaire Instrument used to collect self-reported psychological data from study subjects using pen and paper.

quota sample Nonprobability sample that is conveniently selected according to pre-specified characteristics (e.g. gender or ethnicity).

random assignment Placement of subjects into treatment or control groups using techniques that ensure each subject has an equal chance of being in either group.

range The distance between the highest and lowest scores for a variable.

ratio Level of measurement where a variable possesses the same properties as the interval data plus a meaningful zero.

reading level The readability of a specific piece of written material.

reading rate The number of words that can be read in a minute.

reading strategy (method) System that breaks a reading assignment down into manageable parts that are more readily processed.

reasoning Use of logical thought patterns to solve problems. May be inductive or deductive in nature.

recommendation Statement derived from a research study to guide future research about a specified topic.

reference collection Noncirculating materials meant to be used as reference rather than read through (e.g. indexes, encyclopaedias, dictionaries).

reliability (general definition) Dependability and trustworthiness of information.

reliability (as used in qualitative research) Concern with the accuracy and comprehensiveness of collected data.

reliability (as used in quantitative research) Characteristic of a good instrument; the assessed degree of consistency and dependability of that instrument.

replication Conduct of additional research studies on an identified problem to determine whether consistent results can be achieved.

research Systematic process using both inductive and deductive reasoning to confirm and refine existing knowledge and to build new knowledge.

research critique Detailed critical examination and evaluation of the theoretical and methodological merits of a given research study.

research design The overall plan for collecting data in a research study.

research process Orderly series of phases and steps that allow the researcher to move from asking a question to finding an answer.

research question Use of an interrogative format to identify the variables to be studied and possible relationships or differences between those variables.

research reading strategy Five-step process designed to increase comprehension and application of research studies. The steps are survey, examine, critically read, evaluate and visualise.

research utilisation Process of translating research findings into practice. This process is also called evidence-based practice (EBP).

researcher journal Journal kept by a researcher in which thoughts, ideas, feelings and reflections are recorded. Field notes or observations may also be recorded.

retrospective study Quantitative research that collects data on events that have already occurred.

sample Subset of a population selected to participate in a research study.

sampling The process used to select the sample.

saturation Point at which sampling and data collection are stopped in a grounded theory study because the information being collected is redundant and repetitive. Is similar to the concept of theoretical redundancy.

search Use indexes, abstracts and catalogues to find information about a specified subject.

search engine Tool for finding and retrieving specific information on the world wide web (e.g. Yahoo!, Lycos, Google, Altavista, Excite).

server (host) Computer that offers an information service over the internet.

setting The physical location and conditions under which a research study takes place.

shelves (stacks) Library bookshelves.

significance The likelihood that the study results are meaningful (i.e. not due to chance). The statistical r value is used to report significance.

simple random sample Probability sample in which all subjects in a population are numbered, and a sample is selected using a lottery or table of random numbers.
skewness Degree of symmetry or asymmetry of the distribution curve.
special reserve See closed reserve.
speed reading Reading at an increased rate through techniques that encourage fewer eye fixations on the page.
stability Assessment of reliability by correlating the scores obtained when an instrument is administered twice to the same group of subjects over a period of time.
standard deviation The average distance of spread in a frequency distribution.
stratified random sample Probability sample in which the subjects are subdivided into groups according to some characteristic. The subsets are then randomly sampled.
structured observation Specified behaviours are predetermined and listed on a checklist to be counted or checked off during the observation period.
summary Concise recapitulation of previously stated information that captures the main ideas.
survey Step 1 of the research reading strategy. Designed to provide a general overview and feel for the article.
systematic review Scientific study that seeks to answer a structured question by locating and appraising all published and unpublished work on the subject.
systematic sample Probability or nonprobability sample in which every *kth* (e.g. every fifth, or seventh, or twentieth) subject is selected. If the list is in random order, the sample selected is a probability sample. If the list is ordered (e.g. alphabetical), the sample selected is non-probable.

Telnet Software that allows users to log on to another computer from a remote site. It will show only the text, no graphics or pictures.
theoretical framework The theoretical foundation or frame of reference for a research study.
theoretical sampling Procedure used in grounded theory to gather additional data about emerging concepts.
theory Integrated and interrelated set of concepts used to explain some phenomenon.
thesis Research treatise written by a graduate student as part or all of the degree requirement.
tradition The handing down of knowledge from one generation to the next.
treatment The intervention in an experimental study that is being manipulated.
treatment group The group of subjects in an experimental study that receive the treatment.
trial and error The process of trying a succession of alternative solutions until one solves the problem at hand.
triangulation The use of both quantitative and qualitative research methodologies in a study or series of studies.

uniform resource locator (URL) The address system used by the internet to assist in locating a web page or file.
unstructured observation Method of observation in which behaviours are described and recorded as or after they occur using a journal, diary or field notes.

upload Transfer a file from your computer to another computer, using the internet.

user Client that communicates via computer and uses internet services offered by servers or hosts.

user name The name you use to identify your computer to another computer or computer system.

utilisation criteria Criteria used to evaluate whether research findings can be adapted for use in the clinical arena.

validity (as used in qualitative research) The credibility of a study. For example, does the interpretation of data match the recorded description of the data?

validity (as used in quantitative research) Characteristic of a good instrument; the extent of an instrument's ability to measure what it purports to measure.

variable Concept, characteristic or trait that varies (e.g. takes on measurably different values) within an identified population in a research study.

variance The average area of spread under a frequency distribution curve.

visualise Step 5 in the research reading strategy. Designed to apply research results to practice.

volume Single book or bound sequence of issues of a periodical.

web page One screen on a website.

website Sequence of web pages created by an organisation or an individual for conveying information.

world wide web (www) A collection of computers on the internet that are interconnected by hypertext and store websites.

Index

A
abstracting 58–9
abstracts (databases) 13, 15
    electronic 15–16
    manual 15
abstracts (research articles) 58, 159
abuses of research subjects 115–16
academic libraries 6
accuracy (information) 60
adequacy (information) 60
administrators 275–6
adolescent research *see* children and adolescent research
adults, care of *see* care of adults
ageing *see* care of older adults
ANCOVA tests 123
ANOVA tests 123
applied research 94
archives 9
audioconferencing 41, 46
audiovisual centre 9
Australian Journal of Advanced Nursing 78
Australian Nursing Council (ANC) competencies 77
    and how they relate to research 84–5
Australian Nursing Federation (ANF) 78, 79
Australian Research Council (ARC) 79
authority, knowledge derived from 72
author's credentials 61

B
background (journal article) 159–60
balance (information) 60
Belmont Report 116–17
Boolean operators 20

C
call numbers 7
care of adults
    clinical nursing journal articles 235–40
    nursing research journal articles 230–5
    reading and evaluating research articles 244–6
    research literature approaches 225–6
        addressing clinical and research priorities 226–7
        scanning available resources 229–30
        using issues that arise from clinical practice 227–9
    research resources 224–5
    summarising and using scanning results 240–4
care of older adults
    clinical nursing journal articles 260–4
    nursing research journal articles 256–60
    reading and evaluating research articles 267
    research literature approaches 251
        addressing clinical and research priorities 251–4
        scanning available resources 256
        using issues that arise from clinical practice 254–6
    research resources 250–1
    summarising and using scanning results 264–6
case study method 137, 141, 149
catalogues 11
    electronic 12–13
    manual 11
categorical variables 101
CD-ROM catalogue 12
CD-ROM databases 15, 16
chat rooms 40, 41

children and adolescent research
    clinical nursing journal articles 211–15
    miscellaneous nursing journal articles 216–17
    nursing research journal articles 208–11
    reading and evaluating research articles on children 219–20
    research literature approaches 203
        addressing clinical and research priorities 203–5
        scanning available resources 207
        using issues arising from clinical practice 205–6
    resources 202–3
    summarising and using scanning results 217–19
CINAHL 14, 15, 18, 43, 186, 206, 227, 229, 230, 254
classification system
    libraries 7
    qualitative research 133–4
    quantitative research 93–4
clients 274
clinical and research priorities 82–3, 182, 203–5, 226, 251–4, 272
clinical environment, assessment of 282
clinical merit and applicability 279–80
clinical nursing journal articles
    care of adults 235–40
    care of older adults 260–4
    children and adolescent research 211–15
    maternal–infant nursing research 190–4
clinical nursing journals 156–8, 180–1, 202–3, 224, 251
clinical nursing research 76
clinical practice issues 183–4, 205–6, 227–9
clinical relevance 278–9
clinicians 275
coding 136
collective case study 137
communicating on the net 30, 38–41, 45

comprehension 51, 53, 54
    guidelines to aid
        qualitative research 164
        quantitative research 163
conceiving the study (qualitative research) 139–41
    identification of phenomenon 139
    literature review 139–40
    research aims 140–1
conceiving the study (quantitative research) 97
    formulate variables 101–4
    literature review 98–100
    problem statement 98
    theoretical framework 100–1
concepts 93
conceptual definition 102
conceptual framework 100
conclusion (journal article) 161
conducting the study (qualitative research) 146–7
conducting the study (quantitative research)
    collecting data 118, 146
    gaining approval to use human subjects 115–17
    recruiting subjects 117–18
constant comparative method 148
constants 101
construct validity 114
constructivist–interpretive research 134
content validity 114
continuing education 46
continuous variables 101
control 102
control groups 106
convenience sampling 143
correlation 123
correlational studies 96
credibility 146
criterion validity 114
critical case sampling 143
critical research 134
cross-sectional studies 94

Cumulative Index to Nursing and Allied Health Literature see CINAHL
currency (information) 60, 62
custom, knowledge derived from 71

D

data 111
data analysis (qualitative research) 148
  findings 149
  methods 148–9
data analysis (quantitative research) 118–20
  answering the research question 122–4
  describing the sample 120–2
  interpreting the results 124
data collection (qualitative research) 146, 147
data collection (quantitative research) 118
  methods 111–13
data immersion 148
databases 12, 15–16, 44
declarative form (problem statement) 98
deductive reasoning 74
dependent variable 102, 105–6
descriptive statistics 120–2
descriptive studies 95
Dewey Decimal Classification 7
discussion (journal article) 161
disseminating results 125, 150, 156–61
dissertations/theses 15
distance education 45
downloading 39

E

education, via internet 45
effective reading 51
  strategies 55–7
  tips for 57–8
elderly *see* care of older adults
electronic catalogues 12–13
electronic databases 12, 15–16, 44
electronic journals 43
electronic nursing journals 43
email 30, 38–40
email address 38–9
epistemology 70
equivalence 114
ethical standards, human research 116–17, 146
ethics, manipulation of variables 107–8
ethics committees 117, 146, 147
ethnographical studies 135, 140, 142, 148–9
evaluating information 60–3
  factors affecting information quality 60–1
evaluating research studies 165–6
evaluation skills 62
evidence-based nursing 273
evidence-based practice 77
experimental design 105–6
experimental research 95
explanatory studies 95
exploratory studies 95
extraneous variable 102, 105
extreme sampling 143

F

F tests 123
field notes 145
file transfer protocols (FTP) 30, 41
findings (journal article) 160–1
findings (qualitative research) 149
findings (quantitative research) 93
frequencies 120–1
frequency distribution 121
full-text databases 19
funding of research 79–80, 83

G

generalisation 109
glossary 287–96
grounded theory research 135–6, 140, 141, 142, 143, 148
Gunning Fox Index 52–3

H

Health Research Council of New Zealand 80, 116
highlighting, while reading 56
historical method research 136–7, 140, 141, 143, 149
holdings (periodicals) 9
human research
　ethical standards 116–17, 146
　historical abuses 115–16
hypertext links 29, 34–5
hypotheses 102, 103–4, 122, 124

I

identifying the problem 98
implementation possibilities 280–1
implications of research for practice 125
independent variable 102
　non-manipulation 106–7
Index Medicus see MEDLINE
indexes (to periodical articles) 13–15
　choosing appropriate 18–19
　comparison of manual and electronic 17
　electronic 15–16
　manual 15
inductive reasoning 74
informants 147
information desk 8
information quality, factors affecting 60–1
information searching 99
　internet 35–8, 42–5
　libraries 18–21
informed consent 117–18, 146–7
institutional ethics committee (IEC) 117, 146, 147
institutional research support systems 283
instruments 111, 113
　quality evaluation 113–15
intensity sampling 143
interlibrary loan 13
internal consistency 114

internet
　communicating on the net 30, 38–41, 45
　education and learning possibilities 45
　professional information access 42–5
　services available 29–30
　traditional services 30, 41–2
　usage of 31–42
　what is it? 28–9
Internet Explorer 31
internet service provider (ISP) 31, 39
interpreting the results 124
interrogative form (problem statement) 98
interval categories 119
interval data 119, 120–1
interviews 113, 144–5
introduction (journal article) 159–60
intuition 74

J

journal article format 158–9
　discussion/conclusion 161
　introduction/background 159–60
　methodology or methods 160
　references 161
　results/findings 160–1
　title, abstract and key words 159

K

key words (journal articles) 159
knowledge
　sources of 71–5
　what is it? 70
kurtosis 122

L

libraries
　classification schemes 7
　maintaining ties with 281
　searching for information 18–19
　types of 6–7
　using 11–17

library collections 6, 8–9
Library of Congress classification 7
Likert scale 112–13
listservs 40
literature review 98–100, 139–40
lived experiences 134
loans desk 8
log on 31
longitudinal studies 94

M

manipulation 105, 106
  and non-manipulation 106–7
  ethical factors 107–8
manual catalogues 11
manual indexes/abstracts 15
maternal–infant nursing research
  clinical nursing journal articles 190–4
  miscellaneous nursing journal articles 194
  nursing research journal articles 187–90
  reading and evaluating research articles 196
  research literature approaches 181
    addressing clinical and research priorities 182
    scanning available resources 185–6
    using issues that arise from clinical practice 183–4
    resources 180–1
    summarising and using scanning results 194–5
maximum variety sampling 143
mean 121
measurement 119
measures of central tendency 121
measures of dispersion 121–2
measures of shape 122
median 121
MEDLINE 14, 15, 16, 18, 43, 186, 229
merit and applicability 279–80
metasearch tools 37
methodology 160

methods (journal article) 148, 160
mode 121
monographs 6
multivariate statistics 123

N

National Health and Medical Research Council (NH&MRC) 79
  ethical standards 116–17
  Strategic and Priority Driven Research objectives 182, 226
National Institute of Nursing Research 82, 182
  research opportunities 84
navigating the web
  hypertext links 34–5
  search engines 35–8
  uniform resource locator 32–3
Netscape Navigator 31
New Zealand Nurses Organisation (NZNO) 79, 80
newsgroups 30, 40–1
nominal data 120
nominal variables 119
nonexperimental design 106–8
nonexperimental research 96
nonprobability sampling 109, 110
nurse educators 276
nurse managers 275–6
nursing colleague involvement 282
nursing education 78
Nursing Education and Research Foundation (NERF) 80
nursing in Australia, timeline 80–1
nursing journal articles
  children and adolescent research 216–17
  maternal–infant research 194
  see also clinical nursing journal articles; nursing research journal articles
nursing journals *see* clinical nursing journals; nursing research journals

nursing research
  future of 82–3
  historical perspective 77–82
  importance of 76–7
  in Australia 78–81
  what is it? 76
  who is involved? 84–5
nursing research journal articles
  care of adults 230–5
  care of older adults 256–60
  children and adolescent research 208–11
  maternal–infant nursing research 187–90
nursing research journals 43, 78, 157
  care of adults 224–5
  care of older adults 250–1
  children and adolescents 202–3
  maternal–infant care 180–1, 187–90
  see also clinical nursing journals
nursing theories 78

O

observation 111, 144
older adults, care of *see* care of older adults
online catalogues 12
online databases 15–16
online service 31, 39
operational definition 102
oral history 136, 137
ordinal data 120
ordinal measurement 119

P

p values 123
paediatric research *see* children and adolescent research
participants 147
patients 274
peer reviewed journals 61
percentages 120
periodicals section 8
personal experience, knowledge derived from 73–4

phenomenological studies 134–5, 139, 140, 142, 148
population 108
postpositivist research 134
poststructural research 134
practice-related research 78
predictive studies 95
PREMEDLINE 43
presentation (information) 60, 62
primary sources 62
probabilistic searching 19–20
probability sampling 109, 110
problem solving 70
problem statements 98, 103
professional information access, internet 42–5
prospective studies 94
psychological measurements 112
public libraries 6
purposive sampling 143

Q

qualitative research 75
  classification system 133–7
  combining with quantitative 150–1
  differences from quantitative research 132
  guidelines to aid comprehension 164
  what is it? 131–3
qualitative research article
  reading strategy 172
    critical reading 174–5
    evaluation and visualisation 175–6
    survey and examination 172–4
qualitative research process 138
  phase 1: conceive the study 139–41
  phase 2: design the study 141–6
  phase 3: conduct the study 146–7
  phase 4: analyse the study 148–9
  phase 5: use the study 150
qualitative variables 101
quality of information, factors affecting 60–1

quantitative research 75
    classification system 93–4
    combining with qualitative 150–1
    differences from qualitative research 132
    guidelines to aid comprehension 163
    purpose 94–5
    reasons for 94
    research design 95–6
    time span and point of data collection 94
    what is it? 92–3
quantitative research article
    reading strategy 166
        critical reading 169–71
        evaluation and visualisation 171–2
        examining 167–9
        surveying 166–7
quantitative research process 96–7
    phase 1: conceive the study 97–104
    phase 2: design the study 105–15
    phase 3: conduct the study 115–18
    phase 4: analyse the study 118–24
    phase 5: use the study 125
quantitative variables 101
quasi-experimental design 106
questionnaires 112

R

r (correlation) 123
random assignment 106
random selection 109
range 121
ratio data 119, 120–1
reading level 52–3
reading rate 51, 52, 53–5
reading research articles 162, 164–6
    care of adults 244–6
    care of older adults 267
    children 219–20
    guidelines to aid comprehension 163–4
    maternal–infant care 196
    qualitative research example 172–6
    quantitative research example 166–72

reading strategies 55–7
    see also research reading strategies
reasoning 74–5
recommendations for further research 125, 150
recruit subjects 117–18
reference collection 8
reference desk 8
references (journal article) 161
relevance 278–9
reliability (information) 60
reliability (instrument) 114
reliability (qualitative research) 145
reliable instrument 113
reporting research, research and clinical journals 156–8
research
    how is it used in practice? 277–83
    importance of 68–9, 76–7
    what is it? 70, 75
research aims (qualitative research) 140–1
research articles
    format 158–61
    guidelines to aid comprehension 163–4
    reading 162, 164–76, 196, 219–30, 244–6, 267
research critique 165
research design (qualitative research) 134
    case studies 137
    data collection methods 144–6
    ethnography 135
    grounded theory 135–6
    historical method 136–7
    phenomenology 134–5
    samples and sampling 142–3
    setting 141–2

research design (quantitative research) 95–6, 105–15
  data collection methods 111–13
  experimental design 105–6
  instrument quality evaluation 113–15
  nonexperimental design 106–8
  sample selection 108–11
  setting 108
research funding 79–80, 83
research journal article format *see* journal article format
research journals *see* nursing research journals
research learning opportunities 281–2
research literature
  approaches for reviewing 181–6, 203–7, 225–30, 251–6
  plan for timely perusal of 282
research method 70
research priorities 82–3, 182, 203–5, 226, 251–4, 277
research process
  qualitative 138–50
  quantitative 96–125
research questions 102–3
  answering 122–4
research reading strategies 162, 164–6, 196, 219–20, 244–5, 267
  qualitative research example 172–6
  quantitative research example 166–72
research resources
  care of adults 229–30
  care of older adults 250–1
  children and adolescents 202–3
  maternal–infant care 180–1
research results 125, 150
  dissemination 125, 150
  further research 125
  recommendations 125, 150
research review nursing journals 157
research settings 108, 141–2
research subjects, historical abuses 115–16

research utilisation 272–3
  approaches to 277–8
  barriers to 273–4
  criteria for 278–81
  strategies to strengthen utilisation potential 281–3
  who is involved? 274–7
researchers 274
reserve section (libraries) 9
results (journal article) 160–1
retrospective studies 94
Royal College of Nursing Australia (RCNA) 78–9

S

sample size 110–11
samples 108, 109, 142–3
  nonprobability 109, 110
  probability 109, 110
sampling 108–9, 142–3
saturation 143
scales 112–13
scanning available resources 185–6, 207, 229–30, 256
search engines 35–8
  metasearch tools 37
  speciality search engines 37
search limits 19–20
search operators 20
search parameters 19
search results 20–1
searching for information 99
  internet 42–5, 35–8
  libraries 18–21
    choose appropriate indexes 18–19
    choose appropriate resources 18
    define your mission 18
secondary sources 62
sequential triangulation 151
setting 108, 141–2
shareware 41
shelves (libraries) 9
significance 123

simultaneous triangulation 151
skewness 122
snowball sampling 143
special collections (libraries) 9
special libraries 6–7
speed-reading 54
stability 114
stacks 9
standard deviation 122
statistical analysis 122–4
statistical hypotheses 123
statistical measures 119, 120–2
statistical tests 123
study design *see* research design
summarising 58–9, 194–5, 217–19, 240–4, 264–6

T

t tests 123, 124
Telnet 30, 42
theoretical framework 100–1
theoretical perspective (qualitative research) 134
theoretical sampling 143
theory 100
time span and point of data collection 94
timeliness of information 60, 62
title 159
tradition, knowledge derived from 71
trial and error 73
triangulation 150–1

U

uncooperative behaviour scale 111
uniform resource locator (URL) 32–3
  and type of organisation sponsoring the site 61
  elements of 33
uploading 39
user name 38–9

utilisation criteria 278
  implementation 280–1
  merit and applicability 279–80
  relevance 278–9
utilisation potential, strategies to strengthen
  assess your clinical environment 282
  exploit additional research learning opportunities 281–2
  explore institutional research support systems 283
  get other nurses involved 282
  maintain ties with library resources 281
  plan for timely perusal of research literature 282

V

valid instrument 113
validity (instrument) 114
validity (qualitative research) 145–6
  variables 101–4
measurement 119
variance 122
videoconferencing 41, 45

W

web browsers 31
web pages 29, 34
websites 29
  professional 44
world wide web (www) 29
  navigating the web 31–8

Z

zipped file 41